AND
THOU SHALT HONOR

"*And Thou Shalt Honor* will help make the challenges of caregiving part of our national dialogue."

—**David Tillman, M.D.,** chief executive officer of the Motion Picture and Television Fund in Woodland Hills, California

"Doctors and other health care providers cannot do the work of caregiving, nor do they often or adequately educate caregivers about their critical role in the health care system. That's why *And Thou Shalt Honor* is such an important contribution to the field of caregiving."

—**Howard M. Fillit, M.D.,** executive director of the Institute for the Study of Aging in New York City

"As our population ages, as the cost of health care escalates, and as older parents express an intense desire to remain at home and not be warehoused elsewhere, the demands on adult children—who will provide an increasing amount of hands-on assistance—is a certainty. Thanks to *And Thou Shalt Honor*, responsible sons and daughters will have the opportunity to develop strategies based upon the successful experiences of others. What a wonderful step in improving intrafamily relations this will be!"

—**Rabbi Allen Freehling,** senior rabbi of University Synagogue in Los Angeles

"Families across the country will benefit from *And Thou Shalt Honor*. I encourage caregivers—and those who support them—to read this book and keep it close at hand for future reference."

—**Donna Wagner, Ph.D.,** director of gerontology at Towson University in Maryland

"*And Thou Shalt Honor* is a must-purchase for everyone over 40 for all of the valuable material it includes."

—**William E. Arnold, Ph.D.,** director of the gerontology program at Arizona State University in Tempe

"*And Thou Shalt Honor* will help our country's caregiving heroes to navigate rough terrain, giving them useful information and support."

—**Alan Solomont,** founder of HouseWorks, a Newton, Massachusetts–based organization that helps seniors stay independent

"*And Thou Shalt Honor* brings sensitivity and common sense to a complex and compelling subject. Hopefully, it will serve as a wake-up call to all generations."

—**Susan Friedman,** executive director of the Grotta Foundation in South Orange, New Jersey

"Reading *And Thou Shalt Honor*, I felt as though my most trusted friend was sitting with me, guiding me gently through the issues involved in caregiving—helping me understand where to begin, telling me where to find more information, making me feel confident that I was doing just fine and that I was doing my best for my loved one . . . and letting me know that keeping a sense of humor doesn't hurt, either."

—**Nancy P. Morith, C.L.U.,** president of N. P. Morith, Inc., in Princeton, New Jersey

AND THOU SHALT HONOR

The Caregiver's Companion

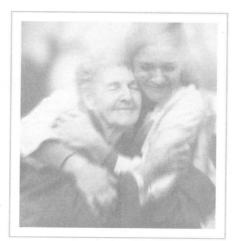

Edited by

BETH WITROGEN McLEOD

Pulitzer Prize–Nominated Author of
Caregiving: The Spiritual Journey of Love, Loss, and Renewal

Foreword by

ROSALYNN CARTER

RODALE®

Printed in the United States of America
Rodale Inc. makes every effort to use acid-free ∞, recycled paper ♻.

Cover and interior design by Carol Angstadt

Interior photographs courtesy of Wiland-Bell Productions, except p. 1, © John Riley/Getty Images/Stone; p. 25, © Peter Mason/Getty Images/The Image Bank; pp. 75 and 411, © A. Menashe/humanistic-photography.com; p. 125, © Ken Fisher/Getty Images/Stone; p. 229, © Bruce Ayres/Getty Images/Stone; p. 281, © Bill Market/Stock Connection/PictureQuest; p. 345, © Anthony Nagelmann/Getty Images/FPG

The "See It On PBS" logo is a trademark of the Public Broadcasting Service and is used with permission.

Credit for the Caregiver's Checklist on page 30 is given to the CaregiverPA Web site (http://caregiverpa.psu.edu) developed by the Pennsylvania State University Gerontology Center, University Park, Pennsylvania, using funding from the Administration on Aging provided through the SPRY Foundation, Washington, D.C.

"Protecting the Rights of Nursing Home Residents" on page 275 is reprinted from *Nursing Homes: Getting Good Care There* (2nd edition), © 2001 by Sarah Greene Burger, et al., and the National Citizens' Coalition for Nursing Home Reform. Reproduced by Rodale by permission of Impact Publishers, Inc., PO Box 6016, Atascadero, CA 93423. Further reproduction prohibited.

Library of Congress Cataloging-in-Publication Data

And thou shalt honor : the caregiver's companion / edited by Beth Witrogen McLeod.
    p.   cm.
  Includes bibliographical references and index.
    ISBN 1–57954–558–0 hardcover
    1. Caregivers.   2. Home health aides.   I. McLeod, Beth Witrogen, date.
    RA645.3 .A53 2002
362.1—dc21   2002006520

Distributed to the book trade by St. Martin's Press

2 4 6 8 10 9 7 5 3 1 hardcover

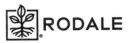

RODALE

WE INSPIRE AND ENABLE PEOPLE TO IMPROVE
THEIR LIVES AND THE WORLD AROUND THEM

FOR MORE OF OUR PRODUCTS
WWW.RODALESTORE.COM
(800) 848-4735

Notice

This book is intended as a reference volume only, not as a medical manual. The information given here is designed to help you make informed decisions about your health and the health of those in your care. It is not intended as a substitute for any treatment that may have been prescribed by a doctor. If you suspect that you or someone in your care has a medical problem, we urge you to seek competent medical help.

Mention of specific companies, organizations, or authorities in this book does not imply endorsement by the publisher, nor does mention of specific companies, organizations, or authorities imply that they endorse this book.

Internet addresses and telephone numbers given in this book were accurate at the time it went to press.

Board of Advisors for the PBS Special *And Thou Shalt Honor*

William E. Arnold, Ph.D., director of the gerontology program at Arizona State University in Tempe

Chad Boult, M.D., M.P.H., M.B.A., professor and director of the Lipitz Center for Integrated Health Care at Johns Hopkins University in Baltimore

Robert N. Butler, M.D., chief executive officer and president of the International Longevity Center and professor of geriatrics at Mount Sinai School of Medicine in New York City

Laura Carstensen, Ph.D., professor of psychology and the former Barbara D. Finberg Director at the Institute for Research on Women and Gender at Stanford University

Gloria Cavanaugh, president and chief executive officer of the American Society on Aging, based in San Francisco

Joseph F. Coughlin, Ph.D., founding director of the AgeLab at the Massachusetts Institute of Technology in Cambridge

Donald Davis, vice president of the workforce development division of the National Council on the Aging

Steve Dawson, president of the Paraprofessional Healthcare Institute in Bronx, New York

Rose Dobrof, D.S.W., Brookdale professor of gerontology at the Brookdale Center on Aging at Hunter College in New York City

Brian Duke, president of the board of directors of Children of Aging Parents

Lynn Friss Feinberg, deputy director of the National Center on Caregiving at the Family Caregiver Alliance in San Francisco

Mike Fenton, president of Fenton-Cowitt Casting in Encino, California

Howard Fillit, M.D., executive director of the Institute for the Study of Aging in New York City

Rabbi Allen Freehling, senior rabbi of University Synagogue in Los Angeles

Susan Friedman, executive director of the Grotta Foundation in South Orange, New Jersey

Deborah Glik, professor of community health sciences at the UCLA School of Public Health

Jennie Chin Hansen, executive director of OnLok in San Francisco

Gail Hunt, executive director of the National Alliance for Caregiving, based in Bethesda, Maryland

Carol Levine, project director for the families and healthcare project at the United Hospital Fund of New York City

Beth Witrogen McLeod, author of *Caregiving: The Spiritual Journey of Love, Loss, and Renewal*

Roy W. Menninger, M.D., chairman emeritus of the Menninger Foundation in Topeka, Kansas

Suzanne Mintz, cofounder and president of the National Family Caregivers Association, based in Kensington, Maryland

Mary Mittelman, Dr.P.H., director of the caregiver research program of the Silberstein Institute for Aging and Dementia of the New York University School of Medicine

Nancy P. Morith, CLU, president of N P Morith, Inc., in Princeton, New Jersey

Phyllis Mutschler, Ph.D., executive director of the National Center on Women and Aging, Heller School of Social Policy and Management, at Brandeis University in Waltham, Massachusetts

David B. Reuben, M.D., professor of medicine and chief of the division of geriatrics at the UCLA School of Medicine

Janet Sainer, special consultant for the Brookdale Foundation Group in New York City

Patricia Schroeder, president and chief executive officer of the Association of American Publishers

Alan Solomont, founder of HouseWorks, a Newton, Massachusetts–based organization that helps seniors stay independent

Percil Stanford, Ph.D., director of the Center on Aging at San Diego State University

Peter J. Strauss, Esq., elder law and trust and estates attorney, author, and adjunct professor of law at New York Law School in New York City

Ronda C. Talley, Ph.D., M.P.H., executive director and professor of the Rosalynn Carter Institute for Human Development at Georgia Southwestern State University in Americus

David Tillman, M.D., chief executive officer of the Motion Picture and Television Fund in Woodland Hills, California

Fernando Torres-Gil, associate dean for academic affairs at the UCLA School of Public Policy and Social Research

Donna Wagner, Ph.D., director of gerontology at Towson University in Maryland

CONTENTS

FOREWORD

When I first became involved with care-giving on a national scale, few groups were focusing on it as a major public health issue. That has changed dramatically over the last decade. Today the needs of caregivers increasingly are being recognized as an important part of our nation's health agenda and are receiving much-deserved attention from concerned individuals and organizations.

Caregiving has been a familiar part of my life since I was 12 years old and my father became terminally ill with leukemia. I was one of four children, and because I was the oldest and a daughter, my 34-year-old mother depended on me. Since Jimmy and I came home from the White House, we have witnessed firsthand the importance of caregiving as his mother, brother, and two sisters struggled with terminal cancer. And I helped take care of my mother until she died in 2000 at age 94. I have had plenty of opportunities to appreciate the many dimensions of caregiving.

My work on this issue has continued through the Rosalynn Carter Institute for Human Development, which was established in 1987 at my alma mater, Georgia Southwestern State University. We began by reaching out to family members of loved ones with mental illnesses, but our efforts quickly expanded to include those who care for individuals with any kind of illness or disability, including the frail elderly. Now in its 15th year, the institute conducts research and engages in education and training to advance its mission: to promote the mental health and well-being of individuals, families,

and professional caregivers; to promulgate effective caregiving practices; to build public awareness of caregiving needs; and to advance public and social policies that enhance caring communities. We are working in Georgia and throughout the nation to promote quality caregiving for all Americans.

Our experiences at the Rosalynn Carter Institute have led us to build support systems that provide communities of caring for caregivers. With funding from the Administration on Aging of the U.S. Department of Health and Human Services, we are developing a Caregiving Community Capacity Index, an instrument that can be used by community leaders to assess and improve their caregiving infrastructures. We have created community-based networks called CARE-NETs that enable family and professional caregivers, representatives of local, state, and federal government agencies, members of religious communities, and advocates to meet on a regular basis. They discuss the needs of caregivers in their areas and plan strategies to address their concerns. Another of our programs, *Caring for You, Caring for Me*, addresses the psychosocial needs of caregivers.

During the past year, we have convened seven expert panels on various caregiving topics and launched a book series to advance knowledge and answer the questions of "what's known and what's needed" in caregiving. We've even established a new professional role, the family caregiving consultant.

While much has been done to bring national

attention to the need for quality professional and family care, much remains to be done. The PBS special *And Thou Shalt Honor* and its companion book present timely and essential information on the lives of the millions of Americans who provide both paid and unpaid care for those who need it. The reference from Exodus 20:12, "honor thy father and thy mother," expresses a point of faith, calling all of us to act respectfully and compassionately toward our families, our neighbors, and our communities.

I strongly commend *And Thou Shalt Honor: The Caregiver's Companion* to caregivers and those who support them. Caregiving can be very challenging and rewarding. Since we will either be caregivers or need caregivers at various life stages, this book will do much to inform us all.

—Rosalynn Carter
President, Board of Directors
Rosalynn Carter Institute
for Human Development

PREFACE

And Thou Shalt Honor came to be *after* our parents died. Neither Harry's dad, affected by Alzheimer's disease, nor Dale's mom or dad would be surprised that their deaths years ago have created a historic journey for their respective sons. As young men from vastly different backgrounds, we were brought up inspired by one common mission: to make a difference, to persevere, to ask the proverbial "Why not?"

Today, 3½ years after we began our journey, we've taken what we learned caring for our respective parents, found out what we *didn't* know, and used it as the foundation for the first national public television broadcast and companion outreach campaign for caregivers. Initially, we imagined ourselves placing our ideas for a caregiving project into corked bottles; after setting the bottles afloat in the vast archipelago of foundations and media, we waited, never knowing if they would land or where, or whether they would ever be opened and their ideas read—and funded.

Fortunately for us, one bottle managed to find a shoreline in landlocked Emmaus, Pennsylvania. More precisely, it was delivered to the doors of Rodale Inc. by Frank X. Malone. From there, it became a symbol of hope in the fulfillment of a dream. Now, many months later, this book—along with our PBS special and Web site (www.thoushalthonor.org), as well as a coalition of outreach partners—stands poised to launch caregiving into the national consciousness, and to empower all those on the front line of the caregiving movement.

The journey could not have been undertaken without the help of many. To begin, we want to recognize all those at Rodale who shared our vision and provided invaluable wisdom and encouragement throughout our project: Tami Booth, Michele Murphy, Cindy Ratzlaff, Amy Rhodes, Lisa Dolin, Gregg Michaelson, Mariska Van Aalst, Mary Lengle, Tom Mulderick, Leslie Schneider, Dana Bacher, Lorraine Rodriguez, Stephanie Hamerstone, and Pam Boyer. And we're very grateful to the editorial team that contributed its time and talents to the creation of this book: Michael Castleman, David Tuller, Arden Moore, Betty Liddick, Bob Condor, and the inspirational Beth Witrogen McLeod; and from Rodale, Susan Berg, Amy Kovalski, Carol Angstadt, Gale Maleskey, Jennifer Bright, Kathy Dvorsky, Darlene Schneck, Madeleine Adams, and Marilyn Hauptly.

Former First Lady Rosalynn Carter, who has done such seminal work on behalf of caregivers, graciously took time from her busy schedule to write a foreword for the book. And award-winning actor Joe Montegna contributed his time and talents as on-camera host of the PBS special. To both of them, we extend our heartfelt appreciation.

The original vision for our Web site was easily surpassed by that of our wry and elegant webmaster, Jim Hood, and his editor, Dave Egner. Mike Ballard, Catherine Smith, and their group—wise allies all—organized and implemented our nationwide outreach campaign. Karen Salerno and Colby Kelly have brought national attention to our project through their stimulating publicity efforts. Gail Gibson Hunt has been unswerving in her advice on all components of the project. Sage Bill Jersey led us to Dave Davis and the Oregon Public Broadcasting team, who've been so generous with their support. At critical points along the way, Francine Lynch and Kay Carlson exemplified courage; Doug Levinson, tenacity; Martin Richards, initiative; Di Nelson, astuteness; Holly Wiland, steadfastness; Jay Shanker, patience; Sandy Heberer, encouragement; David Liu, affirmation; David Tillman and Ken Scherer, camaraderie; Teresa Rogers, allegiance; Allen Freehling, solace; and—for Dale—Larry and Virginia Keene, refuge.

But without the trust of Susan Friedman, Rose Dobrof, Lorin, our board of advisors, our underwriters, Bob Harrison and Bob Baylis, Vivian Greenberg and Connie Ford, and Rona Bartlestone, our project might never have been born. They were the first to open the bottles that we had set adrift on the stormy seas of fundraising. To all, and to our marvelous staff at Wiland-Bell Productions—Teresa Modnick, Yasha Husain, Ada Shaw, Emily Steinberg, Katie Lyon, David O'Dell, Kelsey Namara, Raheem Dawson, Brigitte Anderson, Teri Koenig, David Loeb and Gary Griffin, Elliot Tyson, and the extraordinarily gifted Beverly Baroff—we give our everlasting thanks.

Thanks as well to our freelance teams in the field, and most of all, to the caregivers and their loved ones who invited us into their homes and their lives. Their stories truly are an inspiration; they will be in our hearts and thoughts always.

And finally, to Lillian, Nathan, Michael, Julia, Holly, Winona, Lady, Hugo, Anne, Jonathan, David, Andrew, Linda, and Reave: for their continuous support, our love.

—Harry Wiland and Dale Bell
Executive producers, *And Thou Shalt Honor*

UNDERWRITERS FOR THE PBS SPECIAL
AND THOU SHALT HONOR

Administration on Aging (AoA), U.S.
  Department of Health and Human Services
Ahmanson Foundation
Atlantic Philanthropies
AXA Foundation
Care There, Inc.
Corporation for Public Broadcasting (CPB)
Joseph Drown Foundation
Entertainment Industry Foundation (EIF)
FJC, A Foundation of Donor Advised Funds
Grotta Foundation

Independent Television Service (ITVS)
Jewish Healthcare Foundation
The Jacob and Valeria Langeloth Foundation
Mellon Financial Corporation Foundation
Motion Picture & Television Fund
Mt. Sinai Health Care Foundation
Northwest Health Foundation
School Sisters of Notre Dame
Service Employees International Union (SEIU)
John Vestri

INTRODUCTION

As they say, "If only I knew then what I know now."

When I was 43, my life as I knew it was swept away. My father was succumbing to a rare recurring cancer at the same time that my mother was unexpectedly diagnosed with amyotrophic lateral sclerosis—Lou Gehrig's disease—and Alzheimer's disease. Everything that was familiar abruptly vanished.

For the next 2 years, during which I was my parents' primary long-distance caregiver, I never knew which end was up. I tumbled through a never-ending free fall of medical and financial crises, the nursing home decision, legal minefields, and relentless depression. I didn't know anything about taking care of two dying parents. All I could do was stay focused on the love.

I do wish I had known more about the mechanics of caring for my parents; that alone would have mitigated many emotional and financial ravages. But these memories have no power today. In learning to negotiate this major life change, I discovered not only my own resilience but that of every other caregiver as well.

Because of caregiving, I have been blessed with the opportunity to discover what really matters. I have been witness to personal transformation in the midst of suffering. I have seen the spirit of humankind shine bright, again and again, as families rise to the challenge and create positive change. These unexpected rewards, and so many more, come from the land of the not-yet-known, the terrain of long-term health care for the elderly. These gifts are the light in the darkness of caregiving.

Often I've been asked what one thing I would have done differently "if only I knew then." Honestly, there is no one thing. I wish I had known that services for the aging—many free or low-cost—can provide education, respite, and support. I wish I had known that many talented professionals are ready and able to help. I wish I had known that I was not weak or incompetent just because I was unable to be all things to all people. I wish I had known that my feelings of guilt and exhaustion were not mine alone but are shared universally in the caregiving arena. I wish I had known that what I was experiencing was the leading edge of an unprecedented and historic phenomenon, not merely my personal cross to bear.

Indeed, informal family care has become so pervasive that it is the new midlife rite of passage. We are living longer and generally in better health. But because of this longevity, we also are subject to a higher incidence of disabling conditions that can last for decades. Consider that more than 100 million Americans suffer from chronic illnesses such as arthritis and diabetes. Realistically, every family faces the prospect of being in a caregiving situation someday. So caregiving has become a national issue, requiring broad and bold new public policy to ensure that families are supported rather than sacrificed.

Although caregiving is not an easy journey, it need not be defined by hardship and negativity. We must remember that it's not something to just "get through." It is not a competition or a pathology. Rather, it is a normal event in the cycle of life. There is no right or wrong way to do it; there is only the necessity of being present.

To take on this mantle with grace, we need to be mindful of what is involved in caring for our loved ones. We need to maintain optimum health physically, mentally, and spiritually, or we risk limiting our own lives in the process. For it is not just the physical tasks that take a toll, but especially the emotional and psychological stresses that sneak up on caregivers and burn them out.

Many a caregiver has said, "I just want my life back." And therein lies the journey's greatest challenge: To give good care to others, we first must take care of ourselves. We can become handicapped as caregivers not because we lack knowledge about durable powers of attorney or long-term care insurance—expertise that can be acquired or paid for—but because we exclude ourselves from the care equation. We've been called to tend to others, not to martyr ourselves in the process. If we don't give kindness to ourselves and accept support from others, then we risk becoming disenchanted with the caregiving role when we could be blessed by it instead. Even the Lone Ranger relied on Tonto.

Today more than ever, caregivers have an array of options for making their situations work well. You do not have to reinvent the wheel. In this book, for example, you'll find helpful information and guidance—whether your questions are about medical care, housing, financial and legal planning, end-of-life issues, family dynamics, or some other caregiving issue. Each chapter is structured to stand alone, with a summary of its key points, plus action plans, checklists, and resources. Refer to each chapter as necessary, or read the book from beginning to end, like a mystery or romance novel. On every page, you will find support for the length and breadth of your caregiving journey.

This can be a precious time if we approach the caregiving role as a calling rather than as an obstacle to achieving personal goals. Caregiving truly is a spiritual practice, a nonlinear path with heart. We are asked to expand ourselves and be open to change. We are asked to comfort, to guide, to love. We are asked to listen, to reassure, to advocate. Most of all, we are asked to trust life in a way we never thought possible.

What makes caregiving appear difficult is the inner journey, the one that requires us to summon the courage and flexibility to relate to life in an unfamiliar but more expansive way. This is new territory for most of us; it shows us where we have closed down to what life has to offer, and how much work is necessary to care for ourselves while caring for others. Whether love means learning to set limits or to not take things so personally—these and many other new ways of being in the world are lessons to enrich a lifetime. And all are worth the journey.

Caregiving has heart and meaning because it changes us for the better. Many caregivers say they have deeper compassion, as well as more patience with others and greater faith in their ability to handle difficult situations. Families come together in new ways, healing old rifts and misunderstandings. They have less fear of illness and death because they know how rich this time can be. And just successfully negotiating financial or housing matters—these are no small victories.

When we look at the potential for living more fully through facing our fears, we discover that what we as caregivers do matters deeply. It matters because we learn to honor life by allowing it to unfold on its own. It matters because we learn to be more appreciative of every moment. It matters because caregiving demands from us the best we have—body, mind, and soul.

And this is what ultimately endures, what we take from this journey: the understanding that caring for a loved one ennobles every life it touches. Our caring exceeds our personal story lines and builds community. At the bedside of each needful loved one, we are creating a better world. We pass on our knowledge, with compassion.

All of us are like snowflakes, individually dancing yet together part of the same drifting. Caregiving connects us. No matter what our ethnicity, geographic location, economic situation, religious or political beliefs, we share this human experience with amazing similarity and purpose. We may be diverse on the outside, but in our hearts we are one, and we can all help each other.

Of course, you must decide the meaning this rite of passage has for you. Caregiving is your journey, and yours alone. Only you have your special skills, your family's history, your fears, and your dreams. Your experience can be as individual and light as a beautiful snowflake, or as complex and turbulent as a heavy blizzard. Whatever path you choose, please remember this: You are never alone. Every act of kindness counts. Love is always stronger than fear.

If you are among those in search of answers to the stresses and confusions inherent in caregiving, I say: This *is* your life now. Live it fully in the present. Stay connected to love, which is the heart of caregiving, and your journey will be rewarded many times over.

—Beth Witrogen McLeod

PART ONE

Caregiving:
A Rite of Passage

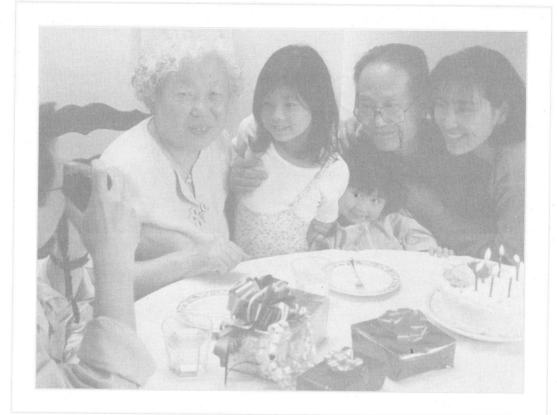

CHAPTER 1

CONTINUING THE TRADITION

What You Need to Know

- Caregiving is a uniquely human act with a history that spans centuries. It will touch almost everyone in the years ahead, whether they become caregivers or care recipients.

- The demand for caregiving services has increased dramatically through the beginning of the 21st century. The aging of the population, combined with the shortage of professional care providers, has made caregiving one of our nation's most pressing public policy issues.

- Whether you are a caregiver or you expect to become one, you're in a unique position to help forge change. What you learn through your own experience can help shape caregiving for future generations.

Because you're reading this book, chances are you've already become a caregiver, or you expect to become one in the not-too-distant future. If so, you're carrying on a long-standing tradition, one that spans generations and cultures the world over. In fact, caregiving falls into the category of behaviors that defines us humans as . . . well, human. While all mammals care for their young, we're the only species to nurture our elderly and frail.

Why do we do it? Certainly we're driven by a sense of responsibility and duty. But that's only part of the answer. If we dig a little deeper, we're bound to touch on even more compelling reasons, like a desire to demonstrate our love, gratitude, and honor for those in our care.

Honor. The word might be equated with obligation, as in "Thou shalt honor thy father and thy mother." Indeed, many of us first become caregivers by default—a family member suddenly requires some kind of assistance, and we're the only ones willing or able to provide it. But even if we're thrust into our caregiving roles, the very act of providing care becomes symbolic of a powerful emotional bond between us and our loved ones. Honor is the heart and soul of that bond.

Of course, each of us defines honor according to our respective caregiving experiences. We connect to those in our care—our parents, spouses, siblings, children, and close friends—in myriad highly individualized ways. They can be physical, emotional, or spiritual, or a combination of all three. They shape our perception of honor and make it a palpable facet of the caregiving role.

While honor drives the relationship between caregiver and care recipient, it tends to get lost among the values of our society as a whole. More often than not, honoring someone is a very public display. It's the stuff of awards shows, civic ceremonies, and high-school assemblies.

But in caregiving, honor is typically more subdued, and certainly more private. Helping a loved one bathe or dress might not earn a golden statuette, but it's a no less remarkable act. Perhaps it's rewarded with a simple "thank you," or a smile, or a loving caress.

Honor is a genuine, heartfelt commitment to one another that can sustain both caregiver and care recipient through the most challenging times. It's a source of focus and determination. It fuels every conversation, every decision, every task that involves providing care.

We need to be mindful of when we're losing sight of honor and becoming complacent about its place in the caregiving relationship. When that happens, we deny ourselves the joy and satisfaction that's so vital to thriving in the caregiving role.

That's not to suggest caregiving doesn't have its downside. It can be exhausting and thankless work, especially if the caregiver isn't getting much-needed support from family and friends. Indeed, the phrase "emotional roller coaster" seems to have been invented just to describe the caregiving experience. But when honor maintains a strong presence in that experience, the ups most certainly can outweigh the downs. Consider the results of a

Kaiser Family Foundation survey, which found that 96 percent of caregivers feel loved, while 90 percent feel appreciated. And 84 percent describe themselves as proud of their caregiver status. These statistics are nothing short of remarkable.

But for a moment, think beyond the numbers to the women and men they represent. They could be people you know, or the people whose stories appear throughout this book. These caregivers undoubtedly would tell you that they've had their share of hardships and frustrations. But they also would point out that the caregiving role has brought unexpected rewards, that it has strengthened their relationships with their loved ones, that it has given new purpose to their own lives. So in providing care, they honor not just their loved ones but also themselves.

You can reap these benefits as well, if you approach caregiving with the right mindset. Think of it as a journey that may test your physical and emotional limits but ultimately will strengthen your sense of self—not to mention the bond between you and your loved one.

Understandably, you may have moments when you feel overwhelmed by a situation you face, or uncertain about a decision you must make. At those moments, use this book as your guide. It offers insightful information and nuts-and-bolts advice from respected caregiving professionals, as well as from real-life caregivers. Their words can help whether you want to learn practical caregiving skills, identify caregiving resources, or find inspiration for your caregiving journey.

For now, pause to acknowledge your place in the caregiving movement, following those who've gone before and blazing the trail for those who are yet to come. Understand that you can help shape the future of caregiving, whether within your own family or on a national or global scale.

Realize, too, that the knowledge you gain now can help you plan for a time when you may require care yourself. Former First Lady Rosalynn Carter—chair of the Rosalynn Carter Institute for Human Development, which specializes in caregiving issues— once shared this quote from a colleague: "There are only four kinds of people in the world—those who have been caregivers, those who currently are caregivers, those who will be caregivers, and those who will need caregivers."

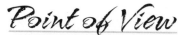

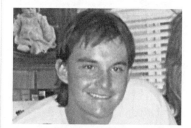

"Honor is a very strong word. I honor the relationship that I have with my grandfather. My grandfather has done everything in the world for me, from taking me on vacation to giving me moral support, to helping me with my homework, to just being there. I feel like I owe him for my whole life, and if that means taking care of him for the rest of my life, I will. Even though it's frustrating sometimes, I realize that he's done so much for me. Now I need to be there for him."

—NICHOLAS LINSK,
Mesa, Arizona

A CAREGIVING NATION

Before we begin delving into the issues that you may encounter on your caregiving journey, you might want to learn a bit more about where you stand and what lies ahead in terms of your caregiver role. The first thing you need to know is that you have plenty of company. A 2000 survey by the Kensington, Maryland–based National Family Caregivers Association found that more than 54 million Americans spend between 18 and 20 hours a week, on average, caring for an adult loved one. Most of these people remain caregivers for 1 to 4 years, though for some—20 percent—the commitment lasts longer.

These figures become even more significant when you consider how rapidly the caregiving population is growing. Back in 1987, when AARP and the Travelers Insurance Company conducted the first formal study of caregivers in the United States, the number of caregiving households totaled about 7 million nationwide. Within a decade, the count more than tripled to 22.4 million. By 2007, it could reach 39 million, according to projections from AARP and the Bethesda, Maryland–based National Alliance for Caregiving.

One reason for the rapid upturn is the abundance of baby boomers who will grow older and live longer with illnesses that can be managed better than in past decades. Heart disease, diabetes, arthritis, and even certain cancers won't cause the premature deaths common in previous generations.

As people live longer, the entire U.S. population will skew older. Whether it will have enough caregivers to look after those who require care remains to be seen. One thing is certain: Professional care providers won't be filling the entire gap. Nursing experts say that their profession already is experiencing shortages that will become even more critical in the next few decades.

Already the vast majority of care is provided not by professionals but by family caregivers—that is, relatives as well as close friends. Some 25 years ago, 80 percent of caregiving took place in the home. According to the latest research, that figure actually has risen, to 90 percent. What's more, the number of people who receive home care is more than four times the number who reside in facilities such as nursing homes.

Given statistics like these, you can see why caregiving has been identified as a major public health issue for the 21st century. With more people requiring care and not enough professionals to provide it, caregiving responsibilities will continue to fall to family members. And families, in turn, will demand more public and private resources to support them in their caregiver roles.

Who Is Giving Care?

As the caregiving population has grown over the years, the definition of "caregiver" has changed. Indeed, deciding who is a caregiver can be a bit of a challenge, partly because the term is used to describe both professional care providers and unpaid, "informal" care providers—usually spouses and adult children. It also can apply to community volunteers, clergy, and others who sometimes step into the caregiver role.

For the purposes of this book, we've adopted the definition first proposed by the San Francisco–based Family Caregiver Alliance: "Caregivers are family, friends, and neighbors who stand by those they love as they face chronic illness, disability, or death. Caregivers are a diverse group of people of all ages and from all walks of life—some new to caregiving, some just anticipating becoming caregivers, and others for whom providing care has become a way of life."

The services that caregivers provide can vary considerably based on individual circumstances. One person may spend Saturday mornings running errands for a parent; another may provide round-the-clock care for a bedridden spouse. "Much of what goes on in the bedrooms and bathrooms of caregiving households involves tasks that the able-bodied and mentally competent take for granted—showering, toileting, dressing, moving, and in some cases, even breathing," notes Suzanne Mintz, cofounder and president of the National Family Caregivers Association.

The typical caregiver is a 46-year-old woman who works outside the home and devotes about 18 hours a week to caregiving tasks. But according to the 2000 survey by Mintz's organization, more men are stepping into caregiving roles. The survey found that the oft-quoted ratio of 75 percent female caregivers to 25 percent male caregivers is more like 56 percent to 44 percent.

Yet even though a growing number of men are involved in hands-on care, in many cases, women automatically become the

EXPERT OPINION

"Caring for our elders is not an industry. And making it an industry perverts the real value in it. We have to move decisively away from care as a big business, as a business opportunity. And I think we can do that by moving away from the idea that care for frail elders has to be localized in buildings we call nursing homes."

—**WILLIAM H. THOMAS, M.D.**, caregiving advocate and founder of the Eden Alternative in Sherbourne, New York (www.edenalternative.com)

"designated caregivers," notes Gail Hunt, executive director of the National Alliance for Caregiving. In some families, the designated caregiver could be helping several aging parents (including in-laws) and other loved ones all at once.

A growing number of Americans—especially those between ages 45 and 55—have the dual responsibility of caring for both older and younger family members. In fact, about 44 percent of this so-called sandwich generation has living parents as well as children under age 21. About a quarter of these people are care-givers for their parents or in-laws.

In terms of ethnicity, the caregiving population reflects the di-versity of our nation as a whole. A 2001 survey by AARP found that within the 45-to-55 demographic, 19 percent of whites are caregivers, compared with 28 percent of African-Americans, 34 percent of Hispanic-Americans, and 42 percent of Asian-Americans.

The reasons for the range in statistics are numerous and com-plex. Economics certainly plays a role, as does accessibility of ser-vices. But perhaps just as important are each ethnic group's customs and values. Asian-Americans, for example, maintain a tradition of caring for their elders that has been passed from im-migrant parents to their children. Hispanic-Americans have a strong family structure, often living in multigenerational homes. And African-Americans tend to express more positive attitudes toward their elders; women, in particular, view age as a source of dignity and respect.

Without question, the cultures in which we're raised help shape our perceptions of caregiving and our duties as caregivers. This mix of ethnic influences will define the future of caregiving in our country—particularly if, as demographics experts specu-late, the non-white elderly populations become the majority in the next few decades.

What's common among all caregivers—regardless of their gender, age, or ethnic background—is a critical need for support, especially in the later stages of a caregiving situation. In a study of spousal caregivers, Richard Schulz, Ph.D., a psychologist and researcher with the Pittsburgh Veterans Administration, found that while people experience increased self-esteem when they first take on their caregiving roles, they eventually reach a point where they report a lot of strain. That's when they become more vulnerable to health problems. They don't eat right, sleep enough, or see their doctors when necessary. They're more prone to depression. And they don't slow down when they're sick because others are depending on them.

What many caregivers fail to realize is that if they don't look after themselves, they can't possibly look after someone else. That's why getting support—whether from family, friends, community resources, or government agencies—is so important. We'll discuss a full range of options throughout the rest of the book.

Who Is Receiving Care?

The profile of a typical caregiver will continue to evolve as the caregiving population grows. But for the most part, the profile of a typical care recipient remains the same. She's a 77-year-old woman who has a chronic health problem, such as heart disease or osteoporosis. And she most likely lives alone, though close to her primary caregiver.

The fact that care recipients tend to be older makes sense, as the incidence of illness and disability increases with age. Some data suggest that men receive more care from their spouses, compared with women, who receive more care from adult children and other family members. This might be because wives tend to outlive their husbands, and so must turn to their families for help.

One of the more significant predictors of who receives care is living arrangement. In general, older people who reside with their spouses are much more likely to be care recipients than older people who live by themselves. In fact, a 2000 survey by the National Family Caregivers Association found that 36 percent of care recipients who live in the same household as their caregivers are spouses. Another 29 percent are elderly parents or parents-in-law, while 9 percent are children, 9 percent are adult friends, and 8 percent are grandparents.

Who these people receive their care from seems to have at least some correlation to their ethnic backgrounds. A study by the National Academy on an Aging Society revealed that among care recipients age 70 and older, whites are most likely to have their spouses as caregivers, while Hispanic-Americans can expect to

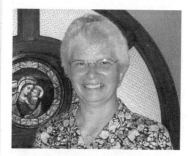

Point of View

"When giving long-term care, you see people in their very vulnerableness; you see them having to let go of so much in their lives—their loved ones, their homes, their possessions. Through my presence and my ministry, I can give them courage, affirmation, and security. In the richness of all of their experience over the years, they give me a sense of God's faithfulness. They are people of dignity.

"The important thing is our constancy with them—to be there, to accept them as they are, to know that they were once vibrant 60-year-old people. Now that they're 85 or 92 or 98, they are at our mercy to be gentle with them and accept them in their illness and their insecurity and their fear of what is yet to come."

—SISTER SUSAN
of the School Sisters of Notre Dame,
Mankato, Minnesota

Point of View

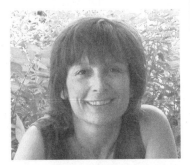

"There isn't anything I wouldn't do for my mom and dad. I just think how lucky I am to have been born to people like them, who sacrificed everything for me. I've had a very wonderful and exciting life. Now it's time for me to give back."

—LORRAINE WATSON,
Sherman Oaks, California

find their adult children in that role. And compared with those two ethnic groups, African-Americans are most likely to get help from someone outside the family.

THE ECONOMIC PERSPECTIVE

For anyone involved in a caregiving situation, whether as caregiver or a care recipient, one of the most pressing concerns is cost. Even if you're relatively new to the caregiving role, you probably have some idea of the potential financial burden you and your loved one are facing, whether you've been pricing nursing homes or shopping for adult diapers.

Fortunately for you, you're becoming a caregiver at a time when the number of caregiving-related products and resources is exploding. You'll find options to suit virtually any budget. As an example, for years the main alternative to caring for a loved one at home was placing the person in a nursing home. Now you can choose from assisted living facilities, continuing care communities, and even home care services—which, with the exception of round-the-clock skilled nursing care, tend to be less expensive than residential care.

Still, depending on the type and duration of care, the bills can stack up quickly. And they don't account for caregiving's "hidden" costs, like the caregiver's donated time and lost income from missed work hours. When a team of researchers at Albert Einstein College of Medicine in New York City factored in these costs, they came up with a price tag for informal (family) caregiving of $196 billion a year. By comparison, formal home health care added up to $32 billion a year, and nursing home care, $83 billion a year.

For caregivers, the lost earnings can hit especially hard. Many are forced to reduce their work hours or even quit their jobs to care for their loved ones, just as caregiving costs are putting the squeeze on family budgets. According to the 2001 study by AARP, nearly 20 percent of sandwich generation caregivers— those between ages 45 and 55—have cut back their work hours, even though they're in their prime earning years. And 27 percent help pay expenses for older family members.

Even when caregivers can stay on the job, their performance

can suffer. Research has shown that 42 percent of caregivers regularly arrive late for work, while 39 percent take sick days. Even when they're at work, they may be distracted by their caregiving responsibilities. All of these factors have an uncalculated impact on future earnings and career opportunities.

Ideally, care recipients will have made arrangements for financing their long-term care, so at least they and their caregivers can limit out-of-pocket expenses. But far too few people plan ahead; instead, the majority expect government programs like Medicare to foot the bill. As many a caregiver has discovered, Medicare covers only short-term stays in nursing homes for patients who are making the transition from hospital to home care. Generally, it doesn't pay for the kind of custodial care required by people with chronic illnesses and disabilities. (We'll talk more about Medicare in chapter 24.)

As a result, older care recipients and their families pay about 44 percent of their long-term care costs out of pocket. What's more, nearly 40 percent of people with chronic illnesses say they can't afford some or all of the services they need. Typically, middle-class caregiving families are hit hardest. Their loved ones don't qualify for Medicaid, yet they can't afford residential care.

To ease caregiving's financial burden, Mintz advises families to talk about finances long before anyone becomes sick and requires care. "We're living longer, and the incidence of chronic illness increases with age," she observes. "The best strategy is to be proactive."

Even if you're already in a caregiving situation, it's not too late to plan ahead. You and your loved one can estimate her long-term care costs, then develop a budget to stretch her savings and safeguard any assets. You also want to be sure that she's taking advantage of all the government programs and private benefits plans for which she's eligible. (We'll delve more deeply into caregiving finances in part 6.)

A GLANCE BEYOND OUR BORDERS

The challenges of caregiving—such as how to pay for it—are far from unique to the United States. Countries around the world are searching for solutions to assist their growing populations of

EXPERT OPINION

"Comparatively, the graying phenomenon is less of an issue in the United States than in many other countries, including Japan, Italy, and the Scandinavian countries. That's largely because we opened our doors to young immigrants who have come and helped to balance the relationship between young and old. Other societies and other cultures are facing a far greater challenge. What I'm seeing around the world is that all industrialized nations are bracing for a coming wave of older adults."

—WILLIAM H. THOMAS, M.D.,
caregiving advocate and founder of the Eden Alternative in Sherbourne, New York (www.edenalternative.com)

caregivers and care recipients. Some have made great strides, whether by supporting and sustaining traditional caregiving practices or by instituting progressive caregiving policies. Others are just beginning to address the population shifts that have precipitated dramatic changes in their nations' caregiving needs. (Incidentally, you'll read more about the world view of caregiving in the Post Cards throughout this book.)

Perhaps the most striking similarity among countries is that for the most part, families are the primary caregivers. In the United States, families provide up to 85 percent of eldercare. That figure is matched or surpassed in Asia, Africa, South America, Latin America, and many parts of Europe. Interestingly, in Canada, which has a nationalized program for medical care, the percentage of caregiving families is slightly smaller—70 percent.

Among the issues facing more economically developed countries in Europe and Asia is the growing number of women in the work force who are taking on caregiving roles, if not leaving their jobs to care for their loved ones. Also of concern to these countries are their rapidly graying populations. In China, where a one-child policy was in place during the 1970s and 1980s, one adult child must care for both parents as well as any surviving grandparents.

The impact of a booming elderly population has been felt not just in China but on a global scale. For example, in Latin American countries, a majority of older female care recipients—64 percent, according to one six-country study—are highly likely to be living in intergenerational homes. This trend is being replicated to a significant degree just about everywhere—including in the United States, where it primarily affects the sandwich generation. Still, traditional intergenerational households are most common in less developed countries.

As yet, no one country has instituted a completely problem-free approach to caregiving. Still, caregivers around the world can help each other and learn from one another as we unite in a global drive for change. As individuals, communities, and nations confront the challenges of caregiving in the years ahead, all of us can take comfort in knowing that we are not alone.

FACING CHALLENGE, FORGING CHANGE

For any kind of social challenge, solutions often find their voice through those in the trenches dealing with the fallout. That's certainly true in caregiving, where caregivers and care recipients alike are coming together to forge change.

"We are already at a point where caregiving is a major societal problem," states Dr. Schulz. "If we look ahead to the year 2005, 2010, 2020, or 2030, the demands for care will increase tremendously.

"Baby boomers do not have as many children as their parents did. So the caregiving load, which is considerably greater, will have to be carried by a relatively smaller number of people—unless we're able to address the issue on a societal level," Dr. Schulz adds. "Whatever solution we come up with, someone will have to bear the costs, whether they're monetary, physical, or psychological."

One potential boost for all caregivers is the increased awareness and involvement of the federal government. Caregiving advocates are succeeding in getting their messages heard by legislators. The long struggle to lobby for some new laws—and funding—is beginning to pay a small measure of dividends.

The National Family Caregiver Support Program, created in 2001, is the first substantial recognition of the caregiving movement by Congress. The program provides the following:

- Information about health problems, resources, and community-based long-term care services

- Assistance in finding help

- Counseling, support groups, and caregiver training to help families make decisions and solve problems

- Respite care to temporarily relieve caregivers of their responsibilities

- Limited supplemental services, including home modifications, incontinence supplies, and nutrition counseling

The program, and the $125 million allocated for it in 2001, is just a start. But caregiving advocates feel it's a significant step

Point of View

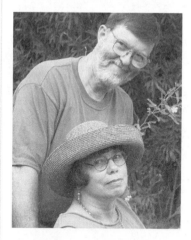

"Caregiving is calling each other into life, isn't it? Having my husband George participate in my care and having other people do the same calls me into life. It says, 'Despite your losses, despite your limitations, you belong here with us and we want you to stay.'

"Perhaps that's the fundamental goal of caregiving: to enable another person to want to be in the world. Not just enable them to be, but to enable them to want to be in the world when not being alive would be easier."

—NANCY MAIRS,
Tucson

forward in getting caregivers and care recipients the support and services they need.

While government action can help initiate much-needed changes in our nation's caregiving policies and practices, it isn't enough by itself. The push for caregiving reform must come from all sides—public agencies and private organizations, individuals and communities.

William H. Thomas, M.D., is one caregiving advocate who's ahead of this curve. He foresees a day when traditional nursing homes will be fazed out and replaced by a myriad of choices, including facilities influenced by his Eden Alternative movement, a consulting group that educates caregivers and managers of caregiving facilities.

After working as a physician in a nursing home for a number of years, Dr. Thomas started spinning his own version of an "eldertopia" in his head. Then he acted on it by founding the Eden Alternative. The concept already has been introduced in 450 residential care facilities around the country.

"I want an alternative to the institution," Dr. Thomas explains. "The best alternative I can think of is a garden. I believe when we make a place that's worthy of our elders, we make a place that enriches all of our lives—caregivers, family members, and elders alike. So the Eden Alternative provides a reinterpretation of the environment elders live in, going from an institution to a garden. That's why we call it the Eden Alternative."

Dr. Thomas is pleased when visitors to the "cream of the crop" facilities trained by Eden Alternative seem perplexed by what they see. "I want people to ask themselves, 'What kind of a place is this?'" he says. "There are kids running around and playing. There are dogs and cats and birds, and there are gardens and plants. I want people to think that this can't be a nursing home. Which it isn't—it's an alternative to a nursing home."

Instead of traditional nursing homes, Dr. Thomas envisions diffusing elders through the community in different places and different ways. To accomplish that, he says, caregivers will need to "think outside the box." But he's optimistic. He fully expects today's baby boomers to reinvent tomorrow's caregiving.

"The baby boom generation will completely wipe out the nursing home as we know it," he says. "The best way to understand what will happen is to think back to when baby boomers were kids. Ice cream came in just three flavors then—that's it. But the baby boomers wanted more choices. By the time they got done with ice cream, they had a thousand flavors. Well, right now, long-term care for the elderly comes in just three flavors. When the baby boomers get done, they'll have a thousand flavors. And that's the way it should be.

"The future of caregiving," Dr. Thomas concludes, "belongs to people and organizations who can dream new dreams about how to care for our elders." That's how all of us—the current generation of caregivers—can make a difference.

CHAPTER 2

PROFILES IN CARING

What You Need to Know

- Though each story is unique, all caregivers share similar joys and frustrations. Connecting with others who've taken on caregiving roles can help you feel less alone.

- Beyond emotional support, much wisdom can be gained from those who are currently caregivers and those who have been in the past. The insight and advice they can share can help shape your caregiving experience.

When you need help, you go to an expert, someone with the knowledge and experience to offer reasoned, responsible advice. In caregiving, you could seek counsel from physicians, geriatricians, geriatric care managers, social workers, and other professionals trained to support caregivers and care recipients alike. But for some issues, you might learn just as much from those in the trenches—the spouses, sons, daughters, and others who provide care for their ailing loved ones day in and day out.

To that end, you're about to meet several caregivers whose stories are featured in the PBS special *And Thou Shalt Honor*, upon which this book is based. Though each person's circumstances are unique, you'll find threads of common experience that tie the stories to each other—and, more than likely, to your own situation. These people have chosen to share their own struggles and successes to help those who follow in their footsteps. In their words, and the words of caregivers featured in the Point of View sidebars throughout this book, may you find comfort, strength, and hope.

LIVING THEIR OWN LOVE STORY

According to Mary Ann Nation of Franklin, Ohio, her caregiving story is "a lot better than some and a lot worse than others." Mary Ann serves as caregiver for her husband of 35 years, Harlan.

In March 1999, Harlan was diagnosed with a rare and incurable brain virus. He lost his ability to communicate orally and needs to use a wheelchair. Mary Ann has chosen not to put her husband in a nursing home or other care facility. Instead, she is responsible for his round-the-clock care.

This is not what Mary Ann imagined when the two young lovers married and quickly had three children. "The kids were our whole life. We put the three of them through college," she recalls. "Once they got married and started their own lives, we thought, 'Now it's our time.' We were going to do anything and everything we wanted."

But without warning, their lives would turn upside down.

When Mary Ann arrived home from work one night, she saw that Harlan was ill. She suspected he might be having a stroke.

"Why didn't you go to the hospital?" Mary Ann asked.

"I didn't know where it was," Harlan replied.

"Why didn't you call me at work?"

"I couldn't remember where you worked. I just knew this was home and you would be here pretty soon."

At first, doctors suspected Harlan had a tumor and suggested waiting to see if it would grow or move in direction. But then Harlan started experiencing severe, violent seizures. After one episode, which included an extremely hard fall, he was rushed to the hospital, where doctors performed emergency surgery to remove a hematoma from his brain. They didn't find a tumor, which seemed like good news—until they told Mary Ann that Harlan appeared to have a brain virus so rare they knew little about it.

Harlan has fared better than expected, says his doctor, Thomas Wantanbe, M.D., a rehabilitation specialist at the Drake Center in Cincinnati. According to Dr. Wantanbe, Harlan's life expectancy is normal, but his quality of life—and Mary Ann's—has undergone profound changes.

"Harlan needs assistance with the most basic tasks, like toileting, bathing, dressing, getting in and out of the car, going anywhere," Dr. Wantanbe explains. "For Mary Ann, it's quite a burden. She isn't working at this point, because Harlan requires a lot of care. Obviously, if we can maximize Harlan's function as much as possible, then we can ease Mary Ann's situation as well."

Despite the heavy workload, Mary Ann found hope in the smallest signs of recovery. "Little by little, he'd get better," she says. "When I first brought him home, he was scared to death. He came out of surgery and he couldn't talk, walk, or move his arm. He didn't know what was going on around him.

"One night, after I got the two of us ready for bed, I kept watching Harlan. I could sense something was different, but every time I looked at him, he would look at me blankly. I didn't know what to expect, and I was scared.

"So I crawled into bed beside him, and he started laughing. I didn't know what was going on. Then he showed me that he could move his toe the slightest bit. It was like, 'Hallelujah!' Moving that toe was the greatest thing in the world. He didn't want the kids to know for a day or two, until he could move his toes at will."

For her part, Mary Ann decided that she'd do what she could to keep her husband as active as possible. She worried that in becoming housebound, Harlan would grow accustomed to not seeing people and would eventually prefer not to go out. So she began taking him on regular outings, even when her sons questioned the wisdom of the trips or she herself was tempted to take the easier route of setting him up in a comfy chair or in bed.

"The disability itself is demeaning enough without having to beg people for help," Mary Ann says. "I've spent a lot of time thinking about this, and I've decided that you just have to make a life for yourself [as a caregiver and care recipient]. You just have to do things."

Still, some days test her resolve more than others. "Sometimes I load Harlan in the car and we'll go do something, even if I don't feel like doing it," Mary Ann says. "I'll take him to visit people that I really don't want to see. I'm kind of mad at them, kind of hurt. But it's not about me, it's about Harlan. He needs that."

As for Mary Ann, she doesn't regret a single minute of her caregiving experience. The Nations are living their own love story, the strongest kind, every day.

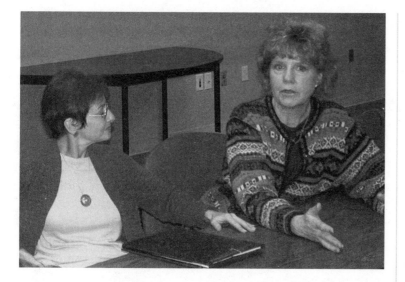

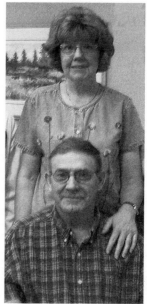

Above: Mary Ann Nation and her husband, Harlan.

Above left: Mary Ann discusses her caregiving experience with Suzanne Mintz, cofounder and president of the National Family Caregivers Association, based in Kensington, Maryland.

"Putting my husband in a home is not an option," Mary Ann says. "As long as he knows who I am, as long as he has memories of what we had together, and as long as he has feelings for what we have together now, it's not an option.

"I'm not saying putting a loved one in a home is wrong, because it's not. The time may come when I have to consider it, but not right now. Not as long as I can make him smile and he can make me smile.

"You know, when I was 18 and standing before that judge to get married, I really wasn't thinking about the vows I was taking. I didn't say to myself, 'Oh, man, this is for life, in sickness and health.' But it is. It's sickness and health. His and mine. You don't rewrite that. It's perfect the way it is."

A BLESSING IN DISGUISE

"Being a caregiver is valuable, rewarding, frustrating, draining—and I wouldn't have it any other way," says Ethelinn Block, a schoolteacher in Mesa, Arizona. She's the primary caregiver for her father, who has Alzheimer's disease. Her brother Brian lives five doors down the street and pitches in when he can. So does Ethelinn's son, along with a niece and nephew. Two other siblings, who live farther away, have not played active roles in their father's care.

"I know what I give to caregiving, but one of my concerns is what it's taking from me," Ethelinn says. "I give in a multitude of ways. I'm the mother, the confidant, the nurse. I'm the person who soothes my dad when he's sick; I figure out what needs to be done to help him get better. I deal not only with my own frustrations, but also with my father's and my family's. It's a lot of work."

Coping with the constant physical and emotional demands isn't easy. But Ethelinn finds strength in being able to honor her father by providing for his care. "What I am doing is what most anyone would do [in similar circumstances]," she says. "It is part of being a family. My father has nothing left except the respect he gets from his kids and grandkids. That's important to me."

Every night, before he falls asleep, Ethelinn's father says thank you. It is a small but treasured token of appreciation for the long hours Ethelinn puts in, and the lost opportunities she must confront.

Despite the sacrifices she has made, Ethelinn is quick to acknowledge all she has gained from her caregiving experience. "I am a more accepting, compassionate person," she notes. "I am also more flexible. For example, instead of insisting that my father adapt to my hours, I have adapted my schedule to his."

In Ethelinn's eyes, the rewards of being her father's caregiver more than outweigh the responsibilities. Still, she can't help but wish the rest of her family would help her out more.

Ethelinn Block is the primary caregiver for her father, Arthur. But she gets a much-needed helping hand from her brother, Brian, and his family, who live close by. Clockwise from right: Ethelinn; her father, Arthur; her niece, Brittany; her son, Nicholas; her sister-in-law, Vickie; her nephew, Tyler; and Brian.

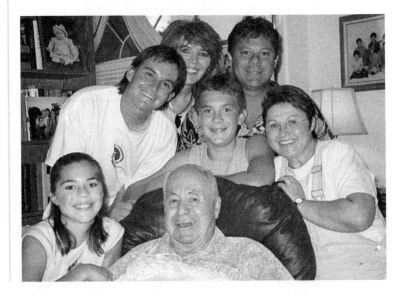

"I never imagined caregiving would be like this," she admits. "When my siblings and I decided that our father would move into my home, I thought we would be sharing the responsibilities. I was shocked and disappointed to realize it wouldn't be like that at all. Now I have one brother I can count on.

"Sometimes I feel jealous of the siblings who aren't helping me," she adds. "They can go out to dinner, run errands, and take vacations, and never worry about who's taking care of Dad. I'm always watching the clock. The home aide leaves at 4 in the afternoon. I have to be there. If an emergency arises, I have to leave work.

"I'm sure that somewhere in their hearts, my brother and my sister are grateful that I'm taking care of Dad and they're not. They're happy."

At least Ethelinn has her brother Brian and his family to count on. For that, she feels truly blessed. "We have stayed close through all of this," she says. "It shows that what we are doing is good and and strong and positive. It shows that we're a family."

SIBLINGS FORM A CAREGIVING TEAM

Mattie Boykin lives in Georgia, but not in one place for more than 4 months at a time. She would rather settle in one home, but "feels fine" about her frequent address changes.

Mattie raised six children. Three of them, Gladys Platt, Milton (Ray) Boykin, and Larry Stegall, decided to share the caregiving duties for their mother after she was hospitalized for a stroke in 1996. They didn't want to place Mattie in residential care, but none of the three were able to take her full-time. So they settled on a rotation.

"Actually, we started out with five or six caregivers," Larry recalls. "But people went their own ways, until only three of us were left.

"When you become a caregiver, you have to rearrange your life. The other three [siblings] weren't ready to commit to that," Larry says. "But we were willing, and all of us have jobs with a little bit of flexibility, so we could do it."

With their shared goal of giving back to their mother, the two brothers and their sister have never felt closer to one another. "We

EXPERT OPINION

"If we want to improve life for everybody in our society, one of the very best places to begin is to change how we think about, care for, and honor our elders. That thread, if you trace it all the way back, is woven through the whole context of our social lives, our families, our churches, our communities. If we can master the art of caring for our elders, we can make a better society for everybody to live in."

—WILLIAM H. THOMAS, M.D., caregiving advocate and founder of the Eden Alternative in Sherbourne, New York (www.edenalternative.com)

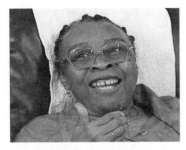

Above: Mattie Boykin.

Right: Mattie's care is a priority for her children—Milton Boykin, Gladys Platt, and Larry Stegall (left to right).

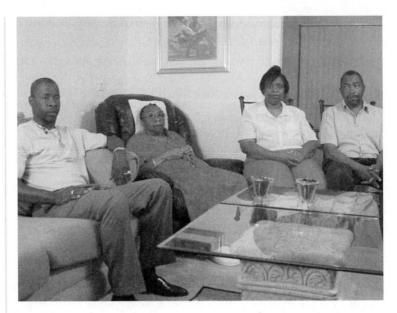

work together and depend on each other," Ray says. "We have disagreements; it isn't always peaches and cream. But we realize that all of us just want to look out for our mother. That outweighs everything."

Like her brothers, Gladys says she doesn't think she is doing anything special. For her, looking after an aging parent just seems right.

"It can be hard, especially on my social life, since I'm single," Gladys says. "But my mom and I, we sit together, we go to the doctor together. She's like my partner."

Fortunately, Gladys has an understanding employer, which is no small matter for caregivers. "If my brothers call with an emergency, I talk to my boss," Gladys says. "At one point, I said to him, 'I think I have to step down so that I can care for my mom.' I was willing to take a lower position just so I wouldn't have to let my mama go in a home.

"But my boss said, 'Let's see if we can work something out.' That's what he has been doing ever since—working things out for me. If I need to take time off, if I need to bring my mama to work, he's fine with that. It relieves a lot of stress for me."

When she's with her mother, Gladys often thinks back to her youth, and to Mattie's commitment to her family. "We were very,

very poor, but Mama did whatever she had to do to take care of us," Gladys says. "I remember a time around my graduation, when I needed a dress but she couldn't afford to buy one. She did anyway. I found out later that she used the rent money to pay for it. That made me so proud.

"Mama has this incredible inner strength," Gladys continues. "When she was under pressure, we would never see it; we would never see her stressed. She did what she felt she had to do to make sure I got my dress. It all comes down to 'whatever it takes.'"

Mattie's children have that same "whatever it takes" attitude, a valuable reserve for any caregiver. "Mama has done so much not just for me but for my family," Gladys says. "She honored me, so I will honor her."

A STUNNING DIAGNOSIS CHANGES LIFE FOR NEWLYWEDS

You never think it will happen to you. Bill Deutsch surely didn't.

Within a year of marrying his wife, Marisol, in the lush surroundings of Jamaica, the 57-year-old physician from Staten Island, New York, noticed he was having difficulty recalling his patients'

Marisol Deutsch is the primary caregiver for her husband, Bill, who's in the early stages of Alzheimer's disease.

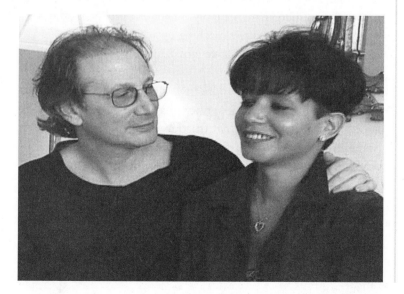

names and medications. He couldn't concentrate as well. He would walk into a room, then not remember why he went there.

Bill consulted fellow physicians about his symptoms. He wondered whether a recent change in medications might be causing them. One doctor ordered an MRI to determine whether Bill had suffered a stroke without realizing it. The test turned out negative.

Then a neurologist recommended a brain scan. The results were staggering. They showed changes in Bill's brain consistent with the early stages of Alzheimer's disease. The doctor immediately prescribed three medications, plus daily vitamin E supplements, to try to slow the cognitive impairment.

Catching the disease early provides some hope to the Deutsches. Still, Marisol has been thrust into the role of caregiver sooner than she might ever have anticipated. Bill has stopped working. He forgets certain things, like whether he took his medications or how to get to a doctor's office.

"I take care of everything," says Marisol, who had worked for Bill before moving away in the mid-1990s, only to return when he courted and then married her. "I do the errands, pay the bills, and schedule the appointments."

For Marisol, coping with the changes in her husband's behavior hasn't been easy. "He's not the same person I used to know," she says. "He's not as outgoing. It's difficult."

In fact, Bill's situation has taken a toll on Marisol's health, triggering the reemergence of a long-quelled ulcer. "I guess the stress of what's going on is really catching up with me," she says. "I just hate seeing the person I love not functioning in the way he should."

"At one point, I had so many appointments for physical therapy and recovery from surgery that she couldn't even think about herself," says Bill. "I get frustrated and she gets frustrated. Sometimes the two of us, you know, we get excited, but then we manage to calm down. She's been very supportive and understanding. When we got married, I didn't know I had anything like this. I'm sure this was as much a surprise to her as it was to me."

Like many caregivers, Marisol takes one day at a time. "You just have to hold on," she says.

PART TWO

When a Loved One Needs Care

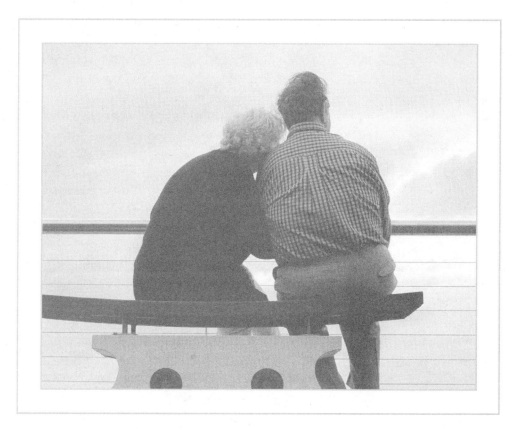

CHAPTER 3

"SHOULD I INTERVENE?"

What You Need to Know

- Entering into a caregiving relationship can be stressful for everyone involved—but it doesn't *need* to be. The key is to manage change well.

- Before you intervene in a loved one's care, assess the person's health and lifestyle. You may realize that he needs only minimal help with specific tasks.

- Don't overreact to your loved one's situation. Occasional memory lapses and other minor behavioral changes should be expected with age or illness.

- If your loved one hasn't already done so, encourage him to undergo a complete physical and cognitive evaluation.

- The first steps toward intervention can be the most difficult. It gets easier with experience.

To intervene or not to intervene: It's a potentially life-altering question. And it comes with no easy answer, no definitive formula for making a decision. Whichever path you choose, you may have second thoughts.

This is to be expected; after all, you're entering unfamiliar territory. Whenever you're feeling unsure of yourself, just remember: *There is no right or wrong way to give care.* As long as you have your loved one's best interests at heart, that's all anyone can ask or expect.

To be sure, intervening can mean major changes for you and your loved one. By its very nature, change involves uncertainty, anxiety, and varying degrees of stress. But it also presents an opportunity to learn skills and to improve relationships.

Signs to Watch For

While the decision to intervene in a loved one's care is seldom clear-cut, certain physical and behavioral changes are definitely cause for concern. Keep a watchful eye for the following red flags.

- Appreciable weight loss or gain
- Sudden paranoia, combativeness, aggression, or hallucinations
- Disturbing changes in attitude and self-esteem
- A noticeable decline in hygiene and grooming
- Excuses for skipping routine tasks like going to the doctor, the barber, or the grocery store
- Lack of interest in friends, hobbies, and activities
- Social isolation
- Unpaid bills, or notices about utilities being shut off
- Unsafe behaviors such as leaving food burning on the stove
- Frequent falls
- Frequent memory lapses
- Getting lost on familiar, well-traveled routes

Keep in mind, too, that in caregiving—as in so many other aspects of life—change is constant. At first, your loved one may need help only with specific tasks, like running errands or fall-proofing his home. But the level of care needed may increase over time.

That's why the initial intervention can feel so difficult: It raises the prospect of a loved one gradually losing the ability to look after himself. And if that person perceives your intervention as interference, he may lash out, saying, "How dare you! You have no right!" when you broach the idea of hiring a home health aide or assuming responsibility for financial matters. Other family members may side with your loved one, saying you're out of line.

Deciding to intervene means wrestling with some very complex and surprising emotions. It means bouncing back and forth between the convictions "I shouldn't" and "I must." It means taking charge and then wondering whether you should have.

But sometimes you have no choice. Sometimes you have to step in and help.

In the event of a sudden medical crisis, such as a stroke or a broken hip, the need for someone to assume a caregiving role is quite clear. By comparison, a slow decline in health can be more difficult to contend with. The need for care is less apparent and more a judgment call. And family members often disagree on what's best.

Take Action... ASSESS THE NEED FOR CARE

Before you intervene, you must ask yourself why you're concerned about your loved one's welfare. The occasional uncharacteristic act—missing an appointment or stumbling on a flight of stairs—shouldn't sound any alarms. But if such behaviors become more frequent, or get worse over time, that's your cue to take action.

The Caregiver's Checklist on page 30, adapted from the Daily Tasks Appraisal for Caregivers on the CaregiverPA Web site (http://caregiverpa.psu.edu), can help you evaluate a loved one's need for care. To complete it, follow these instructions.

X Make several copies of the checklist so you can use it more than once.

✗ Do your first assessment as soon as you suspect your loved one might need help.

✗ Be discreet. You don't want the person to feel you're spying.

✗ Be kind. You and your loved one are embarking on an emotionally challenging journey. Be as gracious and accommodating as possible. Treat the person with dignity and respect. If the two of you have experienced problems in your relationship, now is the time to mend fences. Intervening is much easier when your loved one trusts you and believes you have his best interests at heart.

✗ Distribute the checklist to other family members and request their assistance in monitoring your loved one. The checklist may help them notice subtle changes in your loved one's behavior. If they agree that intervention is necessary, they can lend support when you approach your loved one about your concerns.

✗ Reassess the person every few months.

✗ Date each checklist so you can identify and track any decline in function.

Through this exercise, you may realize that your loved one is faring better than you expected, or needs help only in certain areas. Even if the situation is more urgent or serious, you have valuable information to prioritize your next steps—the first of which should be asking your loved one to get a thorough medical evaluation.

Take Action... GET A PHYSICIAN'S OPINION

In chapter 8, you'll learn about the various health professionals—geriatricians, geriatric care managers, social workers, and the like—who can guide you and your loved one through important caregiving decisions. Long before the two of you get that far, you *must* make sure your loved one sees a doctor for a complete physical and cognitive evaluation.

Here's why: When an older person shows gradual but unmistakable signs of decline, we tend to assume that person must have Alzheimer's disease. We'll talk more about Alzheimer's disease in

(continued on page 33)

EXPERT OPINION

"When missteps in judgment, self-care, or safety are readily apparent, family members rarely disagree about intervening. The trickier, more common scenarios involve subtle slips that escape casual notice. As long as there's no risk to others, I advise families to give an older person 'room to fail' by providing the least restrictive alternative available."

—MARK S. LACHS, M.D., M.P.H., chief of geriatrics and gerontology at New York Hospital in Manhattan

Does Your Loved One Require Care?

In each of the 20 categories below, place a check mark next to the description that best fits your loved one. An A response means all is well, while a B suggests that intervention might be necessary. If you choose C, your loved one clearly requires help, though the nature and scope of that care can vary. A D response means the person requires full-time assistance, perhaps from a home health aide or in an assisted living facility.

Of course, real life is seldom as clear-cut as the choices in this checklist. You may give your loved one an A in some categories but a B or C in others. Even so, the checklist can be a valuable tool when discussing the need for care with your loved one and other family members. Just as important, it can provide some welcome reinforcement and reassurance, should you decide to intervene.

1. Communication

____ **A.** No difficulty speaking, reading, writing, or comprehending.

____ **B.** Occasional trouble recalling words. Reads less. Handwriting is not as legible. Sometimes requests that information be repeated, then comprehends.

____ **C.** Frequent trouble recalling words. Avoids reading; needs help with restaurant menus. Handwriting deteriorates noticeably. Frequently requests that information be repeated, but still may not comprehend.

____ **D.** Significant problems with word recall, reading, writing, and comprehension. Struggles to maintain a conversation.

2. Mental Function

____ **A.** Exercises good judgment. Makes appropriate decisions. No trouble recalling people, places, appointments, directions, or recent events.

____ **B.** Exercises reasonably good judgment, but requires some help or prompting. Experiences occasional memory lapses.

____ **C.** Has noticeable difficulty with judgment. Frequently needs help making decisions. Shows significant memory impairment. Often appears confused.

____ **D.** Judgment and memory substantially unreliable. Needs considerable help making decisions.

3. Mood

____ **A.** Reasonably good morale and self-esteem.

Copes well with everyday stress. Grieves losses, then bounces back and carries on with life.

____ **B.** Displays occasional anxiety, depression, irritability, or fear that may interfere with normal functioning.

____ **C.** Increasing problems with anxiety, depression, irritability, or fear.

____ **D.** Mood problems take over. Becomes unmanageable and may cause harm to himself or others.

4. Behavior

____ **A.** Acts as usual in social situations.

____ **B.** Occasionally acts in an unusual way—for example, wearing the same clothes day after day. Finds unreasonable fault with others.

____ **C.** Frequently acts in disturbing ways that draw the attention of others. You avoid social situations with the person because of the potential for erratic behavior.

____ **D.** Erratic behavior predominates. The person no longer can function socially.

5. Mobility

____ **A.** Walks satisfactorily for a person of that age. Needs no help with stairs, escalators, or revolving doors.

____ **B.** Noticeably slower when walking or climbing stairs. Occasionally needs help with escalators and revolving doors.

____ **C.** Avoids walking. Frequently needs assistance;

may use a cane or a walker. Climbing stairs is increasingly difficult.

___ **D.** Cannot walk unassisted. Climbing stairs is difficult to impossible.

6. Medications

___ **A.** Takes own medications as directed, with few, if any, lapses.

___ **B.** Sometimes is confused about which medications to take when. Occasionally takes the wrong one(s).

___ **C.** Needs regular supervision to take medications correctly.

___ **D.** Depends on others to manage medications.

7. Meals

___ **A.** Prepares meals satisfactorily. Eats well without assistance.

___ **B.** Eats without assistance but occasionally has difficulty preparing meals. Sometimes lets refrigerator and pantry become bare or allows food to spoil.

___ **C.** Needs some help preparing meals and eating. Cannot maintain refrigerator and pantry without assistance; frequently allows food to spoil.

___ **D.** Unable to prepare meals. Cannot eat unaided.

8. Alcohol Use

___ **A.** Not an issue. Drinks moderately in social situations, if at all.

___ **B.** Liquor bottles appear in the garbage or elsewhere in the home with disturbing frequency, but the person seems unimpaired.

___ **C.** Signs of alcohol use increase. The person smells of liquor and appears drunk.

___ **D.** Alcohol use is out of control. Person displays disruptive behavior.

9. Finances

___ **A.** Needs no help with banking, paying bills, or balancing the checkbook.

___ **B.** Easily makes routine purchases but occasionally struggles with other financial matters, such as paying bills or balancing the checkbook.

___ **C.** Needs help to manage personal finances.

___ **D.** Incapable of managing personal finances.

10. Safety

___ **A.** Maintains a safe lifestyle; remembers to lock doors, turn off the oven, and fasten seat belt.

___ **B.** Experiences occasional safety lapses.

___ **C.** Experiences more frequent safety lapses.

___ **D.** Lacks awareness of safety issues, potentially posing a danger to self and others.

11. Housekeeping

___ **A.** Maintains home at usual levels of neatness and cleanliness.

___ **B.** Can perform most housekeeping tasks, but with occasional lapses in neatness; for example, may allow garbage, mail, and newspapers to pile up.

___ **C.** Housekeeping skills are deteriorating. Needs help to maintain home at usual levels of neatness and cleanliness.

___ **D.** Unable to perform housekeeping tasks. Seems unconcerned about neatness and cleanliness or overwhelmed by the inability to maintain home.

12. Social Life

___ **A.** Maintains usual level of interpersonal relations with family and friends.

___ **B.** Occasionally has difficulty with relationships. May act insensitive or fail to observe expected social graces.

___ **C.** Needs prompting and assistance to maintain usual level of interpersonal relations.

___ **D.** Little remaining aptitude for relationships. Not interested in or concerned about others.

13. Transportation

___ **A.** Travels independently. Drives or arranges for other transportation.

___ **B.** Experiences some lapses in judgment behind the wheel. Sometimes ignores stop signs and traffic lights. Has gotten tickets and/or has been

(continued)

Caregiver's Checklist
continued

involved in minor accidents. Sometimes struggles to arrange for other transportation.

___ **C.** Experiences frequent lapses in judgment behind the wheel. Makes passengers feel unsafe, especially when driving at night. Often needs help arranging for other transportation.

___ **D.** Can no longer drive safely. Always needs help arranging for other transportation.

14. Toileting

___ **A.** Needs no help.

___ **B.** Occasional accidents; needs some help.

___ **C.** Frequent incidents of wetting and soiling; needs more help.

___ **D.** Can no longer toilet alone.

15. Bathing

___ **A.** Bathes satisfactorily without assistance.

___ **B.** Reports difficulty with bathing. Needs help getting into and out of the tub or shower.

___ **C.** Needs regular assistance with bathing. May try to avoid it.

___ **D.** Cannot bathe satisfactorily, even with considerable help. Seems unconcerned about personal cleanliness.

16. Grooming

___ **A.** Grooms satisfactorily without assistance.

___ **B.** Experiences occasional lapses in grooming; may neglect to comb hair, or may have trouble shaving, brushing teeth, or caring for dentures or glasses.

___ **C.** Needs considerable help with grooming.

___ **D.** Cannot groom without assistance. Seems unconcerned about appearance.

17. Dressing

___ **A.** Dresses without assistance. Makes appropriate choices in clothing.

___ **B.** May struggle with buttons, jewelry, and/or neckties. May need help selecting clothes.

___ **C.** Dresses with assistance. May seem intimidated by the choices in a closet full of clothes and shoes. May rely on someone else to put together outfits.

___ **D.** Needs help with nearly all aspects of dressing.

18. Grocery Shopping

___ **A.** Purchases groceries without assistance.

___ **B.** Less able to shop independently. May forget items, which results in more frequent trips to the supermarket. Pantry may lack some staples but contain multiples of others.

___ **C.** Needs help to shop. Seems intimidated by the supermarket and more forgetful. Pantry is in a worsening state of disarray.

___ **D.** Unable to shop even with assistance.

19. Laundry

___ **A.** Does own laundry satisfactorily. Takes care of clothing without assistance.

___ **B.** Has some trouble identifying items that need to be hand-washed or dry-cleaned.

___ **C.** Needs help to do laundry; seems confused by the task.

___ **D.** Unable to do laundry even with assistance. Relies on someone else to wash clothes.

20. Telephone Use

___ **A.** Converses appropriately. Looks up telephone numbers, maintains a personal phone/address book satisfactorily. Able to manage a cordless phone.

___ **B.** Occasionally seems distracted or confused during conversations. Sometimes has difficulty looking up telephone numbers and keeping track of them. Occasionally misplaces a cordless phone.

___ **C.** Frequently seems distracted or confused during conversations. Shows decline in ability to look up telephone numbers and keep track of them. Frequently forgets to hang up the phone; often misplaces a cordless phone.

___ **D.** Has significant trouble using the phone; may avoid it.

chapter 14. What you need to know now is that many people who seem to have the disease actually don't.

Yes, Alzheimer's is common, but not as common as we might think. One often-cited statistic describes the condition as affecting some 10 percent of Americans over age 65. But according to a federal government analysis, only 2 percent of the U.S. population between ages 64 and 74 have Alzheimer's disease. The incidence rises to 7 to 10 percent among people ages 75 to 84, and 35 to 45 percent among those 85 and older. In other words, even among the oldest Americans, fewer than half develop Alzheimer's.

The fact is, many conditions can cause changes in mental and physical function that can be mistaken for Alzheimer's disease, especially to the untrained eye. So finding out exactly what's behind your loved one's decline is critical. "It might not be dementia," notes Mark S. Lachs, M.D., M.P.H., chief of geriatrics and gerontology at New York Hospital in Manhattan. "It might be something treatable."

The only way to determine the cause of your loved one's symptoms is through a comprehensive physical and cognitive assessment. In the grand scheme of caregiving, asking your loved one to schedule such a checkup isn't nearly as stressful as, say, taking away the person's car keys. You get to try your hand at intervening, while your loved one can experience the respect and trust essential to a caregiving relationship.

What if your loved one refuses to undergo a medical evaluation? You cannot force a legally competent adult to consult a physician, explain Joseph Ilardo, Ph.D., L.C.S.W., and Carole Rothman, Ph.D., in their book *Are Your Parents Driving You Crazy?* But you can try the following, which may change the person's mind.

✗ Ask why your loved one doesn't want to see a doctor—and when the person offers an explanation, say you understand.

✗ Be creative about finding solutions to your loved one's objections. If she says, "I hate that doctor," suggest shopping around for a new one. If "I don't understand him" is the complaint, offer to go along and explain things. And if the response is "I don't want to undress," say you'll talk with the doctor beforehand to make sure it isn't necessary.

FOR MORE INFORMATION

If your loved one has been diagnosed with Alzheimer's disease, you can learn more about the disease—and get much-needed advice and support—through the following organizations.

• Alzheimer's Association, 919 North Michigan Avenue, Suite 1100, Chicago, IL 60611-1676. **(800) 272-3900**; **www.alz.org**.

• Alzheimer's Disease Education and Referral Center, PO Box 8250, Silver Spring, MD 20907-8250. **(800) 438-4380**; **www.alzheimers.org**.

FOR MORE INFORMATION

To contact your local Adult Protective Services office, look in the blue pages of your phone directory, under "Guide to Human Services." If you don't see a listing, then try calling your Area Agency on Aging—also in the blue pages.

Note: Before taking this course of action, be sure to seek knowledgeable counsel, such as an attorney who specializes in elder law.

✗ If your loved one still won't submit to a medical exam, enlist the aid of other relatives, friends, clergy—anyone whom the person holds in high regard.

✗ As a last resort, report the situation to your local Adult Protective Services office, which is responsible for protecting older people from neglect, abuse, and exploitation. Refusal to see a physician is considered self-neglect. Be aware that contacting Adult Protective Services is a serious measure with potentially huge legal, financial, and emotional ramifications. It should be pursued only when your loved one's life is in danger—and even then only with knowledgeable legal counsel.

WHAT THE DOCTOR SHOULD LOOK FOR

Assuming your loved one has a primary-care physician with whom he feels comfortable (and every older person should), that's the best place to begin a medical evaluation. The doctor can make referrals to specialists as necessary, and possibly provide leads on caregiving resources.

You may want to take along the checklist you completed, so the doctor can see the sorts of changes that prompted your concern in the first place. They may be signs of an underlying problem, such as:

Medication side effects and interactions. Many drugs for heart disease, high blood pressure, anxiety, depression, and other conditions produce side effects that might be interpreted as mental or behavioral decline. In fact, *any* new medication should be viewed as a possible culprit. Perhaps the dose is too high, or maybe the new drug is interacting with other pills—not just prescription and over-the-counter pharmaceuticals, but also herbal and nutritional supplements. That's why the doctor needs to know everything your loved one is taking. Be sure to make a list for the doctor's reference. (For more information about drug interactions, see chapter 15.)

Alcohol intolerance. As a person gets older, alcohol becomes more impairing, says Anne Simons, M.D., assistant clinical professor of family and community medicine at the University of California, San Francisco, Medical Center. "The drink or two your loved one could handle easily at age 60 might cause confusion and other behavioral changes at age 75," Dr. Simons explains.

Depression. Generally, depression is defined as profound sadness, coupled with feelings of helplessness and hopelessness. In older people, however, the condition can manifest itself quite differently. Rather than being sad, a person may appear agitated, hostile, or disoriented. (For more information about depression, see chapter 12.)

Transient ischemic attacks (TIAs). While these may be referred to as mini-strokes, they bear little resemblance to full-blown strokes. A stroke occurs suddenly and produces very distinctive symptoms: slurred speech, loss of balance, paralysis. Sometimes it can lead to death. By comparison, a TIA isn't nearly so dramatic. Its only symptom may be a brief period of disorientation, confusion, or "spacing out." Though this may seem benign enough, TIAs are cause for concern. They can increase in frequency, and they can become precursors to more serious medical conditions.

Caregiving around the World

In Sweden, about 7,400 people are granted a paid leave of absence each year, for an average of 10 days, to care for a close relative or friend who is seriously ill or dying. These payments are called close person's allowances and are social insurance benefits.

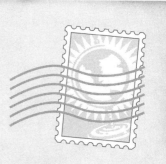

POST CARD

FROM SWEDEN

EXPERT OPINION

"Anyone can get on the wrong bus, or misplace the cordless phone, or forget to stock up on toilet paper. Nobody's perfect. In assessing a loved one's deterioration, look for repeated patterns of declining ability, especially those that might endanger the person or others. Give your loved one the benefit of the doubt. Too many elderly have their autonomy taken away before it's really necessary."

—**GLORIA CAVANAUGH,** president and chief executive officer of the American Society on Aging, based in San Francisco

Post-surgical impairment. A study by University of Florida researchers found that 25 percent of elderly patients develop memory and concentration problems after any surgery involving general anesthesia. In 10 percent, the problems can last for several months. Few people realize that this impairment can occur, which means they may mistake it for the onset of Alzheimer's disease. Cancer chemotherapy also affects mental function.

Nutrient deficiencies. Many older people run low on key nutrients, the result of poor eating habits, an imbalanced diet, and inefficient metabolism. Shortages of the B vitamins—in particular, B_1 (thiamin), B_3 (niacin), folate, and B_{12}—can lead to memory and coordination problems, according to New York City clinical nutritionist Shari Lieberman, Ph.D. (Chapter 13 takes a more in-depth look at diet and nutrition for older people.)

Inadequate hydration. In older people especially, the thirst mechanism may not function all that well. A lack of fluids can contribute to a number of health problems, including dizziness and confusion.

Indoor air pollution. Has your loved one recently moved into a newly constructed or renovated home? The chemicals released by new carpeting and furnishings (formaldehyde) and by new paint, finishes, and wall coverings (volatile organic compounds) can trigger confusion, disorientation, and mental decline. These chemicals are much more likely to affect the older population than younger people. If the doctor thinks indoor air pollution might be the culprit, you can arrange for your loved one to stay elsewhere for about a month, and see if the person's mental function improves.

Endocrine (hormone) imbalances. An underactive thyroid can produce symptoms that might mimic dementia, Dr. Lachs notes. The same is true for undiagnosed diabetes. Your loved one's doctor should order tests to check for an endocrine imbalance. If one is found, it likely can be managed with medication or alternative treatments, or some combination of the two.

Seizures. Most people associate seizures with loss of consciousness and muscle spasms. But as Dr. Lachs explains, some cause only unusual behavior. For example, someone who's having a seizure may move his jaw as if chewing or fumble with his clothes for an extended period of time, or simply appear "spaced out." In many cases, seizures can be controlled with medication.

Brain tumors. A brain tumor can produce physical symptoms like muscle weakness, as well as mental and behavioral symptoms like disorientation, speech impairment, and personality changes. Any of these might be mistaken for signs of Alzheimer's disease, especially since the risk of developing a brain tumor increases with age. Make sure your loved one receives a CT scan as part of the medical evaluation.

Intervening from Afar

An estimated 4 percent of the American workforce cares for loved ones who live more than 2 hours away. "Even from a distance, support can make a significant difference," says Ellen Rubenson, M.S.W., a social worker at Providence Medford Medical Center in Medford, Oregon, and author of *When Aging Parents Can't Live Alone.* "While the actual time spent with your loved one may be limited, the effort to stay in close contact is very important." Here's what you can do.

- Visit as often as you can.
- Phone frequently. You may even want to set up a schedule, so your loved one knows when to expect your calls. If the person is hearing-impaired, you can obtain special telephone equipment for him from the Deaf and Disabled Telecommunications Program. Write to 1939 Harrison Street, Suite 520, Oakland, CA 94612, or call (800) 867-4323.
- Encourage other family members to phone, too, perhaps setting up a calling rotation so someone is always checking in.
- Organize local support. Perhaps a neighbor or friend would be willing to look in on your loved one regularly. Or members of your loved one's religious community might be able to help.
- Utilize community resources. Senior centers, meal delivery programs, transportation services, and adult day care are just some of the resources that can improve your loved one's life—and reassure you. And in many communities, public- and private-sector employees such as mail carriers, meter readers, bank tellers, and grocery clerks are trained to watch for signs of trouble (for example, mail piling up uncollected). This service is coordinated through the Area Agency on Aging.
- Consider installing a personal emergency response system in your loved one's home. The system is hooked up to a central monitoring station, whose staff maintains contact with your loved one and can call in rescue personnel in the event of a true emergency. Some systems offer additional services such as medication management and telephone reassurance.
- Hire a geriatric care manager (GCM) to organize and manage those aspects of your loved one's care that you cannot handle yourself. GCMs receive diverse training that enables them to serve as social worker, nurse, counselor, and financial advisor. Look for one who is certified by the National Association of Professional Geriatric Case Managers. For a referral, write to the NAPGCM at 1604 North Country Club Road, Tucson, AZ 85716, or check the organization's Web site at www.caremanager.org.

EXPERT OPINION

"Honor is a way of expressing the sacred in a human being. Why do we care for the old and the frail? Why do we honor them? We do it because we can see through the withered husk of the body. We can see the human spirit still pure, still complete, still beautiful. And when we commit ourselves to the work of caring for that person, we honor the true essence of that human being."

—**WILLIAM H. THOMAS, M.D.,**
caregiving advocate and founder of the Eden Alternative in Sherbourne, New York (www.edenalternative.com)

WHERE YOU'LL GO FROM HERE

While several of the problems mentioned above are serious, the good news is that all of them are treatable to some degree. Your loved one may not require assistance after all—at least not yet. The two of you (and other family members, as appropriate) would be wise to seize on the opportunity to plan ahead, so you're prepared to make the transition into a caregiving relationship if and when the time comes.

Even if your loved one needs care now, you may have intervened early enough so that you can work with the person to lay out a comprehensive caregiving plan. Admittedly, this can be a challenge. Your loved one may resent your "intrusion," or may fear becoming "a burden." Family members may dispute the need for care or disagree with your plan of action. You yourself may feel conflicted or guilty, especially if your loved one remains capable of making most of his own decisions.

Indeed, as long as the person remains reasonably competent—earning mostly A's and B's on the Caregiver's Checklist—he has every legal and moral right to chart his own course. Everyone needs to respect this. "After all, your loved one still has the wisdom of many active, productive years," notes Ellen Rubenson, M.S.W., a social worker at Providence Medford Medical Center in Medford, Oregon, and author of *When Aging Parents Can't Live Alone.* "In an early intervention, remember that your goal is to make the person happy, comfortable, and safe."

If your loved one won't accept your help just yet, use this time to research community resources, so you'll know what's available when the person is ready to discuss it. And be sure to stay in touch with other family members. That way, they'll feel their input matters—and you'll get a sense of who's willing to pitch in and provide support.

As your loved one becomes more dependent, you may notice that the person is less cantankerous about receiving assistance—and you feel less conflicted about providing it. What's more, those family members who once resisted intervention now may realize its necessity. Everyone can move forward with clear heads, open hearts—and a mutual understanding that giving care is the right thing to do.

CHAPTER 4

BUILDING BRIDGES

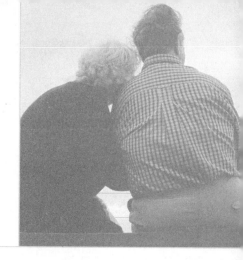

What You Need to Know

- Caregiving can be very demanding, especially if you're doing it alone. Don't feel ashamed or guilty about asking for help.

- Begin enlisting the aid of others by contacting community agencies and finding out about the services they provide.

- Schedule a family meeting and invite any relatives who could be involved in making decisions or providing care for your loved one.

- Find ways to involve your spouse, your children, and even close friends in the caregiving process.

From the outset of your caregiving experience, take to heart the well-known words of the English poet and clergyman John Donne: "No man [or woman] is an island." You need the physical and emotional support of others, especially if you're the primary caregiver. You get that support by reaching out to family and friends—in essence, by building bridges between the islands.

These bridges are crucial if you want to thrive in your caregiving role. As Gloria Cavanaugh, president and chief executive officer of the San Francisco–based American Society on Aging, observes, "Caregiving is one of the most challenging tasks a person can take on, especially if the situation lasts for more than a few months. You can't do it all yourself. You need help, and lots of it."

Many caregivers try to manage on their own. That's how we humans are socialized. We prize our personal independence, our self-reliance, our ability to accomplish things for ourselves. We don't want to be dependent on anyone else.

Point of View

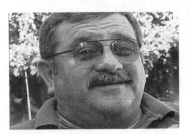

"My sister and I lived in the same town as our parents. Our other siblings moved away. We communicated all the time by phone, so my sister and I weren't doing everything.

"But caregiving gets to you. We were exhausted, catching colds all the time. Finally, we called a family meeting.

"Everyone said they'd help. And they did. But my sister and I were dealing with Dad every day. He'd wander off. Once he was lost all night.

"We talked to our siblings about placing Dad in a nursing home. It wasn't easy, but we found a place that cared for people with Alzheimer's.

"Now my sister and I can sleep at night knowing that he's being taken care of.

"You grow up hearing about how family members took care of other family members. But today, everyone works. To me, honoring Dad means knowing he's well taken care of, even if it's in a nursing home."

—CHARLES FIGUEROA,
Santa Barbara, California

But the American image of the totally self-sufficient "rugged individual" is an illusion. In virtually every aspect of our lives, notes Claire Berman, author of *Caring for Yourself While Caring for Your Aging Parents*, we're involved with others—and we count on them. Even if you live alone and do all of your housekeeping yourself, you most likely call a plumber when your sink gets clogged, a mechanic when your car breaks down, or the electric company when your power shuts off. That's true for the vast majority of us.

As caregivers, we're dealing with loved ones who are becoming more dependent on us over time. So we, in turn, must become more dependent on the family members and friends who help us and comfort us.

Unfortunately, many of us cling to the belief that asking for assistance is a sign of weakness, a personal failing. That's not so, says Virginia Morris, author of *How to Care for Aging Parents*. Total independence is an unrealistic notion, and an unhealthy one at that. We need to separate ourselves from it, or risk being overwhelmed by our caregiving roles. We must change our habitual ways of relating to the world around us, just as our loved ones are changing theirs.

As a caregiver, you're going to develop a whole new set of skills, not the least of which is reaching out to others. It may feel uncomfortable at first, but with practice, it will build courage and self-confidence. Sure, you might get no for an answer, but you'll learn to be flexible and to look elsewhere for the help you need. You'll also learn not to take every "no" personally.

Perhaps you want to ask for help, but you don't know how. You can learn. Consider it a caregiver's rite of passage.

Take Action... FIGURE OUT WHAT OTHERS CAN DO FOR YOU

As your loved one's situation evolves, so will your caregiving role. Certain tasks the person can manage herself now may require a helping hand down the road. That's okay, because you'll have planned ahead for them. And you'll have gotten some practice at asking others to pitch in.

Your immediate assignment is to figure out what sort of support your loved one needs right away or in the very near future, and what services you—or possibly community agencies—can provide. That way, when you approach other family members for help, you can be very explicit about which tasks they might take on. And you may feel more comfortable asking for their help once you see just how much you're doing and what remains to be done.

As you assemble your caregiving to-do list for your family, experts recommend following these steps. (If you'd like, you can make notes on the form on page 42.)

✗ Write down everything—including household chores, transportation, personal finances, and tasks of daily living (like dressing and grooming)—with which your loved one currently requires assistance. Be sure to gather as much input from your loved one as she's able to provide. Another good source of information is the Caregiver's Checklist you completed in chapter 3.

✗ Determine how often each task must be performed, getting as specific as you can. For example, your loved one may need a hand with mowing the lawn every week, or with paying the bills once a month. If you're caring for the person in your home, you might want someone to drive her to the senior center every Wednesday, while you're at work.

✗ Gather information about caregiving resources in your or your loved one's community, such as Meals on Wheels, transportation services, adult day care, and respite care. We'll explore these services in detail in chapters 19 and 20. For now, be aware that many agencies and organizations exist for the sole purpose of aiding caregivers like you. "Contact just one office to start," Cavanaugh advises. "The person there can direct you to other places, as necessary. You can make a lot of valuable connections with very little time and effort."

✗ Once you know what various agencies and organizations can offer, go back to your caregiving to-do list and mark which tasks they're able to take on, such as phone check-ins or grocery delivery. Be sure to keep contact information for everyone you've dealt with, in case you have additional questions once you've consulted your family.

FOR MORE INFORMATION

Perhaps the best place to start your search for community caregiving resources is with the Area Agency on Aging. The staff there can tell you about the services available locally, and can put you in touch with representatives of other agencies and organizations. To contact the office nearest you, look in the blue pages of your telephone directory, under "Guide to Human Services." You can also check the Eldercare Locator, a nationwide service sponsored by the U.S. Administration on Aging. Call **(800) 677-1116**, or visit the Eldercare Locator Web site at **www.eldercare.gov**.

Caregiver's Checklist

What Does Your Loved One Need?

Use this form to help track the various caregiving tasks with which your loved one—and you—could use a helping hand. As family members volunteer to help out, you can add their names to the "Who's Responsible" column, then make copies of the form for their reference. If an agency or organization is picking up a particular task, be sure to note the name and phone number of the person with whom you spoke under "Contact Information."

Task	How Often	Who's Responsible	Contact Information

✗ Make plans to share your list with your loved one, and with others in her caregiving circle. This might best be done at a family meeting, which we'll discuss next. However you decide to move forward, you'll know you've done your homework, thoroughly researching community resources and all of the services they provide. You've done everything you can without your family's involvement. Now all of you must decide on your respective roles in your loved one's care.

Take Action... PLAN A FAMILY MEETING

A family meeting allows all those who might want a say in a loved one's care, including the loved one herself, to gather for a frank discussion of the person's circumstances and needs. Attendees have equal opportunity to express their opinions about what needs to be done, by when, and by whom. If the meeting achieves its purpose, everyone will pull together to support the primary caregiver and ease the physical and emotional demands of giving care.

There is no "best" time to arrange the first meeting. Some families choose to convene before a loved one requires considerable support, so they can plan ahead. But for many others, a medical crisis forces the issue. Even then, experts say, getting together can help organize caregiving efforts—and maintain family harmony.

To ensure that your meeting goes smoothly and achieves its purpose, caregiving experts offer these tips.

✗ Invite *everyone* who is affected by a loved one's situation— family members as well as close friends (with your loved one's approval, when possible). If some people can't attend in person, make arrangements for them to call in on a speakerphone, so they can hear everything that's being discussed. Another option is to go online. Today, many families conduct meetings in private chat rooms on the Internet.

✗ Don't forget your loved one, whose attendance at the meeting is especially important. If the person is hospitalized but able to take part, you may want to make arrangements to gather at the hospital (though in that case, you

---

FOR MORE INFORMATION

If you're not comfortable running a family meeting on your own, or if family members can't agree on certain aspects of a loved one's care, consider asking a third-party professional to step in on your behalf. Potential facilitators include the family cleric, a psychologist, a social worker, or a geriatric care manager.

The National Association of Social Workers can provide a referral to a qualified social worker in your area. You can contact the organization by calling **(800) 638-8799** or visiting their Web site at **www.socialworkers.org**.

To find a geriatric care manager in your area, get in touch with the National Association of Professional Geriatric Care Managers, which also offers a referral service. The phone number is **(520) 881-8008**; the Web address is **www.caremanager.org**.

If You're an Only Child

Siblings who have been embroiled in a disagreement about a parent's care may envy the caregiver who is an only child. While being an "only" might seem to simplify the decision-making process, it also puts all the caregiving responsibilities squarely on the shoulders of one person. If that person is you, you're going to need extra support. What can you do?

- Take full advantage of community resources, including government agencies, senior centers, and church and fraternal organizations.
- Involve your immediate family—spouse and children—as much as possible.
- Reach out to your extended family—aunts, uncles, and cousins—as well as to friends and neighbors. They may be willing to help.
- For your own well-being, join a support group, either in your community or online.

might need to limit the invitees to just immediate family). In the event your loved one can't participate because of cognitive or functional impairment, hold the meeting anyway, then report back to the person afterward. Provide options that encourage her to make decisions about her own care, to the extent she is able.

✗ For the first meeting, keep your expectations realistic. Emotions may run high as family members adjust to their loved one's situation and that person contemplates the prospect of needing care. Under the circumstances, just getting together is a major achievement. In effect, everyone acknowledges they have something important to discuss.

✗ Create and circulate an agenda before the meeting. List the most important items first, so they're sure to get covered in case you run short on time. You can always reconvene later if you need to. Along with your agenda, you might want to distribute a copy of the Caregiver's Checklist you completed earlier, so everyone can see the tasks and resources you've identified so far.

✗ At the start of the meeting, get everyone to agree to stay on the subject—namely, your loved one's care—and not to bring up other family matters. If the discussion strays off course, gently remind everyone to stick with the agenda.

✗ Make sure everyone has an opportunity to speak without interruption. In family meetings, as in business meetings, some people may be long-winded, while others say barely a word. To prevent any one person from dominating the discussion, you might want to go around the room and invite each person to voice her opinion in turn. You could even set a time limit of, say, 5 minutes per person.

✗ Encourage speakers to make "I" statements when expressing how they feel and what they think should be done: "I believe Mom is doing remarkably well for a woman of 84. But I'm concerned that she has had two fender-benders in the past 2 months. I wonder if it's time for her to stop driving. I can take her some places. And I've already checked into transportation services for seniors."

✗ Caution against making "you" statements, which tend to sound accusatory: "You need to be more careful about Dad's wandering. You should keep the doors locked."

✗ Address big issues by divvying up the solutions. Suppose your father can no longer shop or cook for himself. Making sure he's eating properly can seem like a daunting task. But it becomes quite manageable if one person does the grocery shopping every week, and four other people prepare a day's worth of meals each, and Meals on Wheels comes around the remaining 3 days.

✗ At the end of the meeting, choose a date when everyone can get together again. And make sure those family members who didn't attend the meeting are made aware of all that has happened so far. If you don't have time to pass on the information, ask someone else to do it.

✗ If anyone in your family chooses not to take part in discussions of your loved one's care, don't try to force the issue. Just keep the person in the loop as best you can, without asking anything of her. Eventually, she may change her mind about getting involved. (We'll talk more about dealing with family conflict and uncooperativeness in chapter 5.)

Take Action... ENLIST YOUR SPOUSE'S HELP

As your loved one's situation changes and the family meetings continue, all of the participants can decide for themselves how and when they want to contribute to the person's care. Everyone, that is, but your spouse, whose level of involvement is pretty much dictated by your own. And that can take a toll on even the healthiest of marriages.

While spouses promise to care for one another in sickness and in health, that vow generally doesn't apply to the in-laws. Still, you need your partner's understanding and support, perhaps now more than ever. How do you get it? These strategies might help. (For more, see chapter 27.)

✗ Explain to your spouse that caring for your loved one means a great deal to you—as does sustaining your marriage. From the outset, promise you'll make every effort to

That's What Friends Are For

While family members may assume primary responsibility for a loved one's care, close friends may offer to pitch in, too. Take them up on it; you'll welcome the extra physical and emotional support—for your loved one and for yourself.

What can friends do for you? Kay Marshall Strom, author of *A Caregiver's Survival Guide*, offers the following ideas.

- Shop for groceries
- Prepare a meal
- Wash your car
- Mow your lawn
- Watch your children for an afternoon
- Keep you company while you care for your loved one
- Bring a pet to visit your loved one
- Sit with your loved one while you take a break
- Help research caregiving resources within your community
- Continue to include you in their lives, even if your caregiving responsibilities prevent you from accepting all of their invitations

Caring across the Miles

If you and your loved one live far apart, you may not be able to help out with the day-to-day caregiving tasks. But you can stay involved in other ways. Some suggestions:

- Participate in family meetings by phone or online.
- Call the primary caregiver often to offer emotional support.
- Contribute financially as you're able.
- Identify caregiving tasks you can take on, even at a distance. For example, you could research community resources, manage your loved one's finances, or call other family members with updates on your loved one's situation. Ask the primary caregiver what you can do.
- Visit your loved one as often as possible. If she's living with the primary caregiver, plan your trips so that person can take a welcome break.

minimize the impact of your caregiving responsibilities on your relationship.

✗ Discuss your spouse's role in caring for your loved one. He or she most likely won't be as involved as you are. That said, some partners feel comfortable pitching in with caregiving tasks. Others prefer to remain in the background, picking up more responsibilities at home to ease the burden on their husbands or wives.

✗ If you ask your spouse for help, be very specific about what you want—whether it's making dinner on Monday nights, driving the kids to soccer practice Saturday mornings, or doing the laundry once a week.

✗ When your spouse does lend a hand, be sure to express your gratitude—sincerely and often.

✗ Make plans for just the two of you. You and your spouse need time alone, away from the demands of giving care. Go to a concert, a movie, a sporting event—whatever you both enjoy. Or get away for an entire weekend. If no one in your family can take over the caregiving responsibilities while you're gone, you might arrange for your loved one to stay overnight in an assisted living facility. Many such facilities offer short-term respite care. (For more information about this service, see chapter 20.)

✗ Surprise your spouse with little gifts he or she will like. This simple gesture shows you're thinking of the person, and of your relationship.

✗ Be sensitive to your spouse's feelings. As time passes, even the saintliest of partners may grow to resent the impact that caregiving has on his or her personal life. Encourage your spouse to express concerns, then work together to find creative solutions.

✗ If caregiving responsibilities are causing a significant rift between you and your spouse, think about consulting a family therapist, marriage counselor, or cleric. Any of these professionals can help the two of you resolve your differences and strengthen your relationship.

Take Action... RECRUIT YOUR KIDS TO PITCH IN

Your caregiving role will affect everyone in your home—not just your spouse but also your children. For the younger family members, the issues are logistical ("If you're staying at Grandma's on Thursday nights, how will I get to my scout meeting?") as well as emotional. After all, kids believe the adults in their lives can fend for themselves. So when someone they love needs care, they may feel confused and frightened.

Involving children in the caregiving process can help them understand their loved one's situation, and perhaps allay their fears. You may want to arrange a special meeting just for them, in which you explain in general, nonjudgmental terms the issues that have come up and any decisions that have been made so far. Some other suggestions:

- Be honest about what's going on. Your openness might encourage youngsters to ask questions and express their feelings without fear.

- Find creative ways to let your children help out. Most kids want to, but they don't know how. Perhaps they can play games with your loved one, or walk around the block with her, or just listen to her while she reminisces. Youngsters can also pitch in with household chores so you're freed up for caregiving.

- Choose tasks for your children that are appropriate for their ages, interests, and needs. You know your kids better than anyone. If both your father and your 11-year-old are passionate about chess, arrange for them to play together. But your 5-year-old might feel more comfortable singing songs with Grandpa.

- Don't force your children to become involved. Young ones, in particular, may not feel comfortable around someone who needs care—at least not right away. They need time to warm up to helping. When they're ready, they'll let you know.

Above all, reassure your children that while your loved one's need for care will change their world, you'll do all that you can to keep their lives as normal as possible. This lets them know they're important to you—and often that's all they want to hear.

Point of View

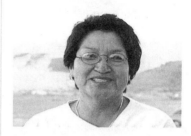

"While Mom was in the hospital, my brother and sister and I went through training so we could manage her personal needs, help her exercise, transfer her from the bed to the wheelchair—everything.

"Initially, my idea was that we would rotate the caring, 1 month each. We'd live in her house with her. We did that for 8 months. But we got burned out.

"So we had another family meeting and decided on 2 weeks at a time. That worked well for several months. Then my sister [couldn't do it anymore]. Now I'm with Mom for 4 weeks, alternating with my brother, who's with her for 2. I don't have little children, so I can handle 4 weeks. My brother has little kids, so 2 weeks is all he can do.

"My husband helps me. He's so good. His father has Alzheimer's, and we had to put him in a home. We joke that if we ever hit the lottery, we'll build a nursing home to take care of my mom and his dad."

—ARLENE GARCIA,
Moenkopi, Arizona (Hopi Nation)

CHAPTER 5

THE CONFLICT OF CARING

What You Need to Know

- Disagreements can occur in any family when a loved one's well-being is at stake.

- Be realistic with your expectations. Assuming that family members will understand your point of view or offer their assistance can lead to disappointment and anger if they don't.

- If a discussion turns contentious, stay in control by refocusing on the issue at hand—your loved one's care.

- If a serious family dispute arises, consider mediation as a means of resolution.

A family comes together because one of their own needs care. The meeting is productive, with everyone agreeing on the loved one's situation and an appropriate course of action. Then they offer to help, volunteering their time, money, and emotional support.

If only organizing a caregiving plan always proceeded so smoothly. In reality, it sometimes doesn't.

Relationships within families are complicated and often taken for granted. They profoundly influence any discussion or decision about a loved one's need for care, for better or for worse. The primary caregiver may feel family members should volunteer to help without being asked. Some family members may be more than willing to pitch in, but not agree on who should do what. Others may not want to share in the caregiving responsibilities, which can stir feelings of frustration, hostility, and resentment.

How your loved one's situation affects your family dynamic,

and vice versa, very much depends on the people involved. "Caregiving can strengthen relationships. You may develop a new appreciation for your spouse or a closer bond with your siblings," notes Virginia Morris, author of *How to Care for Aging Parents*. "Unfortunately, it can also drive a sharp wedge into relationships. And the people we are closest to—the ones we have known longest and most intimately—are the ones who can most infuriate, hurt, and disappoint us."

Our reactions to those who are less cooperative than we expect or desire can be amplified by the realization that we have no control over their actions—or their inaction, as the case may be. All of us like to maintain some sense of order and structure in our lives. That can be a challenge in a caregiving situation, in which we're taking our cues from someone else's needs and wishes. Instinctively, we turn to other family members to anchor and support us. But they have needs and wishes of their own.

When you're dealing with family members who either disagree about caregiving plans or want nothing to do with them, Leslie Plooster, M.A., program associate for the Bethesda, Maryland–based National Alliance for Caregiving, suggests you remember this: "The only thing really in your control is your reaction to what's going on around you." You can lash out at others for their stubbornness, or you can change your own patterns of judgment, even accepting the views of those around you philosophically. This doesn't mean you allow them to call all the shots. You work to let go of the resentments that exhaust you and interfere with your caregiving role, not to mention the rest of your life.

Making peace with the realities of your situation can foster optimism and hope. A family member who's being difficult now very well may have a change of heart in the future. If he does, you want to encourage his involvement, not shut him out. After all, as a caregiver, you're going to need all the help you can muster. Why not hope for the best?

Take Action... BRING THE FAMILY TOGETHER

As explained in chapter 4, once you've made the determination that your loved one needs care (or will in the near future),

EXPERT OPINION

"Some of the most difficult situations in life involve dealing with family. When loved ones won't help, of course you feel angry and resentful. That's natural. But try not to take their resistance personally. Don't denounce them. If you leave the door open to them, they may help later."

—GLORIA CAVANAUGH, president and chief executive officer of the American Society on Aging, based in San Francisco

your best bet is to call a family meeting to lay the foundation for a caregiving plan. Of course, depending on the circumstances within your family, you may have reservations about bringing everyone together for what can be a very emotional discussion. Your concerns are understandable, but experts suggest that you try for at least one meeting. Then you can find out what each person is thinking about your loved one's situation. They may not say what you want to hear, but it's better than being in the dark.

Chapter 4 offers some general guidelines for organizing a family meeting. If your family has issues that could complicate talks about your loved one's care, you may want to consider these strategies as well.

X Before you actually schedule a meeting, contact each family member to explain what you're doing and why. Some may say up front that they don't want to participate. On the other hand, people often forget—or at least temporarily suspend—their grudges to deal with a family crisis.

X If some family members want to get together but others don't, move ahead with the meeting anyway. Some discussion and planning is better than none.

X Consider bringing in a third-party professional—such as a psychologist, a social worker, a geriatric care manager, or a member of the clergy—to run your meeting. Some family members may object, believing the matter is private family business and others shouldn't be involved. If so, you can explain that the facilitator won't be making decisions on the family's behalf; she's there primarily to keep the discussion on track and to give everyone the opportunity to voice their opinions. Besides, family members may be less likely to argue when an outsider is present. (To determine whether your family meeting might benefit from a facilitator, complete the Caregiver's Checklist on page 51.)

X Whether you or a third-party professional runs the meeting, make sure the discussion stays focused on the main issue: your loved one's care. You have a lot of ground to cover, even if your goal is simply to identify the next

FOR MORE INFORMATION

If you're thinking about asking someone else to facilitate your family meeting, the following organizations can refer you to a qualified professional in your area.

• National Association of Professional Geriatric Care Managers, 1604 North Country Club Road, Tucson, AZ 85716. **(520) 881-8008;** **www.caremanager.org.**

• National Association of Social Workers, 750 First Street NE, Suite 700, Washington, DC 20002. **(800) 638-8799;** **www.socialworkers.org.**

steps toward developing a comprehensive caregiving plan. You don't want to waste time criticizing the people who didn't attend, or hashing out other family matters.

✗ If any family members decline to attend your meeting, don't write them off for good. You're going to need physical and emotional support, and they may be willing to provide it—just not right now. "Initially, some family members may resist getting involved in a loved one's care because they're not ready to accept the person's declining health," explains Mark S. Lachs, M.D., M.P.H., chief of geriatrics and gerontology at New York Hospital in Manhattan. "If you're understanding about the challenge of facing up to your loved one's situation, you have an excellent chance of eventually getting the help you need."

Take Action... HANDLE DETRACTORS DIPLOMATICALLY

Of course, being understanding isn't easy if a family member becomes stubborn or insolent to the point of hindering discus-

---

Caregiver's Checklist

Do You Need an Outside Facilitator?

Answer each of the following questions by placing a check mark in one of the boxes to the left. If you have even one "yes" response, you may want to think about bringing in a third-party professional to facilitate your family meeting.

☐ yes ☐ no   Are you dreading your meeting because you fear that family members will be argumentative or disrespectful with one another?

☐ yes ☐ no   Even before the meeting, does your family seem divided about the best approach to your loved one's care?

☐ yes ☐ no   Has any previous family gathering turned contentious?

☐ yes ☐ no   Has any previous family gathering left you feeling angry, uncomfortable, or disappointed?

sions about a loved one's care. Even in the most close-knit of families, personalities can clash and disagreements can flare when everyone has their own opinions about what's best for a loved one and who should be responsible for various caregiving tasks.

How do you deal with people whose words and actions may seem more hurtful than helpful? Above all else, try to remain calm and rational. It may take a lot of effort on your part, but an even-keel response can defuse some of the stress you're feeling. What's more, it just might foster greater cooperation and self-control among those around you.

Here are some additional strategies for coping with difficult family members without losing sight of the real issue—your loved one's care.

- Accept that your family isn't obligated to help. You may feel that caring for your loved one is "the right thing to do," but others may not share your opinion. They're entitled to say no when you ask them to pitch in. By preparing yourself for that, you're less likely to feel disappointed, angry, or resentful if they decline to lend a hand. And you're more likely to appreciate any offers of assistance you do receive.

- Expect differences of opinion when making decisions about a loved one's care. Every family member has a unique relationship with your loved one, and it influences each person's perception of what's best in terms of care. In most cases, you can find opportunities for compromise.

- When disagreements arise, let family members know that you respect their viewpoints. You may not see eye-to-eye on particular issues, but you're united by your concern for your loved one and your desire to make sure that person receives the care he needs.

- Express appreciation to your family members for any help they provide. This might be a challenge if they pitch in infrequently or grudgingly. But as the saying goes, you draw more flies with honey than with vinegar.

- Ask friends and neighbors to lend a hand when family members can't or won't. Recruiting people from outside the family can work very well, because usually they don't have the emotional ties to a loved one's situation that your relatives do. And often they're eager to help out. Just be sure your loved one knows about their involvement and feels comfortable with it. Get the person's approval, if that's possible.

✗ Take full advantage of community caregiving resources such as telephone reassurance, transportation services, and adult day care. They'll assume responsibility for a variety of caregiving tasks, helping to pare down your to-do list—and your reliance on family intervention. You'll learn more about the agencies and organizations that provide caregiving services in chapters 19 and 20.

✗ Even if family members decline to help out, let them know what's going on with brief updates on a regular basis— weekly, biweekly, or monthly. This practice can give you peace of mind by keeping everyone in the loop about your loved one's situation and giving them the opportunity to provide input. Over time, your updates might trigger a change of heart and persuade others to pitch in.

✗ Forgive family members who choose not to get involved in a loved one's care. It may not be easy; you may feel angry or resentful because the rest of the family isn't doing as much as you are. But carrying around those negative emotions is no good for your own physical and emotional health. To free yourself from them, try thinking about all that you'll gain from giving care. You'll have a chance to reassess your priorities and decide what really matters in your life. You'll be spending precious time with someone you love. You'll experience moments of grace and beauty that you'll always cherish. Once you're able to focus on caregiving's gifts, you may find forgiveness that much easier.

✗ If you can't seem to let go of your negative emotions, consider getting counseling. Chronic anger and resentment gnaws at your soul, interfering with your ability to care for your loved one—and yourself. Venting to a professional usually helps you let go of a hardened perspective.

FOR MORE INFORMATION

The Area Agency on Aging that serves every county in the United States can provide information about local caregiving resources. It's a good place to start planning for your loved one's care. To contact the office in your area, look in the blue pages of your telephone directory, under "Guide to Human Services." You can also check the Eldercare Locator, a nationwide service sponsored by the U.S. Administration on Aging. Call **(800) 677-1116**, or visit the Eldercare Locator Web site at **www.eldercare.gov.**

Take Action... TRY OTHER WAYS OF COMMUNICATING

In some families, caregiving issues strain relationships so much that face-to-face conversations become almost impossible. Still, family members need to know about their loved one's situation, whether or not they're involved in the person's care. With time, their emotions and attitudes may change, paving the way for more compassionate, productive interactions.

As long as in-person discussions remain difficult, other means of communication are your best bet. These days, you have lots of options. Here's what experts recommend.

✗ Ideally, use e-mail. You can prepare your messages quickly and revise them easily, to get just the right tone and wording. Consider running your messages by someone else before sending them, so you're certain not to say anything that others might find offensive or accusatory.

✗ If you or your family doesn't have access to e-mail, then write a letter instead. Revising it may not go as quickly, and it won't reach its recipients as fast. On the other hand, by its nature, writing allows time for reflection about tone and word choice. As with an e-mail, showing your letter to someone else before sending it is a good idea.

✗ As a last resort, pick up the phone. Calling family members is direct, but it's not without discomfort. You may run the same emotional gauntlet that made face-to-face conversations so difficult—feeling resentful, losing your temper, saying things you regret later.

If you must communicate with your family by phone, these tips can help make it easier.

✗ Relax before you call. Soak in a warm bath. Take a short walk. Say a prayer. Anything you can do to collect your thoughts and control your emotions will help you get through the conversation without losing your cool. You may not be able to let go of your anger or resentment completely, but you can keep it at arm's length for the duration of the call.

✗ Write down what you want to talk about. Having a "script" keeps your mind focused and your conversation on track.

✗ Pick a good time to call. You want to try to reach the person when he's at home and relaxed. Generally, in the evening after dinner is best. When the person answers the phone, say to him, "Do you have a few minutes to talk? It's about Mom, and it's important." If the time is inconvenient, ask when you can call back.

✗ Be matter-of-fact without placing blame or making demands. "Mom hasn't heard from Meals on Wheels yet. Have you been able to get in touch with them?"

✗ If the person becomes defensive or says no to your request, focus on remaining calm. You don't want to trigger a confrontation that may cut off communication for good.

✗ Reach out emotionally, acknowledging the difficulty of the situation and the person's concern for your loved one: "I

Caregiver's Checklist

Should You Hire a Lawyer?

Sometimes family disputes worsen to the point where the only hope for resolution is through legal action. You may want to consider consulting an attorney if you answer "yes" to any of the following questions.

☐ yes ☐ no   Do you have reason to believe that your loved one's health and welfare are in jeopardy because of a family member's actions?

☐ yes ☐ no   Do you have reason to believe that your loved one's financial assets are being misused?

☐ yes ☐ no   Is a family member pursuing a course of action that you strongly oppose? For example, is one of your siblings trying to move your mother into an assisted living facility and sell her home when you and the rest of the family feel that isn't necessary?

☐ yes ☐ no   Has a family business been affected by the dispute?

☐ yes ☐ no   Has a family member sued you, or threatened to?

☐ yes ☐ no   Has a family member hired a lawyer, or threatened to?

know how hard this must be for you, realizing that Mom needs help . . ."

✗ Then return to your main point: ". . . but we need to make arrangements for her meals to be delivered."

✗ Try to get a commitment: "When do you think you'll call Meals on Wheels?"

✗ Provide an out: "Are you sure you have time to do it? If not, I need to know now so I can ask someone else to handle it." Allowing the person to say no may be galling, especially if you're feeling overwhelmed by caregiving responsibilities. But remember, the purpose of your call is not to berate the person, even if you want to. It's to make sure that your loved one is getting the help she needs.

✗ Express thanks. If the person follows through on his promise, let him know that you—and your loved one—appreciate his efforts. Realizing that he made a difference may encourage him to help out more in the future.

✗ If the person doesn't follow through, allow yourself time to deal with any anger or resentment you may experience. You want to have your emotions in check before you approach the person again.

✗ Decide when to stop trying. If a family member repeatedly fails to follow through on his promises to pitch in, you're not obligated to keep giving that person another chance. But before you make a decision one way or another, think through the situation and talk about it with your spouse, a sibling, or a close friend. If you come to the conclusion that you just can't count on the person any longer, then you're free to take him out of the caregiving loop.

IF A SERIOUS DISPUTE ARISES . . .

Sometimes families must deal with problems that simply can't be resolved at a meeting, by e-mail, or on the phone. Perhaps a parent develops nasty bruises on her arms and legs while in her daughter's care. Or she starts getting past-due notices for her bills while her son, who's in charge of her personal finances, is driving around in a brand-new car he could not have afforded before.

FOR MORE INFORMATION

Certain situations may require the intervention of Adult Protective Services. Usually, this agency is listed in the blue pages of the telephone directory, under "Guide to Human Services." If it isn't, you can get a phone number from the Area Agency on Aging that serves your community. That number is in the blue pages as well.

Note: Contacting Adult Protective Services is a last resort, to be pursued only when an older person's health and welfare are at stake—and even then, only with guidance from a professional who is knowledgeable about elder care, such as an attorney specializing in elder law.

Situations of abuse or neglect require special assistance, usually from outside the family. But they must be handled very carefully. Once they're reported, the financial and legal ramifications can be serious. While you have every right to be concerned about your loved one's health and welfare, you don't want to wrongly accuse another family member of inappropriate behavior.

If you have reason to believe an older person in your life is in some sort of danger, you can report the situation to Adult Protective Services, the agency responsible for protecting seniors from neglect, abuse, and exploitation. Usually, complaints can be filed anonymously. Still, experts recommend choosing this course of action only after consulting an attorney who specializes in elder law or another professional with appropriate training and expertise.

Third-party professionals can also help resolve family disputes through various legal means, including mediation, arbitration, and lawsuits.

Mediation. Essentially, this is supervised negotiation. The people involved in the dispute present their points of view before an attorney or another trained mediator, who then helps the parties reach a compromise solution.

Arbitration. Compared with mediation, arbitration is more like a conventional court proceeding. A trained arbitrator hears both sides of a dispute before making a determination that in most cases is legally binding.

Lawsuits. Family members can file civil suits against one another. If settlement isn't reached out of court (or the case isn't thrown out), the parties may go to trial before a judge and jury.

Of these three options, mediation is considered the best choice. Arbitration can be difficult to arrange, and family members may not want to abide by a third party's decision. Lawsuits can linger in the judicial system for years, making them very costly—and very stressful.

To find a qualified mediator in your area, start by checking with your local bar association. Most have referral services, though be aware that they may charge a nominal fee. According to the American Bar Association Section on Dispute Resolution, more than 6,000 member attorneys are trained in mediation. Other potential resources include the National Academy of Elder Law Attorneys and the AARP Legal Services Network.

FOR MORE INFORMATION

The National Academy of Elder Law Attorneys maintains a list of its more than 350 members; the list is available to the public for a nominal fee. The organization also provides referrals to elder law resources. Usually, attorneys who specialize in elder law deal with issues such as estate planning and long-term care. But they may be able to help resolve family disputes, or at least direct you to someone who can. You can contact the National Academy of Elder Law Attorneys by writing to 1604 North Country Club Road, Tucson, AZ 85716, or checking the organization's Web site at **www.naela.org**.

If you belong to AARP, you may want to take advantage of the organization's Legal Services Network. It offers referrals to attorneys who charge reduced rates for AARP members. For more information, write to AARP Legal Services Network, 601 E Street NW, Washington, DC 20049, or log on to **www.aarp.org/lsn**.

IN SICKNESS AND IN HEALTH

What You Need to Know

- Respect your parents' relationship. They understand each other's needs and wishes better than anyone else.

- Realize that spousal caregiving has unique physical and emotional demands, especially for those couples who are up in years.

- Remember that time is on your side. Your parents may not want help now, but they'll become aware that they need it as their functioning declines.

- If one parent continues to refuse help for the other, get involved discreetly, in ways that won't be considered intrusive.

- Intervene assertively only when you feel your loved one—be it the caregiver or the care recipient—is at risk for personal harm.

When couples exchange their marriage vows, they promise to be there for each other "in sickness and in health." But they may not realize the full implication of those words until one partner requires care, whether because of age or illness. Usually, the other partner becomes the primary caregiver—and just like that, the relationship between the two of them is transformed.

In the best of circumstances, caregiving spouses are physically and mentally capable of looking after their loved ones as well as themselves. But sometimes they're not, in which case other family members may feel they need to step in. The caregivers may resist help, though, believing the responsibility for providing care is theirs alone. And family members may hesitate to intervene in marital relationships that have lasted for years.

More often than not, older couples are reluctant to acknowledge—or may not be aware of—the possibility that one of them needs more care than the other can provide. Many a husband and wife have sworn to never place their spouses in nursing homes, usually early in their marriages when they can't imagine themselves in declining health. They may feel bound by that commitment in their later years, even when their spouses might be much better off in a professional caregiving environment.

Intervening in someone else's marriage can be uncomfortable, especially for adult children and their elderly parents. "Adult children can go crazy when one parent can't or won't provide the care the other parent needs, then refuses help besides," says Lois Escobar, M.S.W., a family consultant with the Family Caregiver Alliance in San Francisco. "But as long as the caregiver is mentally competent and the care recipient isn't in any danger, adult children really can't do anything. And that can be difficult to accept."

PARTNERS FIRST, PARENTS SECOND

If one of your parents has begun caring for the other, you need to adapt to their new roles, just as they are. You may be able to handle the situation better by remembering these points, offered by Gail Hunt, executive director of the Bethesda, Maryland–based National Alliance for Caregiving.

You can't change your parents. They've been around a lot longer than you, and they're that much more set in their ways. They can change, but they must do it on their own terms and their own timetable. When they do, give them all the support you can.

Your parents know each other better than you know them. Unless one of them is your stepparent, your mom and dad have a relationship that predates your existence. They've been dealing with each other much longer than they've been dealing with you. That experience can help them make the right decisions for their caregiving situation, even though you might not agree with them.

Your parents may not want you to know everything about them. Even if you're close to your parents, they probably haven't told you all the details of their personal lives, particularly with regard to their finances. They're entitled to some privacy, and you need to respect their autonomy.

EXPERT OPINION

"When I'm working with caregivers, I often tell them about what I call the 11th Commandment: Thou shalt not parent thy parent. In saying that, I'm not suggesting that people stop caring for their parents. But when they 'parent' their parents, they experience subconscious feelings of sadness and frustration as they realize their parents are no longer the immortal figures of their childhood. So they try to do a role reversal—they become the 'parents,' and the parents become the 'children.' I advise caregivers not to dwell on the past but to assess the present situation and identify their parents' needs today, from the perspective of a true caregiver and not a grown child."

—MARK EDINBERG, PH.D., a psychologist and gerontology expert from Fairfield, Connecticut, and author of *Talking with Your Aging Parents*

Outlook

"The biggest challenge in the future will be having enough qualified, committed people to provide services not just in senior facilities but in homes as well. I feel optimistic about the future of caregiving, though, because people are starting to talk about the subject. It seems everywhere I go, everyone has a caregiving story to share. I think people's sensitivities have been sharpened and their awareness heightened to the issue of caregiving. It makes sense, because these days, just about everyone is less than one degree of separation removed from an elderly person needing care."

—**DAVID TILLMAN, M.D.,** chief executive officer of the Motion Picture and Television Fund in Woodland Hills, California

The parent who is giving care needs time to grieve. Caregivers of all ages must come to terms with the fact that their loved ones are no longer able to look after themselves. For older caregivers, in particular, this can mean facing a loved one's mortality as well as their own. Feelings of grief and loss can be especially intense for spousal caregivers, who may cling to their caregiving roles as part of their marital vows.

When one spouse starts taking care of the other, it changes the entire complexion of their partnership. These two people shared dreams and overcame adversity together. Now they must redefine their marital roles and prepare for an uncertain future. As they do, they will grieve for their unrealized plans, for their loss of companionship and intimacy, for the end of a daily routine that has endured for years. As many a caregiver has said, "I'm not just losing my spouse. I'm losing part of myself." The same sentiment of regret over a changing relationship can hold true for a daughter caring for her mother, or a son for his father.

You can help your parents help themselves. If you're concerned about a particular aspect of your parent's care, raise the issue by asking questions rather than making "should" statements. For example, don't say to your mother "You shouldn't let Dad near the checkbook. He can't manage money anymore." Instead, ask her "Does Dad need my help with the checkbook? He seems to be having trouble managing money." A "should" statement invites resistance; a question, on the other hand, opens the door to explanation. Your mother may tell you that your father has always taken great pride in his ability to handle their financial affairs, so she allows him to think he's in charge. In reality, she writes all the checks and pays all the bills.

WHEN CARING BECOMES TOO MUCH

Respecting your parents' caregiving relationship is important. If you don't try to micromanage every detail, they'll know you're there for them. As they'll soon discover, spousal caregiving presents a set of physical and emotional challenges all its own—because the caregiving is occurring within the framework of a marriage, and because most spousal caregivers are at midlife or beyond.

Older caregivers, in particular, may feel overwhelmed by the responsibilities they face, especially if their physical stamina and psychological resilience have declined over the years. And while all caregivers must face "anticipatory grieving"—that is, coming to terms with a loved one's eventual death—the elderly can be exceptionally stressed by it. This further undermines their ability to cope, both physically and emotionally.

In several studies, scientists determined that levels of stress-related hormones in the blood tend to be significantly higher in older people who are caring for their spouses than in older people who are not. Research has also shown the following:

Older spousal caregivers are at unusually high risk for depression. According to the National Institute of Mental Health, between 2 and 4 percent of the general population suffers from significant depression (known medically as clinical or major depression) at any given time. But a study at Stanford University found that rate to be significantly higher—more like 20 percent—among spousal caregivers. In older people, depression may manifest not as profound sadness but as unusual irritability or anxiety. Be alert to these behavioral changes in your caregiving parent.

Older spousal caregivers are prone to declines in immune function. Stress and depression can compromise the body's disease defenses no matter what a person's age. But in older people, the effects can be especially debilitating. Several studies have monitored immune performance among elderly spousal caregivers after they received various vaccinations. These shots stimulate the immune system to produce antibodies that provide protection against certain diseases. Compared with older people who are not caring for their spouses, those who are get significantly less protection from vaccinations because they have lower antibody production, the result of poorer immune function.

Older spousal caregivers are particularly vulnerable to illness. If the body's immune system isn't functioning as it should, it can't fend off disease as it should. Caregivers of all ages seem to get sick more frequently than the general population. Older spousal caregivers are at even greater risk, since their immunity can be weakened not just by stress but also by the aging process itself, if they haven't maintained optimum health through the years.

Point of View

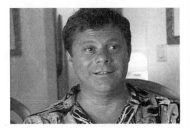

"If my dad had to go into a home, we would agonize over it so much. When my mom was around, she would say, 'Let me die before you let me go to a home.' So now I think doing that to my dad would be the worst thing."

—**BRIAN BLOCK,**
Mesa, Arizona

Older spousal caregivers have a higher death rate than non-caregivers. Just as poor immune function opens the door to common ailments like colds and flu, it also raises the risk of more serious illness. Researchers at the University of Pittsburgh tracked more than 800 elderly people, about half of whom were caring for a spouse. During the 5 years of the study, the death rate was 63 percent higher among the caregivers than among the non-caregivers.

What does all of this mean for you, if one of your parents is caring for the other? In terms of your getting involved in the caregiving process, "time is on your side," Escobar says. "Even caregivers who steadfastly resist help eventually may have a change of heart." Whether because of declining physical health, mental burnout, or financial concerns, they may become more comfortable reaching out—and will come to understand that asking for help is not a betrayal of their marriage vows.

Escobar's advice? "Be patient," she says. "Refrain from providing assistance that your caregiving parent doesn't want. As the weeks and months pass, you'll be asked to do more. And what you do will be very much appreciated."

Take Action... RECOGNIZE OPPORTUNITIES TO STEP IN

Of course, some parents may continue to refuse help, even when they seem to need it. As mentioned earlier, unless the caregiver is mentally incompetent or the care recipient is in danger (showing signs of abuse or neglect), you can't force your parents to accept your assistance. But they might be more open to it if you approach it in a respectful way. These strategies can help.

- Look for little things you can do. Offering to pick up a prescription or prepare a meal is much less intrusive and controlling than, say, taking charge of the checkbook. Once your parents realize you just want to make their lives easier, they may feel more comfortable asking you to pitch in.

- Support your parents even when they turn down your assistance. Don't let frustration drive you away. Remember that over time, the parent who's providing care may become overwhelmed to the point where he or she has to reach out for help. In the meantime, you can pitch in from the sidelines by monitoring your parents' situation for any risks to their health and safety.

✗ Express praise for a job well done. Caring for a spouse is not easy. If your father has assumed the caregiving role, he may be taking on household chores that he has never dealt with before, like meal preparation. If your mother is the caregiver, she may be learning new tasks as well, like money management. Acknowledge your parent's commitment and adaptability, and recognize his or her accomplishments.

✗ Allow the parent who's providing care to make his or her own decisions, even if you don't agree with some of them. As long as they don't jeopardize anyone's health or safety, they're a good way to learn. And if they don't produce the expected results, they may convince your parent to ask for help.

✗ Be sensitive in deciding when to intervene. If the parent who's providing care has trouble with a particular caregiving situation, your instinct may be to jump in and "make things right." Don't, unless your help is requested. Let your

Keeping a Close Watch from Far Away

If you're like a lot of people, you live miles from your parents, which means you can't check in on them in person as often as you'd like. But with a little resourcefulness, you can keep tabs on their caregiving situation, even long-distance.

- Call and visit your parents as often as you can. And recruit others in their circle—friends, neighbors, members of their church congregation—to do the same.
- Find out about check-in services, in which someone will call or stop by your parents' home to make sure they're okay. You may need to pay

a nominal fee for some of these services, though many are free. For more information, contact the Area Agency on Aging in your parents' community.

- Ask people who see your parents regularly to pay attention for signs of problems. The pharmacist, the hairdresser, the newspaper carrier, the bank teller—anyone who does business with your parents or provides services for them can help. Ask these people to alert you (or the appropriate authorities, in the event of an emergency) if they notice any unusual behavior.

FOR MORE INFORMATION

These days, many agencies and organizations offer services that enable people in need of care to stay in their own homes, rather than moving into nursing homes. Here are two you may want to check into on your parents' behalf.

• The National Adult Day Services Association. Phone: **(866) 890-7357**; Internet address: **www.ncoa.org/nadsa**. Provides information on adult day care facilities nationwide, including a checklist for evaluating them.

• The Visiting Nurse Associations of America. Phone: **(800) 426-2547**; Internet address: **www.vnaa.org**. Specializes in home-based skilled nursing and personal care and offers referrals.

FOR MORE INFORMATION

The National Association of Social Workers provides referrals to certified professionals nationwide. Call **(800) 638-8799**, or visit **www.socialworkers.org**.

The National Association of Professional Geriatric Care Managers also has a referral service. Call **(520) 881-8008** or log on to **www.caremanager.org**.

parent resolve the problem, then look for an opportunity to discuss it. Perhaps the person will express anger or regret about the situation. That's your chance to mention what you might have done differently, based on information rather than instinct.

✗ Point out that the caregiver's health is a factor in the caregiving equation. As Plooster explains, "After the caregiving parent has suffered through a few bouts of illness, you may sense an opportunity to say, 'Look, if you don't get help, you could be too sick or exhausted to provide care. That's not good for either of you.'"

✗ Discuss caregiving options. Spousal caregivers often worry that their husbands and wives will be taken away and placed in nursing homes. That's one reason why they try so hard to shoulder all of the responsibilities themselves. But according to Mark S. Lachs, M.D., M.P.H., chief of geriatrics and gerontology at New York Hospital in Manhattan, nursing homes no longer are the only alternative to spousal care. In most cases, family members, close friends and neighbors, and community agencies and organizations can provide just the sort of help that will allow the care recipient to stay at home—and give the caregiver much-needed respite. (To learn more about community caregiving resources, see chapters 19 and 20.)

✗ Point out that accepting assistance does not signal weakness or failure on the caregiver's part. No one can provide competent, loving care 24 hours a day, 7 days a week.

✗ Suggest getting a professional's opinion. While the parent who's providing care may brush aside your input, he or she may be willing to listen to someone with expertise, such as a social worker or a geriatric care manager.

✗ For your own sanity, consider joining a support group. Many people are in situations similar to yours—one parent caring for the other, rejecting offers of assistance even though they seem to need it. Talking with others can help disperse some of the frustration you may be feeling. And you'll likely come away with insights and ideas for dealing with your parents' situation.

WHEN YOU MUST INTERVENE

If one parent's ability to provide care declines to a point at which either spouse's health or safety is in jeopardy, you may feel you have no choice but to step in. It's a judgment call, but as long as you've been monitoring your parents' situation, you'll know when they're heading for trouble.

"That's what happened with my grandparents," Plooster says. "My grandfather was caring for my grandmother, and he refused help from my mother and my two aunts. For quite a while, the three of them stayed on the sidelines, providing what little support Granddad would accept. Eventually, they decided Granddad couldn't manage any longer. They sat him down and told him the time had come for them to get more involved. Granddad didn't like it, but he didn't resist."

To ease the intervention process, you might want to call a family meeting to discuss your parents' situation. Be sure to invite both the caregiver and the care recipient, if that person is able to attend. (For tips on organizing a family meeting, see chapter 4.) Another option is to enlist the assistance of someone whom your parents trust—a member of the clergy, a family doctor, an old friend, even a social worker or geriatric care manager.

If the parent who's providing care continues to refuse help, you might want to raise the possibility of reporting the situation to Adult Protective Services, the agency charged with protecting older people from neglect, abuse, and exploitation. The potential embarrassment of an investigation could be enough to change your parent's mind about accepting assistance. On the other hand, you run the risk of infuriating and alienating your parent, which won't benefit anyone. So mention Adult Protective Services only as a next-to-last resort, and make clear that you're doing it because you feel you have no other choice.

Your last resort, as you might guess, is to actually follow through with Adult Protective Services. It's a serious step, with significant financial and legal implications. That's why it should be pursued only when you feel one of your parents is in danger,

FOR MORE INFORMATION

If you're looking for a support group in your area, you may want to start your search with one of the following organizations.

• **Children of Aging Parents.** Call **(800) 227-7294** or visit **www.caps4caregivers.org**. Offers referrals to support groups and other resources for people with parents in caregiving situations.

• **Family Caregiver Alliance.** Call **(800) 445-8106** or visit **www.caregiver.org**. Provides information for families with brain-injured care recipients and can help locate support groups.

• **National Alliance for Caregiving.** Visit **www.caregiving.org**. This organization offers support for caregivers and their families. The Web site features links to many helpful organizations.

Another option is to contact the local chapters of organizations dedicated to specific diseases, such as the Alzheimer's Association or the American Cancer Society. Often they sponsor support groups for patients and their families. Check the blue pages of your phone directory, under "Guide to Human Services."

FOR MORE INFORMATION

Your local Adult Protective Services office should be listed in the blue pages of your phone directory, under "Guide to Human Services." If it isn't, check with the Area Agency on Aging that serves your community. That number should be in the blue pages as well.

Note: Before you file a report with Adult Protective Services, be sure to discuss your parents' situation with a qualified professional, such as an attorney specializing in elder law.

EXPERT OPINION

"Your caregiving parent may not listen to you or other family members. But an old friend may prove more persuasive. Talk with your parents' friends about the caregiver's refusal to accept help. Invite them to visit, to see for themselves, and to encourage the caregiver to accept assistance."

—**GLORIA CAVANAUGH,** president and chief executive officer of the American Society on Aging, based in San Francisco

and only after you've consulted an attorney who specializes in elder law or other knowledgeable counsel.

If you call Adult Protective Services, you'll speak with a trained social worker, who can help determine whether your parents' situation requires official intervention. The social worker will look for risk factors such as physical or mental abuse, abandonment or desertion, impaired mental function, inability to perform tasks of daily living, financial mismanagement, and fiduciary exploitation (abuse of confidence or trust). Based on your consultation, the social worker may decide the situation does not constitute abuse or neglect, but your parents do need assistance—in which case she'll provide information on appropriate services and resources. If abuse or neglect is suspected, Adult Protective Services will investigate further.

Another last-resort option is to initiate legal proceedings to become your parents' guardian or conservator, assuming legal responsibility for them and their property. In some jurisdictions, the terms "guardian" and "conservator" are used interchangeably; in others, the guardian handles all personal matters, while the conservator oversees financial decisions. Like contacting Adult Protective Services, seeking a guardianship or conservatorship is a serious and potentially costly course of action. We'll discuss this option in more detail in chapter 25.

Even when you have the best of intentions, stepping in to help your parents can strain your relationship with them, at least initially. Your parents may infer from your actions that they're no longer whole, contributing members of the family or the community. But any anger or resentment usually subsides with time, as your mom and dad realize that you've acted with their interests at heart. You can nurture this healing process by staying respectful and supportive, by keeping open the lines of communication . . . just by being there.

Remember, your parents are under tremendous stress and dealing with all kinds of emotions that you're not aware of. But through caregiving, the three of you may forge a new bond—one that's defined by love, trust, and understanding.

CHAPTER 7

A FAMILY IN TRANSITION

What You Need to Know

- *Change* happens around you. *Transition* happens inside of you; it's your own internal process for dealing with and accepting change.

- By its nature, caregiving creates change and transition, especially in relationships—affecting not just the caregiver and care recipient but also other family members and even close friends.

- In general, all transitions move through the same three stages: preparing for transition, taking the necessary steps, and establishing the new equilibrium.

- Life means constant changes and, therefore, constant transitions. Instead of fighting them, embrace them.

Taking the crucial first steps in a caregiving situation—deciding whether a loved one needs care, discussing it with other family members, asking them to pitch in—can seem like crossing a fast-moving river on stepping-stones. Before each step, you feel apprehensive; you worry that you might lose your footing and get in over your head. Sure enough, as you ease yourself onto the next stone in your path, it begins to wobble. But with focus and determination, you manage to steady yourself and regain your balance. So you keep moving forward, maneuvering from stone to stone, finding your way through the transitions that are part and parcel of caregiving.

In conversational English, we tend to use the words *change* and *transition* interchangeably. But according to business consultant William Bridges, author of *Managing Transitions*, the two terms

Outlook

have important distinctions. Change, he explains, occurs in the external world. It's your mother needing a live-in helper, or your father-in-law moving into your home. Transition is the internal process of coming to terms with change.

Managing transitions can be challenging; it requires a lot of mindful internal work. This is because transitions are the pivotal point between wanting to hold on to a familiar past and needing to move on to a new but hazy future. Mentally and emotionally, you're being pulled in opposite directions. This creates a lot of anxiety and uncertainty, a sense that you're living on the edge—a place where most people aren't comfortable.

"The transitions involved in caregiving can unbalance you," says Gloria Cavanaugh, president and chief executive officer of the American Society on Aging, based in San Francisco. "You go into the caregiving relationship thinking that you're just looking after someone else. But you quickly discover that you need to look after yourself as well. The big task is to find your balance, and to maintain that balance whenever you experience change."

THE THREE STAGES OF TRANSITION

While everyone experiences transition in their own way, the process usually consists of the following three stages. (These descriptions have been adapted from OregonCares, the caregiving support program of the Oregon Department of Human Services.)

1. Preparing for transition. At this stage, you're facing both an ending and a beginning. The change that put you at this point may not be welcome or expected. Perhaps your mother's vision has deteriorated so much that she can no longer drive, or your spouse has become so forgetful that he or she can't stay home alone.

Whatever the change, recognize it. Don't deny it. Denial is an attempt to freeze time, to preserve a situation as it once was. But time never stands still. It continues to move forward, bringing subsequent changes ever closer.

Of course, denial is a very human emotion. Most of us shrink from change. We'd rather not have to endure it. But it's an essential part of life.

As you acknowledge the change that you're facing, and the transition that it will bring, you can begin letting go of the "old reality"—the situation as it was. Often this involves grieving a loss. Allow yourself to grieve, if you need to; it can help ease the transition process.

In the course of letting go of the old reality, you can open yourself to the new reality. This doesn't mean you need to accept it right away. Usually, acceptance takes time. For now, focus on dealing with any confusion, anxiety, and fear brought on by thoughts of what lies ahead. These emotions are perfectly normal, and like the change you're facing, they shouldn't be denied. Nor should they be dwelled on to the point where they become paralyzing through their own negativity.

2. Taking the necessary steps. This is the stage of greatest uncertainty. To use the river analogy once more, you're going from a stone that feels comfortable to one that doesn't. It may wobble in unexpected ways, making you struggle to stay on course.

If you're having doubts about moving forward, remember that you're not alone. Your loved one is in the same situation, though seeing it from a different perspective. This person may be struggling just as much as you are. You can help each other—and anyone else facing this change—by being supportive, kind, and patient.

3. Establishing the new equilibrium. Once you reach this stage, you've weathered the most challenging part of the transition. You may feel some residual anxiety, but it should subside as you regain your inner balance and embrace your new perspective and deeper emotional strength.

Remember, though, that the next change may be just around the corner. Stay prepared for it, rather than settling into the mindset that this new equilibrium will last forever.

Take Action... STAY ON COURSE THROUGH THE CHALLENGE

Of course, the nature of the change you're facing can have a profound influence on the ease of the transition. You might breeze through it, or you might get stuck and feel overwhelmed. If that happens, the following strategies can help put the situation in perspective and keep you moving forward. (Also see the Caregiver's Checklist on page 72.)

EXPERT OPINION

"When a loved one dies, you grieve and, over time, adjust to the loss. But in caregiving, especially for an elderly parent in decline, the grieving process is ongoing, as you mourn all the losses your loved one—and your family—experiences along the way. You have to do the work of grieving while you're doing the work of caregiving."

—**LOIS ESCOBAR, M.S.W.,** a family consultant with the Family Caregiver Alliance in San Francisco

Point of View

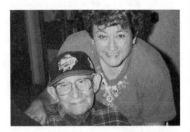

"In Latino culture, we take care of our own. In the old days, the aunts and uncles and cousins were there, taking care of whoever needed help. Even the neighbors pitched in. Nowadays, it's so different. Everyone has to work; no one stays at home. Still, there's a stigma against people who don't take care of their own. Family members who are old school . . . you can explain that things have changed, that we no longer have extended families, but still they don't understand."

—ALICIA FRANCO,
Santa Barbara, California

✗ Allow yourself to observe "silly" fears about the change. What makes fears unsettling is that they seem beyond your control. But they're not; after all, they're only mental perspectives. Instead of berating yourself for letting your fears get the best of you, know that they will pass when you stop giving them so much attention. Take your focus off them and bring it back to the present moment.

✗ Tune in to what's changing now, rather than what hasn't happened yet. This can prevent "worse-case scenario" thinking, in which you imagine the situation to be much worse than it really is. For example, if your mother can no longer drive, you might be telling yourself, "Mom can't live by herself anymore." But that may not be the case. She just needs someone to take her places—to the supermarket, the doctor's office, the beauty salon. Otherwise, she's fine on her own.

✗ Identify the reasons you're uncomfortable with the change. Perhaps you're worried that your mother will be devastated about having to give up driving. Maybe you're upset that you're going to be your mom's primary chauffeur, even though you're working full-time and one of your siblings isn't. These emotions are normal reactions to change, so don't let them overpower you. The best way to keep them in check is to address their causes. Ask your mom how she's feeling about not being able to drive. Help her explore other transportation options, such as community transit services.

✗ Consider the effects of the change on other family members. Because your mom can't drive, she won't be able to pick up your niece after school on those days when your brother works overtime. Helping him find a solution can shift your perspective, allowing you to see beyond the impact of the change on you alone.

✗ Put off "subsidiary" changes that can complicate the transition process. Because your mom won't be driving, she won't be needing her car. The two of you can wait to figure out what to do with it. You have time, and you want to be sure you're making a decision that you're comfortable with. Right now, the car isn't a priority.

✗ Think about the things that haven't been touched by the change. Even though your mother's vision is failing, her mind remains sharp, and she walks without assistance. Recognize that she can still do a lot on her own—like call a cab to the pharmacy, or hitch a ride with a friend to the senior center. In fact, she may want to make these arrangements on her own, without your intervention.

✗ Look for the upside of the change. Now that your mother isn't driving, you don't have to worry about her having an accident. And the money from the eventual sale of her car will bring her some much-needed cash. Most people focus on the negative aspects of change, notes Mark S. Lachs, M.D., M.P.H., chief of geriatrics and gerontology at New York Hospital in Manhattan. But it also has its positives.

✗ Find ways to make the change more tolerable. You or your loved one might resist change because it threatens to take away something you truly enjoy. Don't let it. Even though your mom can't drive to the ice cream shop, one of your siblings can pick up a pint of her favorite flavor. Or you can treat her to lunch at the new café that's within walking distance of her home.

✗ Reach out to others. "Support groups can be especially helpful when you feel you can't go on," says Gail Hunt, executive director of the Bethesda, Maryland–based National Alliance for Caregiving. "There's something deeply comforting about unburdening yourself to people who know exactly what you're going through because they've been there. And they can offer good suggestions for coping and using community resources."

✗ If you're really struggling, consider getting professional help, says Lois Escobar, M.S.W., a family consultant with the Family Caregiver Alliance in San Francisco. "You're not the first person to face a difficult transition," she notes. "Many social workers, psychologists, members of the clergy, and staffs of caregiving organizations have experience

---

FOR MORE INFORMATION

Many organizations can help you find a caregiving support group in your area. A few examples:

• **Children of Aging Parents** offers referrals to support groups, among other services. Phone: **(800) 227-7294**; Internet address: **www.caps4caregivers.org**.

• **Family Caregiver Alliance** specializes in assisting brain-injured care recipients and their families. It can help locate support groups. Phone: **(800) 445-8106**; Internet address: **www.caregiver.org**.

• **National Alliance for Caregiving** provides a variety of services for caregivers, including a Web site with many links for tracking down support groups. Internet address: **www.caregiving.org**.

In addition, many disease-specific organizations—such as the Alzheimer's Association, the American Cancer Society, and the American Diabetes Association—have support groups of their own. To find one that's appropriate for your situation, look in the blue pages of your phone directory, under "Guide to Human Services."

Caregiver's Checklist

How Are You Coping?

As you move through the transition process, you may have moments in which you feel overwhelmed by stress and self-doubt. That's when you need to step back from your situation and ask yourself the following questions. They can help pinpoint any problems and keep your transition on track.

1. Exactly what is changing?

_____

_____

_____

2. What bothers me about this change?

_____

_____

_____

3. How are other family members reacting to this change?

_____

_____

_____

4. Which aspects of this change must be dealt with now, and which can wait until later?

_____

_____

_____

5. What has not been affected by this change?

_____

_____

6. What are the benefits of this change?

_____

_____

7. How can I make this change more tolerable, even pleasurable?

_____

_____

_____

counseling people in situations like yours. They're trained to help. Use them."

X Celebrate your success. Once you get through a transition, take time to acknowledge it. And treat yourself to something special—whether it's dinner at your favorite restaurant, a trip to the bookstore, or a nice long soak in a warm bath.

HELPING OTHERS NAVIGATE CHANGE

The transitions in caregiving have something of a ripple effect, moving outward from the care recipient to the primary caregiver to the larger circle of family and friends. Oftentimes each person has an opportunity to deal with a change individually, on his or her own terms. But sometimes they feel the impact collectively, as when family members are told that Mom can no longer make Thanksgiving dinner for 30 people.

Changes that affect an entire family at once can feel especially difficult because they may foreshadow an evolution in family roles. Mom has been the center of the family, the person who took care of everyone else. Now she needs care herself, and her children are going to provide it. Many caregivers say they didn't feel like full-fledged grown-ups until they began looking after their aging parents.

As you find your way through each transition, be sensitive to the fact that virtually everyone close to you is in a similar situation. You can help each other adjust to change, provided you apply a few basic ground rules.

Understand and accept that everyone copes with change differently. Change can make an anxious person more anxious than you think is appropriate. It can send chronic deniers into denial longer than you might like. It can spur organizers to insist on more organization than you feel is necessary. Their means of coping is no more "wrong" than yours is "right." So allow family members to be themselves—as long as they don't compromise your loved one's health or safety, or their own. And try not to take their reactions personally; change is about living life, not controlling it.

Don't be surprised if some people "overreact" to change, while others "underreact." Overreacting and underreacting are

---

FOR MORE INFORMATION

If you feel you might benefit from professional counseling, either of the following organizations can help locate a certified member in your area.

• The National Association of Professional Geriatric Care Managers. Phone: **(520) 881-8008**; Internet address: **www.caremanager.org**.

• The National Association of Social Workers. Phone: **(800) 638-8799**; Internet address: **www.socialworkers.org**.

Point of View

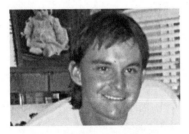

"At first, I felt very confused and frustrated. I didn't know how to deal with my grandfather. I used to get angry because I wanted him to be his old self again. But as time goes on, I'm learning how to cope. He has this disease. He doesn't know any different. This is the way he is now. I have to accept it. I'm slowly beginning to realize that. He's healthy. He's happy. This is the best it's going to be, so we have to live with it."

—NICHOLAS LINSK,
Mesa, Arizona

judgments based on individual perspective. For example, you might think your sister is blowing the situation out of proportion, while she may feel you're not as concerned as you should be. Simply recognizing and respecting differences in transition styles can make supporting one another that much easier.

Watch for emotional reactions that may be signs of grieving. When coming to terms with change, many people go through a period of grieving. It's a normal, natural part of the transition process—and it can color a person's interactions with you. Be aware of grief-driven reactions such as anger, denial, confusion, fear, sadness, depression, and indecisiveness.

TRANSITION AS A WAY OF LIFE

By its nature, caregiving presents many changes and many transitions. Sometimes they happen so quickly that the "new reality" and "old reality" seem like one and the same. That can leave you wondering whether your life ever will be "normal" again.

If you think about it, though, you've been going through changes and transitions from the moment you were born. Some you even celebrated, like getting your driver's license, graduating from high school, marrying your sweetheart, and starting a family. Caring for a loved one is just another marker on life's continuum, although it hasn't yet earned the same recognition as other rites of passage.

Think about how you've made many changes and transitions over the years, and how you've managed to find a new equilibrium with each one. You can use that experience now, as you adjust and readjust to your caregiving role.

In a way, the transitions of caregiving are a gift. They help you learn to nurture your family relationships, and yourself. What's more, they allow you as a caregiver to glimpse your own future, to see the sorts of transitions you may need to make as you get older. In life, change and transition are the only constants.

PART THREE

Preparing to Care

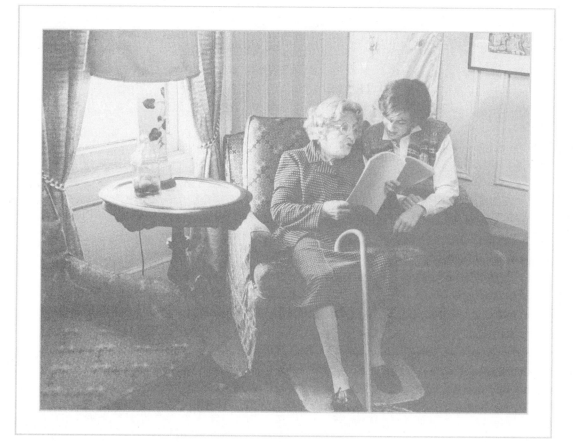

CHAPTER 8

YOUR CAREGIVING SUPPORT NETWORK

What You Need to Know

- A caregiving team is a core group of health professionals who can help develop a comprehensive caregiving plan and oversee certain aspects of your loved one's care.

- Every caregiving team is unique. Whom you choose for yours depends on what your loved one needs, what you can provide, and how much other family members can pitch in.

- Key members of most caregiving teams include primary care physicians, geriatricians, and geriatric care managers, as well as nurses, physical therapists, and social workers.

"My dad lives alone, and he can't cook for himself. How do I go about enrolling him in a meal delivery program?"

"My wife had a stroke and needs assistance with everything. I can't manage by myself anymore. I need help."

"My siblings and I work full-time. How do we find someone who is qualified—and whom we can trust—to provide care for our mother during the day, when we can't be there?"

At this very moment, scenarios like these are playing out all across the United States, for any of the 54 million people actively involved in caregiving. For them—and for you—help is available.

As the American population ages, individuals and organizations are responding by offering formal and informal support for all kinds and levels of caregiving. In this chapter, you'll learn how to tap into these resources by creating a support network that meets your loved one's needs as well as your own.

Identifying the professionals who will make up your support network—your caregiving "team"—may require some legwork up front, but it will pay off in the long run. These people can provide an objective perspective on your loved one's situation. They can help identify which caregiving services are necessary, and who can provide them. Perhaps most important, they can take over some of the caregiving tasks, so you'll be less likely to burn out from attempting to manage all the care yourself. You'll be better able to support your loved one—physically, mentally, and emotionally.

Take Action... ORGANIZE YOUR RECRUITMENT PLAN

Whom you choose for your caregiving team depends primarily on three factors: what sort of help your loved one requires, what sort of help you can provide, and how much the rest of your family is willing to pitch in. Be sure you have this information before you begin scheduling meetings with prospective team members. You want to be able to present a clear picture of your situation to these people, so you're certain to get the support you need right from the start.

To that same end, the following strategies can help as well.

✗ Contact the Area Agency on Aging in your loved one's community. The staff there knows all about the caregiving support services available locally, from meal delivery programs and transportation services to senior centers and adult day care programs. They can direct you to people who can provide more information about these services, if that's necessary. They can also answer questions about health insurance, legal matters, home care, and many other issues that caregivers encounter. (You'll learn more about Area Agencies on Aging, as well as other community caregiving organizations, in chapter 19.)

✗ Call your loved one's primary care physician—especially if he has known your loved one for any length of time. The doctor or his staff may be able to help develop a caregiving plan and recommend other helpful resources, such as in-

FOR MORE INFORMATION

To contact the Area Agency on Aging in your loved one's community, look in the blue pages of the telephone directory, under "Guide to Human Services." Or check the Eldercare Locator, a nationwide service sponsored by the U.S. Administration on Aging. Call **(800) 677-1116**, or visit the Eldercare Locator Web site at **www.eldercare.gov.**

home care. Remember that to qualify for reimbursement from Medicare, Medicaid, or private insurance for services that your loved one requires, a doctor's certification of medical need is essential.

✗ Buy a notebook in which you can write down information during your meetings with prospective members of your caregiving team. Be sure to note the date you speak with each person, as well as a phone number or e-mail address in case you have any follow-up questions.

✗ Also invest in a file folder or binder in which you can keep any letters, brochures, forms, and other documents that you collect during your meetings. Store your folder in a convenient location—perhaps by the telephone, so it's right at hand when calls come in.

✗ Allow ample time to conduct research, gather information, and interview prospective members of your caregiving team. It's an involved process, but it helps ensure that

Your Home Care Information Sheet

If you're expecting your loved one to require some form of in-home care, you can improve your prospects for finding a skilled, reliable caregiver by putting together an information sheet about your loved one's situation. The sheet doesn't have to be especially detailed, but it should include at least the following:

- The care recipient's name, address, and phone number(s)
- Directions to the care recipient's home
- The care recipient's date of birth, height, and weight
- Important points about the care recipient's physical or mental health status—for example, whether your loved one is on medication, incontinent, or forgetful

- Tasks requiring assistance, which can range from light housekeeping and shopping to bathing, dressing, and feeding
- Your name, address, and phone number(s)
- The names and phone numbers of your backup contacts, including family members, neighbors, and the care recipient's physician
- Names and ages of everyone living in the same home as the care recipient
- Names, ages, and species of any pets living in the same home as the care recipient

This information will come in handy as you check into agencies that provide in-home care, because they'll be better able to match their employees and services to your loved one's needs and circumstances.

Point of View

"I cared for my mother at home for the last 10 years of her life. I knew when I retired and moved out to Long Island that I wanted to use my nursing background to help hospice patients. I realize that their time is limited and that many of them know they are dying. I see my role as making their final days pleasant. Sometimes we spend time talking or watching TV. Or I just hold their hands to give them a sense of calm. Being a hospice volunteer makes my day. I do it because I enjoy helping others."

—ROBERTA MULLINER,
Cutchogue, New York

you're finding the right people and services for your particular caregiving situation.

✗ Before you agree to any for-fee services, find out what's covered by your loved one's insurance and what must be paid out-of-pocket. Caregiving bills can add up quickly, while your loved one's financial resources may have to stretch out over years. In some cases, you may be able to find a comparable service that's free of charge or available on a sliding scale.

THE KEY PLAYERS ON YOUR TEAM

As you begin the selection process for your caregiving team, keep in mind that you want people who are good fits for your unique situation—people who can provide the support you need in a manner that you're comfortable with. For this reason, your team may be different from those of other caregivers. In general, though, every "lineup" includes some mix of the following professionals.

- Primary care physician
- Registered nurse
- Geriatrician
- Physical therapist
- Geriatric care manager
- Social worker

Each of these people brings a unique set of skills and knowledge to your caregiving team. Each sees your situation from a slightly different perspective. Some may be called upon only at certain points in your caregiving plan, while others will be involved for the duration.

Beyond this core group of professionals, your caregiving team may have a number of supporting players—people who provide various kinds of assistance, ranging from light housekeeping and meal delivery to medical treatment and respite care. Among the primary advantages of these services, of course, is that they allow your loved one to remain at home. And that in itself has several important benefits, experts say.

- It enables your loved one to maintain a sense of independence and self-worth.
- It reduces the risk for infection and illness, which is higher in nursing homes and hospitals.

* It ensures that your loved one is getting individualized attention in a familiar environment.

* It allows family members to spend "quality time" with their loved one, even if that person is sick.

* It's less expensive than the round-the-clock care provided in nursing homes and hospitals. Experts estimate that typical in-home care costs about one-tenth as much as hospitalization and one-quarter as much as nursing home occupancy.

You'll find more information about caregiving support services in chapters 19 and 20. For now, let's turn our attention to the key players on your core caregiving team, including the training they receive and the help they can provide.

Primary Care Physicians

In professional sports, every team has its own doctor. So should yours. A primary care physician can serve as medical gatekeeper, monitoring your loved one's physical, mental, and emotional health and attending to any emerging concerns promptly. If your loved one doesn't already have a primary care physician, you can find one on your own. But you want to be sure the doctor you choose is a good fit—someone whom you and your loved one are comfortable with.

Before you begin your search, you need to find out whether your loved one's health plan has any guidelines for selecting a primary care physician. For example, if your loved one belongs to an HMO, including Medicare HMO, your choices are limited to the doctors under contract with that plan. What's more, the doctor who becomes your primary care provider will serve as point person in making referrals to medical specialists, such as internists or geriatricians.

Once you know what, if any, guidelines you must follow, you're ready to put together a list of physician candidates from which you and your loved one can choose. How do you go about finding them? First, check with hospitals in your loved one's community; many have physician referral services. Ask family members, friends, and coworkers for their recommendations, including what they like—and dislike—about various doctors. You can even look in the Yellow Pages for leads.

FOR MORE INFORMATION

The American Medical Association (AMA) maintains a database of information on almost every M.D. and D.O. in the country. Check the AMA Web site at **www.ama-assn.org** for a list of board-certified primary care physicians in your area.

Once you have a list of four or five candidates, you and your loved one should schedule an initial consultation with each physician. Among the issues the two of you should consider when making a final decision:

Qualifications. Do you want a primary care physician who is board-certified in many specialty areas, such as geriatric medicine? Actually, HMOs have a policy of hiring only those physicians who are board-certified. The advantage of board certification is that you can be sure the doctor has had additional training in his specialty, and he's taking continuing medical education courses in order to stay certified.

Gender. Some people just feel more comfortable with physicians of their own sex. Others prefer doctors of the opposite sex.

Age. Because they equate age with experience, some people like older physicians. Others seek out younger physicians, who may be more familiar with new medical techniques.

Availability. Be sure to find out how each physician handles patient calls that come in after hours or while he's on vacation. You want a doctor with reliable backups, fellow physicians who will step in and provide care during his absence. You also want a doctor who isn't so busy that you have difficulty scheduling appointments—or spend long periods of time in the waiting room.

Interest in patients. A primary care physician should demonstrate a genuine interest in caring for older people. He should be willing to take the time necessary to perform a thorough examination. He should welcome questions from you and your loved one during office visits.

Of course, the most important consideration in choosing a primary care physician is finding someone whom you trust to care for your loved one. Always remember that if you're dissatisfied with one doctor, you're not obligated to stay with him. You have the right to change physicians at any time, for any reason.

Geriatricians

Like children, older people have medical needs that are different from those of adults at midlife. Geriatricians have the expertise necessary to attend to those needs. Their job is to improve quality of life for the elderly and to keep them functional and independent for as long as possible. In other words, a geriatrician is like a pediatrician, only specializing in issues at the other end of life.

By definition, a geriatrician has completed a residency in either internal medicine or family medicine, followed by 1 to 2 years of training (known as a fellowship) in the medical and psychological problems that affect older adults. This additional training enables the geriatrician to recognize and treat a wide range of health concerns, including memory loss, dementia, depression, pressure sores, weight loss, and drug interactions. This person is also skilled in identifying social and economic issues that may impede care.

Geriatrics is a relatively new medical specialty. The American Medical Association has been granting board certification in this area for only about 2 decades. But the need for geriatricians will continue to grow as baby boomers age. People over age 85 represent the fastest-growing segment of the American population, and living to age 100 is no longer a rarity.

According to a recent study conducted by the Rand Corporation, the United States will need about 35,000 geriatricians by 2020 in order to meet the demand for services. As of 2000, only 20,000 physicians were certified in geriatric care. Finding medical students to specialize in this field has been difficult. It's not the sort of specialty in which physicians necessarily perform heroic measures or save lives. What's more, many medical students go through their entire training without meeting a board-certified geriatrician, so they're not learning about the field. Still, geriatrics can be a gratifying specialty for those dedicated to helping aging Americans.

Should you include a geriatrician in your caregiving team? Possibly, if your loved one fits into one of the following categories.

- The frailest old with multiple medical problems

- Older adults with multiple medical problems and limited social support

- Older adults with medical problems primarily associated with aging, such as heart disease or osteoarthritis

Finding a board-certified geriatrician can take some time and effort. Again, hospital referral services are a good place to start. If your loved one lives in a small town, you may need to broaden your search to include nearby cities. But don't settle on the first person you find. Consider the same issues for your geriatrician as for your primary care physician, and make your decision accordingly.

Geriatric Care Managers

Think of the geriatric care manager as the quarterback of your caregiving team. This person serves as your family's advocate in all kinds of caregiving issues. Geriatric care managers are especially adept at navigating bureaucratic red tape.

Geriatric care managers wear many hats. They perform need and problem assessments, crisis intervention, and family conflict mediation. They can coordinate financial, legal, and medical assistance as well as housekeeping and transportation services. They can make arrangements for adult day care and in-home care. They can even evaluate housing options and help find a suitable nursing home, if that becomes necessary. In essence, their job is to monitor your loved one and oversee every aspect of her care.

"A geriatric care manager can be a family's best asset because this person has no emotional ties to the situation," says Patricia McGinnis, executive director of the California Advocates for Nursing Home Reform in San Francisco. "What's more, this person can be there when family members cannot—when, say, Mom lives on the East Coast but her kids live out west."

In general, geriatric care managers are either nurses or social workers with special training in gerontology. The National Association of Professional Geriatric Care Managers has established voluntary standards of quality and a code of ethics for geriatric care managers. Its members are required to have professional degrees in human services and at least 2 years of geriatric experience.

If you're interested in hiring a geriatric care manager, use the following criteria to find the right person for your situation.

- Your geriatric care manager should have appropriate credentials. Because these managers aren't licensed, their training can range from a bachelor's degree to doctorates in multiple disciplines. The best in the field have experience in gerontology, social work, psychology, and nursing.

FOR MORE INFORMATION

The National Association of Professional Geriatric Care Managers has a referral network that encompasses every part of the country. For a list of current members in each geographic region, you can call the association at **(520) 881-8008**. The list includes each geriatric care manager's areas of expertise. You might also want to check out the organization's Web site at **www.caremanager.org**. Click on "Find a Care Manager," and you'll be able to search for geriatric care managers that meet specific criteria.

- Your geriatric care manager should listen well and find answers to your questions.

- Your geriatric care manager should be willing to solve problems and respond to calls and emergencies.

- Your geriatric care manager should be able to customize a caregiving plan and actively supervise your loved one's care.

- Your geriatric care manager should be familiar with the full range of available caregiving services.

- Your geriatric care manager should be objective and independent when assembling your caregiving team. Be cautious if the person owns or is otherwise affiliated with any in-home service providers.

Caregiver's Checklist

Which Geriatric Care Manager Should You Choose?

For many a caregiver, hiring a geriatric care manager is an absolute lifesaver. But because geriatric care management has no licensing requirements, finding someone who's truly qualified can take a bit of sleuthing. As you interview care managers for your caregiving team, be sure to ask yourself the following questions. (You may want to make extra copies of this checklist, so you have enough.)

☐ yes ☐ no   Does this person share my views on caregiving policies and practices?

☐ yes ☐ no   Does this person seem familiar with all of the caregiving resources available to meet my loved one's needs?

☐ yes ☐ no   Does this person do a satisfactory job of monitoring his clients' care?

☐ yes ☐ no   Is this person thorough in assessing my loved one's needs?

☐ yes ☐ no   Does this person ask appropriate questions about my loved one's physical and mental health status, medications, and lifestyle?

☐ yes ☐ no   Does this person seem knowledgeable about dementia and its associated needs?

☐ yes ☐ no   Does this person charge for short phone consultations, in addition to in-person consultations and long phone consultations?

☐ yes ☐ no   Can this person educate me about my caregiving role?

Point of View

"My mother, Virginia, is 83 years old. She's pretty viable mentally. But a few years ago, she needed a hip replacement. Then she fell and shattered her femur bone. Now she has trouble going up and down stairs, so she lives next door in a ground-floor apartment we own. One of the best things we did was hire a physical therapist, Candy, to come in each week. Candy is like a miracle worker. She helps my mom stretch, eases her sore muscles, and in essence, makes her feel great. A lot of it has to do with Candy's attitude. She is patient and compassionate. My mom looks forward to her visits."

—KAREN HADLEY,
Seal Beach, California

Before you make your final decision, be sure to call your local Better Business Bureau or Consumer Affairs Office to find out whether any complaints have been filed against your prospective geriatric care manager. Also contact the manager's references to get their assessment of his services.

Please note that most geriatric care managers charge on a fee-for-service basis. Generally, their services are not covered by most insurance policies, nor are they recognized as billable by Medicare or Medicaid. You may be able to obtain reimbursement for certain services from your insurance carrier, depending on your specific case.

The fees charged by geriatric care managers vary by geographic location and level of experience. Generally, you can expect to pay between $200 and $350 for the initial assessment, and $30 to $150 per hour for subsequent consultations. Some public and private care management providers assess fees using a sliding scale based on income.

Other Key Players

Depending on your loved one's needs and circumstances, you may decide to expand your caregiving team to include any or all of the following health professionals.

Nurses and physical therapists. If your loved one is ill or recovering from surgery, you can hire a nurse to check up on the person at home. Nurses can attend to a variety of medical needs, such as changing wound dressings, administering injections, dispensing medications, and monitoring vital signs. Similarly, physical therapists can provide in-home rehabilitation services—for example, teaching exercises to speed the post-operative recuperation process.

Generally, these professionals charge about $90 per visit, though the actual fee depends on the length of the visit and the type of care. For nursing care, licensed practical nurses (L.P.N.'s) and certified nursing assistants (C.N.A.'s) charge less than registered nurses (R.N.'s). Some of the cost may be covered by your loved one's Medicare, Medicaid, or supplemental or private insurance.

To begin the process of finding a nurse or physical therapist who provides in-home care, ask your loved one's primary care physician for recommendations. You can also check with local hospital referral services, or look in the Yellow Pages under "Nurses" or "Physical Therapists."

Social workers. Like geriatric care managers, social workers provide a myriad of nonmedical support services for caregivers and care recipients. If you need assistance in navigating the network of social services in your loved one's community, consider hiring a social worker for your caregiving team.

Professionals in the social work field have a broad range of education and training, as illustrated by the alphabet soup of initials that often follow their names. Some caregiving experts say the most important set of initials is N.A.S.W., which indicates licensure by the National Association of Social Workers. Other initials you may see include the following:

- M.S.W.: masters of social work, the traditional degree for qualified social workers

- L.C.S.W.: licensed clinical social worker; used in some states to indicate licensure

- M.Ed.: masters in education, a degree held by many counselors

- L.P.C.: licensed professional counselor

- M.F.C.C.: marriage, family, and child counselor; used in some states to indicate licensure

- M.S. or M.A.: masters of science or masters of arts, the traditional advanced degrees awarded by colleges and universities

- M.Div.: masters of divinity, awarded to ministers who wish to become pastoral counselors

- Ed.S.: educational specialist; indicates training beyond a master's degree but short of a doctorate

Home health aides and homemakers. If your loved one needs some assistance with personal care or housekeeping tasks, you may consider hiring a home health aide or a homemaker. These professionals can help with everything from bathing, grooming, and dressing to meal preparation, grocery shopping, and light housecleaning—though they cannot administer medications or provide other medical care. Their services are described in more detail in chapter 20.

(continued on page 90)

FOR MORE INFORMATION

Caregiving experts recommend hiring a social worker who's licensed by the National Association of Social Workers (NASW). For a referral to a social worker in your area, you can call the NASW at **(800) 638-8799**, or visit the organization's Web site at **www.socialworkers.org**.

FOR MORE INFORMATION

For helpful tips on choosing a home care provider to assist your loved one, visit Homecare Online, the Web site of the National Association for Home Care. Among the site's features is a home care/hospice agency locator. Log on to **www.nahc.org**.

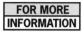

Which Home Care Provider Should You Choose?

The National Association for Home Care advises family members seeking in-home assistance for their loved ones to ask the following questions when interviewing prospective home care providers.

1. How long has the provider been serving the community?

_____

_____

2. Does the provider offer literature explaining its services, eligibility requirements, fees, and funding sources?

_____

_____

3. How does the provider select and train its employees?

_____

_____

_____

_____

4. Does the provider protect its employees with written personnel policies, benefits packages, and malpractice insurance?

_____

_____

5. Do nurses and therapists evaluate the patient's home care needs? Do they consult the patient's physicians and family members?

_____

_____

_____

_____

6. Does the provider consult the patient and family members when developing a caregiving plan?

_____

_____

7. Does the provider document the details of the caregiving plan, assigning specific tasks to each person on the caregiving team?

_____

_____

_____

8. Do the patient and family members receive copies of the caregiving plan, and can it be updated as the patient's needs change?

_____

_____

9. Does the provider take time to educate family members about the care given to the patient?

_____

_____

10. Does the provider assign supervisors to oversee the quality of care given to patients?

_____

_____

11. Whom can the patient and family members contact with questions or complaints? How does the provider follow up on and resolve problems?

_____

_____

_____

_____

12. What are the provider's financial procedures? Does the provider furnish written statements explaining all of the costs and payment options associated with the caregiving plan?

_____

_____

_____

_____

_____

13. How does the provider handle emergencies? Is help available 24 hours a day, 7 days a week?

_____

_____

_____

_____

14. How does the provider ensure patient confidentiality?

_____

_____

_____

_____

FOR MORE INFORMATION

In-Home Support Services usually operates under the jurisdiction of the county Department of Human Services. Check the county government listings in the blue pages of your phone directory.

Fees for home health aides and homemakers range from minimum wage to $18 an hour, and usually, they're not covered by Medicare, Medicaid, or supplemental or private health insurance. But the fees may be waived or adjusted on a sliding scale for people who qualify as low-income. One program, called In-Home Support Services, provides nonmedical personal care for at-risk low-income elderly and disabled people.

Keep in mind, too, that new standardized Medicare supplemental insurance (known as Medigap) provides reimbursement for a very limited range of in-home caregiving services. But not all Medigap plans offer this coverage, and not all applicants qualify. (For more information about Medicare, Medicaid, and Medigap, see chapter 24.)

ANOTHER KIND OF CAREGIVING TEAM

The primary purpose of your caregiving team is to help shape and implement a caregiving plan for your loved one. In this way,

Caregiving around the World

In the Netherlands, the principle of solidarity, or concern for each other, manifests itself in many ways. One example is found within the country's health care system: Many Dutch doctors make house calls, especially for seniors. In fact, about 17 percent of all physicians' primary care occurs in the home. The doctors believe that making house calls helps them provide better care, as they get a welcome glimpse into their patients' living environments and lifestyles.

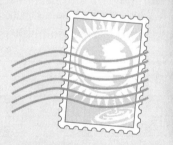

POST CARD

FROM THE NETHERLANDS

it's providing support for you. But you may also need another kind of support, the kind that can help ease the emotional challenges and conflicts of giving care. That's what support groups are for.

"Caregiving can be stressful, emotionally as well as physically," says Larry Lachman, Psy.D., a family psychologist in Carmel, California, who has conducted caregiver support groups for more than 20 years. "Support groups provide a forum in which caregivers can address their feelings of anger, frustration, fear, and depression. In the process, they realize that they are not alone. And the groups help reconfirm the good work the caregivers are doing in caring for their loved ones."

If you're interested in joining a support group, Dr. Lachman recommends looking for a group led by a professional licensed counselor, social worker, or psychologist. A good group leader maintains the structure of the meetings and prevents any one member from monopolizing a discussion.

In his support groups, Dr. Lachman limits membership to no more than seven. He asks members to focus on their own thoughts and feelings, to stay in the present, and to respect the confidentiality of others.

While support groups are not cure-alls for caregivers, Dr. Lachman says the groups have their benefits.

- You can learn to be more effective in your relationships with others, including the loved one for whom you're providing care.

- You can experiment with new behaviors in a controlled and safe environment.

- You can learn about yourself as you're seen through the eyes of others.

- You have the opportunity to bounce ideas off of people outside your family who share in a common situation.

If you're not comfortable participating in a support group in person, or if you can't leave home to attend group meetings, you might want to look into online groups instead. For example, ThirdAge.com sponsors an online chat for caregivers. The chat room is open 24 hours a day, 7 days a week. (For more information on support groups, see chapter 19.)

CHAPTER 9

NO PLACE LIKE HOME

What You Need to Know

- One in five care recipients resides in the same household as the caregiver. Often the care recipients are parents, and the caregivers are adult children.

- The best time to talk with your parents about living arrangements for their elder years is while they're healthy and independent. But no matter when you have the conversation, be respectful of the sensitive nature of the topic. Most older Americans want to spend the rest of their lives in their own homes.

- Whether your parents are on their own or with you, you'll want to accident-proof their living space. Even simple measures like removing throw rugs and installing night-lights can help ensure your mom and dad's safety.

Donna Hickey knew that her mother, Jessie Allen, would move in with her someday. She also knew that her mom, a very independent-minded woman, wouldn't take kindly to the idea of giving up her home. So Donna didn't press the issue.

But after Jessie turned 80, her behavior began changing so noticeably that Donna feared for her mother's safety. Jessie was calling family members by the wrong names, tripping over rugs, and forgetting to turn off her gas stove. Her arms and legs had purple blotches, telltale signs of nasty collisions with the furniture in her home.

Then one spring afternoon, Jessie stumbled while walking through her front lawn. She fell violently, breaking her left hip. In pain and immobilized, she cried out to a young girl who happened to be walking past her home.

"Please call my daughter," Jessie said, giving Donna's number to the girl. "Tell her I fell and I can't move. Tell her I need her."

The girl relayed the message to Donna, who rushed to her mother's side. The incident convinced her that her mom couldn't live alone anymore.

Jessie needed surgery to repair her hip. While she was hospitalized, Donna seized the opportunity to once again invite her mother to move in with her and her husband, Bill. They had the space—their five grown daughters were living on their own—and their three-bedroom home in Hastings, Florida, was just 5 miles from Jessie's place.

Mother and daughter talked, and Jessie finally admitted that she needed help. She had been diagnosed with early-stage Alzheimer's disease. Her asthma had worsened, requiring her to receive breathing treatments three times a day. She was forgetting to take her medications. She felt shaky on her feet.

"My mom never wanted to lose her independence, and I knew that she would totally give up on life if she was placed in a nursing home," Donna says. "I was able to convince her that my home would be the best place for her."

Take Action... DECIDE WHERE "HOME" SHOULD BE

Donna is among a growing legion of adult children now faced with the responsibility of providing shelter, food, and personal care for their aging parents. In fact, 20 percent of care recipients—one in five—share housing with their caregivers, according to a survey by the National Alliance for Caregiving and AARP.

If you're thinking about inviting a parent to move into your home, caregiving experts stress the importance of considering the thoughts and feelings of *everyone* affected by this life-changing decision. It will require a lot of adjustments, some of which will likely be very taxing both physically and emotionally. (But you and your family can take steps to ease the transition, as we'll discuss later.)

Ideally, the best time to discuss your parents' future housing is while they're still healthy and independent. It's far better than making a rushed decision after Mom breaks a hip or Dad suffers

Point of View

"I live in Delaware and my sister, Martha, lives in Louisiana. A few years ago, we needed to place our mother, Mildred, in a nursing facility. She was showing signs of dementia, and she was withering away in my parents' old, drafty farmhouse in Illinois.

"After my mother went into the nursing facility, my sister and I had to work out a living arrangement for our father. We decided he would stay with my wife and me for 2 months in the spring and 2 months in the fall. He lives with my sister and her husband the rest of the year.

"My father is 93. He's still witty, but he can no longer drive a car. We're happy knowing that he's not by himself in an old farmhouse far away. He is here with us, and he is well-fed, warm, and happy."

—KARL SMITH,
Newark, Delaware

Should Your Parent Move In with You?

When considering a parent's living arrangements, be sure to address the following questions. If any gets a "no" response, you may want to discuss that particular issue with your parent and everyone else in the household. Working together, you might find a way to make the situation more comfortable for all involved. If not, you may come to the conclusion that your parent would be better off living elsewhere—perhaps with another family member or in residential care.

☐ yes ☐ no   **Physical space.** Is your home large enough to provide privacy for all family members once your parent moves in?

☐ yes ☐ no   **Relationships.** Does your spouse or partner get along with your parent?

☐ yes ☐ no   **Children.** Are your children mature enough to understand why their grandparent is moving into your home, and to welcome him or her?

☐ yes ☐ no   Will they make adjustments willingly?

☐ yes ☐ no   **Accessibility.** Does your house have wheelchair-accessible entryways and handrails and grab bars by the toilet, bathtub, and shower?

☐ yes ☐ no   **Your job.** Will you be able to maintain your schedule at work and still take care of your parent?

☐ yes ☐ no   Does your workplace have a flextime policy?

☐ yes ☐ no   **Your health status.** Are you willing and able to provide the necessary care for your parent now and in the future?

☐ yes ☐ no   **Lifestyle and values.** Are your lifestyle and values compatible with your parent's?

☐ yes ☐ no   **Family history.** Will you be able to view yourself as a decision-making, in-charge adult and not feel like a child in the presence of your parent?

☐ yes ☐ no   Have you resolved any past conflicts with your parent, and do the two of you get along well now?

☐ yes ☐ no   **Community resources.** Can you depend on other family members and community services to step in and give you an occasional break from caregiving?

☐ yes ☐ no   **Expectations.** Will you feel comfortable asking your parent to pitch in with household chores, finances, and/or childcare, if he or she is able?

a heart attack. Although living arrangements can be an awkward and sensitive topic, expressing your views before the need arises often results in better communication and less conflict.

To help you and your parents feel comfortable with this important conversation, experts offer the following strategies.

- Look for opportunities to bring up the subject. Maybe your dad mentions that he worries about his arthritis getting worse. Or your mom wonders aloud whether she can manage such a big house on her own. Seize upon these openings to nudge your parents into a discussion of their future housing. You can also broach the topic on your own, especially if you know of someone who has been in a similar situation: "I've been thinking about this a lot lately, because a good friend of mine just went through this with his parents. I want to be able to help you when the time comes."

- Select a private time to talk. You can show respect for your parents and avoid a heated tiff by not bringing up the subject at a social gathering like a holiday dinner or a birthday celebration.

- Plan for future conversations. You and your parents won't be able to cover all of the issues surrounding their living arrangements in a single session. It would be too emotionally overwhelming for everyone. But over time, the discussions do get easier. Regard them as an ongoing process.

- See yourself in your parents' shoes. How would you like to be spoken to? This brings greater compassion into your conversations. Remember, too, that most older Americans would prefer to "age in place"—that is, to spend the rest of their lives in their own homes.

Take Action... MAKE THE MOVE EASIER

Even if your parent has already agreed to come live with you, even if Mom or Dad seems to be looking forward to a "change of scenery," you need to be prepared for a very different reaction once the move is complete. Family therapists say that older people, in particular, may show signs of anger, depression, confusion, and

EXPERT OPINION

"As an urgent care physician treating a lot of what I like to call VPs (vintage people), I've learned to recognize some characteristic signs in those who would be better off living with loved ones or in an assisted living facility than by themselves. Some people who live independently don't want to 'bother' their relatives when they get sick, so they put off calling for help for 2, 3, even 4 days. Suddenly, they've developed pneumonia or some other condition that requires hospitalization. Other people might call family members repeatedly with minor problems that don't need medical care. Often the real reason for the call is loneliness, not illness. We need to pay attention to the message behind the call—or risk delaying medical help."

—DALE L. ANDERSON, M.D., an urgent care physician in St. Paul, Minnesota

Point of View

"While my mom was in the hospital recuperating from her hip surgery, my husband and I put most of her furniture into storage. But we moved her bookcase to our home and put it in her new bedroom, making sure to replace all her books in the same order and on the same shelves as she had them. We put her favorite quilt and bedspread on her bed. And we took all the pictures she had in her house and mounted them on her bedroom walls. She must have had about 80 photos; her bedroom looks like a wall-to-wall mural. We wanted her to be surrounded by things familiar to her when she made the move from the hospital into our home."

—DONNA HICKEY,
Hastings, Florida

grief. They might also become disoriented and pine for the homes they left behind. Experts often refer to this as relocation trauma. How can you help your parent cope?

✗ Understand that any negative emotions Mom or Dad is experiencing are perfectly normal. Moving is a major life event under any circumstances. In this case, your parent has been uprooted from a place—and possibly a community—that he or she may have called home for decades. So if Mom or Dad lashes out or sinks into a funk, don't take it personally. It's not you; it's the situation. (But if mood changes persist, be sure your parent sees a doctor. Such changes may be a sign of an underlying health problem.)

✗ Find ways to make your house feel like home. Ask your parent to bring along cherished possessions, like family photos or a favorite chair. Decorating your home with these items can help your parent to feel more comfortable in his or her new surroundings and less fearful of losing his or her independence.

✗ Invite your loved one's close friends and former neighbors to visit. If these people no longer live close by, urge your parent to stay in touch by writing letters, making phone calls, or sending e-mails.

✗ Identify opportunities for your parent to pitch in. Your mom may feel a sense of accomplishment when she bakes her family-favorite apple pie. Or your dad's self-esteem may get a lift when he shows your teenage son how to tune up a bicycle. Helping your parent feel like an integral part of the household is absolutely vital.

✗ Encourage your parent to continue with favorite hobbies. If Mom likes to grow roses, set aside a corner of your flower garden where she can putter. Or clear out some space in the family room or basement so your dad can set up his model trains.

✗ Respect your parent's need for privacy. Regard your dad's or mom's bedroom as his or her private suite, and always knock before entering. Make sure your parent has his or her own closet and, if possible, a private bathroom. Let your mom or dad choose the decor of the rooms, right down to the color of the walls.

Take Action... SAFEGUARD YOUR OWN SANITY

Just as you'll need to help your parent feel welcome and comfortable in his or her new surroundings, you'll need to adjust to the new living arrangement, too. That can bring its own set of tumultuous emotions—frustration, resentment, anger, depression, guilt, and grief. To help you feel better about the situation, the National Family Caregivers Association offers this advice. (We'll discuss more general coping techniques for the emotional demands of caregiving in chapter 26.)

✗ Acknowledge that caregiving is an important but challenging task. Strive to do your best, but don't aim for perfection.

✗ Trust your instincts to lead you in the right direction.

✗ Love, honor, and value yourself. You deserve some personal time, even if it's just 10 minutes for an uninterrupted soak in a warm bath.

✗ Accept help from family members and friends when they offer it. Maintain a "wish list" of tasks that you'd like to pass off to others.

✗ If your parent has an illness, educate yourself about it. Information is empowering.

✗ At the same time, be careful not to let your parent's illness or disability always take center stage and overshadow the rest of your life.

✗ Check out ideas and technologies that can support your parent's independence.

✗ Stand up for your rights as a caregiver. Be your own best advocate for self-care.

✗ Join a formal support group for caregivers or establish your own informal support network. Either way, you'll have a forum for sharing your ideas and releasing pent-up feelings of stress and guilt.

✗ Be alert for early signs of depression, and seek professional help if you need it.

EXPERT OPINION

"In my 30 years of nursing, I've worked with patients and their families in critical care units, intensive care units, cardiac surgical units, public health, and hospice care. Burnout is very common among caregivers. They give so much to so many for so long that they have nothing left.

"My advice: Know thyself. Know what makes you laugh and when you are most likely to laugh. Notice who makes you laugh—your spouse, children, friends, coworkers. Laughter is important. People who are laughing seem to be healthier."

—PATTY WOOTEN, R.N., a registered nurse, therapeutic humorist, and author from Santa Cruz, California

Remember, too, that when you become a caregiver, you're blessed with an opportunity to spend some "quality time" with your parent. The same is true for your children, especially if they're still living at home. They can create some wonderful memories with their grandparent that they'll treasure for a lifetime.

Take Action... REMODEL WITH SAFETY IN MIND

Whether your parents stay in their own home or move into yours, you want to make sure their living space is as safe and accident-proof as possible. They may not feel your decorative nips and tucks are necessary, but in fact, such upgrades can be lifesavers. Mobility, dexterity, and mental function tend to decline with age, which means your parents may become more prone to mishaps over time.

Falling is the most common of these mishaps. One in three adults age 65 and older experiences a serious fall each year. In fact, in this age group, falling is the number one cause of injury-

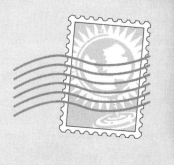

Caregiving around the World

One in four Canadian adults responding to a national survey said that they provide some form of care or support to an elderly family member or friend while trying to balance work and parenting responsibilities. According to the survey, this "sandwich generation" devotes an average of 60 hours a month to meeting the personal care needs of aging loved ones. In order to reduce rising absenteeism rates among caregivers, the Conference Board of Canada—which sponsored the survey—recommends that Canadian companies consider offering their employees flexible work hours, financial assistance, and information on caregiving.

POST CARD

FROM CANADA

related deaths, according to the National Center for Injury Prevention and Control. And 6 in 10 fatal falls happen at home, perhaps caused by a curled-up rug, a steep staircase, or a slippery bathroom floor. If your parent has an illness or disability that affects his or her balance, strength, sight, or judgment, it raises the risk of a fall or another household accident.

Experts on aging say you can make your parents' living space safer and give yourself greater peace of mind without spending a lot of money on costly renovations. At the top of the list: Post emergency phone numbers in a highly visible place, like next to the telephone or on the refrigerator door. Include your parents' home address and phone number; in the panic of an emergency, such details can temporarily be forgotten. Also include the names and phone numbers of family members and others who should be contacted in the event of an emergency.

Other safety measures can be just as inexpensive yet effective. The following examples have been customized to three common caregiving scenarios. If you have additional questions about your specific situation, you may want to consider consulting an occupational therapist. They're trained to assess homes and make recommendations for safety adaptations. Their services may be covered by Medicare and other insurance plans. Ask your loved one's primary care physician for a referral.

Scenario 1: Memory or Judgment Problems

If your parent has dementia or shows signs of declining memory or judgment, these precautions can be especially helpful.

- Install childproof doorknobs and cabinet locks wherever cleaning supplies, insecticides, fertilizers, paint thinners, and other poisonous chemicals are stored.

- Store medications in a locked cabinet and post a list of all the medicines your parent is taking inside the cabinet door.

- Put any small appliances in cupboards and remove the knobs from the stove when your parent is alone and unsupervised.

- Inspect the contents of the refrigerator weekly and remove any spoiled food to prevent food poisoning.

- Dismantle firearms and dangerous tools.

FOR MORE INFORMATION

To check out various devices designed to make living easier and safer for frail older people, visit the Family Caregiver Alliance Web site at **www.caregiver.org/fact sheets/consumerproducts. html.** There you'll find a fact sheet on consumer products and assistive equipment.

FOR MORE INFORMATION

Ageless Design is an independent Web site that provides information and advice on home modifications and resources, especially for people with Alzheimer's disease.

You can visit the Web site at **www.agelessdesign.com**.

✗ Install door alarms, safety locks, and gate locks if you are concerned that your parent might wander away from home.

Scenario 2: Mobility or Balance Problems

Perhaps your mom or dad has difficulty walking or maintaining balance, which increases the risk of a fall. Here's what to do.

✗ Install handrails on stairways and porch steps, or check to make sure existing handrails are securely fastened.

✗ Eliminate clutter on stairs and in hallways.

✗ Put night-lights in bedrooms, bathrooms, and hallways.

✗ Remove throw rugs that are not securely held down.

✗ Keep floors dry, especially in the kitchen and bathrooms. Clean up spills immediately.

✗ Lay a nonskid rubber mat in front of the kitchen sink.

✗ Install nonslip mats and grab bars in the bathrooms.

✗ Remove all loose wires and cords from pathways.

✗ Switch to cordless telephones with chargers to eliminate phone cords.

✗ Make sure your parent has a sturdy, comfortable chair with arms to lean on to steady himself or herself.

✗ Discourage wearing slippers or other loose-fitting shoes, especially if your parent isn't too steady on his or her feet. Sturdy, rubber-soled shoes are best.

✗ Limit your parent's alcohol consumption, especially if Mom or Dad is taking medication. Alcohol could impair the sense of balance.

Scenario 3: Smokers in the Family

Where there's a smoker, there's an increased chance of accidental fire. If your parent—or anyone in the household—smokes, these safety measures are crucial.

✗ Install smoke detectors, especially near all bedrooms. Check them the first of each month to make sure they're in working order.

✗ Replace the smoke detector batteries twice a year. Many

fire safety experts suggest changing the batteries when you reset the clocks in spring and fall.

✗ Install fire extinguishers in the kitchen, basement, and garage. You should have at least one on each floor of the home.

✗ Prohibit smoking in bed. Do a nightly inspection, if necessary.

✗ Ban smoking around oxygen tanks to prevent an explosion.

✗ Create an escape plan and make sure everyone in the household practices it at least twice a year. You could do your run-throughs when you replace the smoke detector batteries in spring and fall.

Caregiver's Checklist

Is Your Living Space Accident-Proof?

If your parent is moving into your home, you'll want to take some precautions to reduce the chances of a mishap. The following measures are recommended by the U.S. Consumer Product Safety Commission. As you complete each one, check the box at left.

Tasks before the Move

☐ Remove throw rugs that are not securely held down and replace them with slip-resistant rugs and runners.

☐ Clear clutter from hallways and stairways.

☐ Make sure stair rails are sturdy and securely fastened.

☐ Put night-lights in bedrooms, bathrooms, hallways, and stairways.

☐ Install grab bars by the bathtub, shower, and toilet to help your parent stand up safely.

☐ Place nonslip mats or textured strips on the shower and bathtub floors.

☐ Install smoke detectors on all levels of your home, especially near bedrooms. Make sure they're not close to air vents.

☐ Install fire extinguishers in the kitchen, garage, and basement and near fireplaces.

Tasks after the Move

☐ Set the temperature on your hot water heater below 120°F to avoid scalding. If you're not sure how to make this adjustment, consult a qualified professional.

☐ Check all electrical cords for signs of fraying. Make sure the cords are tucked away, out of the flow of foot traffic.

☐ Keep space heaters and kerosene lamps away from flammable materials such as curtains and rugs and out of passageways.

☐ Put fire-resistant oven mitts within easy reach of the stove.

☐ Replace appliances with those that feature automatic shut-offs.

CHAPTER 10

TAKING STOCK

What You Need to Know

- Asking your loved one about financial and legal matters can feel awkward. But by compiling and organizing these kinds of documents before a crisis occurs, you'll be prepared when you really need them.

- Create a filing system that's accessible and easy-to-use. You want to keep important papers where you can get to them quickly.

- Consider investing in a home safe or a safety deposit box for originals of legal documents like birth certificates, marriage licenses, deeds, and wills.

- Give photocopies of your loved one's advance directives and other papers for end-of-life planning to a trusted family member, friend, or attorney. That way, you'll have backups in case the originals can't be retrieved.

Managing paperwork is one of those tasks that most of us put off until we just can't avoid it anymore, like when we need to file our income tax returns. But for caregivers, organizing and maintaining a loved one's medical, financial, and legal records ranks among the most important of their responsibilities. Otherwise, when the need arises to find a doctor's bill, an insurance policy, or a copy of the will, the search could go on for hours, even weeks. Worse, the documents could be missing.

"Unfortunately, I see it all the time—families caught unprepared when a crisis strikes, like a parent suffering a stroke or going into a coma," says Mark Edinberg, Ph.D., a psychologist and gerontology expert from Fairfield, Connecticut, and author of *Talking with Your Aging Parents*. "Caregivers suffer much more emotionally than they need to. Being prepared medically, financially, and legally can bring families a sense of calm and togetherness."

Patricia McGinnis, executive director of the California Advocates for Nursing Home Reform in San Francisco, also encourages family members to talk about caregiving issues before a crisis occurs. Once the family settles on a course of action, they can make all the necessary arrangements—including preparing and organizing critical medical, financial, and legal documents—so they're ready when their loved one requires care or when they must make tough decisions.

"The biggest problem is that people wait until the last minute to discuss things like medical care, investments, and wills," McGinnis says. "These topics can be awkward. Parents don't want to talk about them, and adult children want to sweep them under the rug. But the time to take action is *before* the need arises."

McGinnis heeds her own advice. She and her six siblings live all across the United States. Working together, they researched and bought a home health care policy for their mother shortly before her 80th birthday, when the policy premiums would dramatically increase.

"My mother is in great health—she only takes blood pressure medication—but this policy will cover the cost of home health care for so much per day," McGinnis says. "It's good for both medical and nonmedical services."

She and her siblings have made sure their mom is taken care of legally by encouraging her to write her will. And two of the siblings have durable power of attorney—one for health care, the other for finances—on their mother's behalf.

Shortly after her 80th birthday, McGinnis's mother slipped at home. The fall caused a slight crack in her tailbone, which kept her confined to her bed for 6 weeks. McGinnis and her siblings traded phone calls and e-mails and rearranged their vacation time so they could share in their mother's at-home care.

"Mom is very independent, and sometimes she wonders why all of us are taking care of her," McGinnis says. "But we remind her that she spent her life taking care of us. For all of us, she is our hero."

EXPERT OPINION

"The problem in the United States today is that most people do not plan ahead for their long-term care. So when the time comes, their options are very narrow. Unfortunately, too many people end up on Medicaid in publicly financed long-term care programs . . . with only nursing home care as an option. What we would like to see is families . . . saving, investing, or insuring for the risk of long-term care, so that when the time comes and a family member goes into crisis, they have the full range of alternatives available: home care, assisted living, and access to the very best nursing homes."

—STEPHEN MOSES, president of the Center for Long-Term Care Financing in Seattle

| Caregiver's |
| Checklist |

Is Your Loved One's Personal Information in Order?

Make a photocopy of this form and fill in the blanks with the requested information. Then file the paper with the rest of your loved one's important documents, so you can find it when you need it. You might want to make a copy to keep in your purse or briefcase as well.

PERSONAL INFORMATION

Full name _____

Maiden name or other names _____

Home address _____

_____

Phone _____

Date and place of birth _____

Social Security number _____

Driver's license number _____

Military ID number _____

Medications _____

_____

Religious affiliation _____

Church or synagogue _____ Phone _____

Clergy_____ Phone_____

HEALTH CARE CONTACTS

Primary care physician _____ Phone_____

Pharmacist _____ Phone_____

Other health care providers

    Name _____ Phone_____

    Name _____ Phone_____

    Name _____ Phone_____

Hospital _____ Phone_____

LEGAL AND FINANCIAL CONTACTS

Attorney _____ Phone _____

Accountant/tax preparer _____ Phone _____

Financial advisor _____ Phone _____

Insurance agent _____ Phone _____

Banks

   Name _____ Phone _____

   Name _____ Phone _____

EMERGENCY CONTACTS

Police department _____ Phone _____

Fire department _____ Phone _____

Ambulance service _____ Phone _____

Poison control center _____ Phone _____

Family members

   Name _____ Phone _____

   Name _____ Phone _____

   Name _____ Phone _____

   Name _____ Phone _____

Neighbors

   Name _____ Phone _____

   Name _____ Phone _____

   Name _____ Phone _____

Friends

   Name _____ Phone _____

   Name _____ Phone _____

   Name _____ Phone _____

   Name _____ Phone _____

EXPERT OPINION

"Prevention is just as important in the legal arena as in health care. Honor yourself as you would honor your loved one by protecting yourself with the proper documents—trust, will, power of attorney, and other legal instruments."

—**PETER J. STRAUSS, ESQ.**, elder law and trust and estates attorney, author, and adjunct professor of law at New York Law School in New York City

Take Action… PUT PAPERS IN THEIR PLACE

Even before you start thinking about which documents your loved one should have, you need to decide where you're going to store them. Too often, the family "filing system" consists of important papers stashed haphazardly in a shoe box or shoved in a kitchen drawer. Yes, establishing a complete, organized record-keeping plan requires some effort. But once it's in place, all that important information is always at your fingertips.

So where do you begin?

✗ First, caregiving experts say, talk with other family members and decide who will be the chief record-keeper. Often the primary caregiver takes on the task—which makes sense logistically, since that person has the most convenient access to a loved one's paperwork. But perhaps someone in your family has financial, legal, or even administrative expertise that makes him well-suited to the record-keeping role.

✗ After you've chosen your record-keeper, start sorting through your loved one's papers—with your loved one helping out, if that person is able. Create two piles: one to keep, one to toss. To protect your loved one's privacy, be sure to shred or tear up any documents before throwing them in the trash.

✗ Next, designate a desk drawer or file drawer to store business and financial records. Use separate file folders for the various kinds of documents your loved one may have, such as mortgage papers, loan contracts, automobile titles, appliance warranties, insurance policies, and stock certificates.

✗ Invest in a fireproof, burglarproof home safe for legal papers such as birth and death certificates, marriage licenses, deeds, original signed copies of wills and trusts, and funeral and burial instructions. Another option is to rent a safety deposit box at a banking institution. Many older banks still have them.

Once you've sifted through all the paperwork, filing the important documents and discarding the rest, you'll want to take inventory to determine whether your loved one has all of the

Caregiver's Checklist

Do You Have All the Papers You Need?

As you sort through your loved one's paperwork, you can use this inventory to track what's accounted for and what's missing. Mark the "yes" boxes for those documents you're able to find and the "N/A" boxes for those that don't apply to your loved one's situation. By default, the documents marked "no" are the ones you should have but don't. Try to get copies of these, so your files are complete.

☐ yes ☐ no ☐ N/A   Birth certificate

☐ yes ☐ no ☐ N/A   Marriage license

☐ yes ☐ no ☐ N/A   Military discharge certificate

☐ yes ☐ no ☐ N/A   Spouse's death certificate

☐ yes ☐ no ☐ N/A   Divorce record

☐ yes ☐ no ☐ N/A   Medicare benefits information

☐ yes ☐ no ☐ N/A   Medicaid benefits information

☐ yes ☐ no ☐ N/A   Medigap/supplemental insurance policy

☐ yes ☐ no ☐ N/A   Long-term care insurance policy

☐ yes ☐ no ☐ N/A   Last will and testament

☐ yes ☐ no ☐ N/A   Advance medical directive

☐ yes ☐ no ☐ N/A   Prepaid funeral plan

☐ yes ☐ no ☐ N/A   Burial agreement

☐ yes ☐ no ☐ N/A   Auto insurance

☐ yes ☐ no ☐ N/A   Homeowner's insurance

☐ yes ☐ no ☐ N/A   Liability insurance

☐ yes ☐ no ☐ N/A   Disability insurance

☐ yes ☐ no ☐ N/A   Life insurance

☐ yes ☐ no ☐ N/A   Checkbook

☐ yes ☐ no ☐ N/A   Savings account register

☐ yes ☐ no ☐ N/A   Stock and bond certificates

☐ yes ☐ no ☐ N/A   Annuity contracts

☐ yes ☐ no ☐ N/A   Pension plan information

☐ yes ☐ no ☐ N/A   401(k)/IRA documents

☐ yes ☐ no ☐ N/A   Social Security benefits information

☐ yes ☐ no ☐ N/A   Veteran's benefits information

☐ yes ☐ no ☐ N/A   Mortgage papers

☐ yes ☐ no ☐ N/A   Property deed

☐ yes ☐ no ☐ N/A   Home equity loan papers

☐ yes ☐ no ☐ N/A   Vehicle title

☐ yes ☐ no ☐ N/A   Vehicle loan/lease papers

☐ yes ☐ no ☐ N/A   Income tax returns

☐ yes ☐ no ☐ N/A   Contracts

necessary medical, financial, and legal papers. Of course, what's necessary varies from one caregiving situation to the next. We'll discuss the basic must-haves here.

COORDINATING HEALTH INSURANCE INFORMATION

Depending on eligibility, your loved one most likely has some combination of public and private insurance. Determining whether the benefits are sufficient, and which policy pays for what, may require some investigation on your part. But it's well worth the effort, especially if you can close up any gaps in coverage that may be exposing your loved one to significant expense and financial loss.

We'll get into the particulars of various kinds of health insurance and benefits in chapter 24. For your record-keeping purposes, let's briefly review the major health insurance programs.

Medicare. Run by the federal government, Medicare is automatically available to people age 65 and older who qualify for Social Security benefits. In general, Medicare provides reimbursement for some inpatient hospital care and skilled nursing facility stays. For a monthly premium, additional coverage picks up some of the cost of doctor fees and outpatient medical care. Medicare does not reimburse for most types of in-home nonmedical or custodial care, such as personal assistance, meal delivery programs, and housekeeping services.

Medigap. Even though this supplemental coverage is underwritten by private insurers, the policies themselves are fairly standard, with only minor variations. The primary purpose of Medigap is to take care of Medicare's co-payments and deductibles. In some cases, it pays for occasional use of home health aides, occupational therapists, medical social services, and medical supplies and equipment. Generally, though, it doesn't provide any greater reimbursement for home health care or skilled nursing facility stays than Medicare does. More expensive policies will cover the costs of prescription drugs.

Medicaid. This federally funded program, administered through each state's welfare department, provides health insurance for people who are considered low-income. Medicaid covers a portion, if not all, of an eligible individual's nursing home care.

Keep in mind that the regulations governing public health insurance programs can change, as can the provisions of private insurance policies. That's why staying on top of your loved one's insurance paperwork is so important. These tips can help.

- Buy a large accordion-style folder in which you can keep all documents relevant to your loved one's health insurance claims and benefits. Use individual folders to organize bills and benefits statements by the date of service, whether for a doctor's office visit or a hospital stay.

- If you don't already have them, obtain copies of your loved one's Medigap policy and/or private health insurance policies. Keep these in your health insurance folder, so they're handy in case you have questions about your loved one's coverage.

- Take advantage of free booklets and brochures that explain your loved one's Medicare benefits. The federal government's official Medicare Web site, www.medicare.gov, has a number of publications that can be downloaded at no charge. If you don't have Internet access, you can request a copy of Medicare's publications catalog—also at no charge—by calling (800) 633-4227 (800-MEDICARE). File any reference materials you obtain with the rest of your loved one's health insurance information.

- Create an insurance information sheet with your loved one's Medicare or Medicaid claim number, his Medigap policy number, and/or the policy numbers for any other health insurance coverage he may have. Also include the telephone numbers you'd need to call with questions about claims or benefits. That way, you won't need to repeatedly rout through your loved one's papers for this information. Put the sheet in your loved one's health insurance folder for safekeeping.

ORGANIZING FINANCIAL RECORDS

For caregivers, delving into a loved one's finances can be a particularly uncomfortable task. People tend to view handling their own financial matters as a symbol of their independence. They may not want to disclose the particulars of their saving and spending habits, even to other family members.

FOR MORE INFORMATION

For more information about Medicaid, including benefits and eligibility requirements, visit the Centers for Medicare and Medicaid Services Web site at **www.cms.hhs.gov**. The Centers for Medicare and Medicaid Services was previously known as the Health Care Financing Administration.

FOR MORE INFORMATION

AARP offers informative, up-to-date booklets on Medicare, Medicaid, Medigap, long-term insurance, and other health insurance options. You can order the booklets you need by calling AARP at its toll-free number, **(800) 424-3410**, or visiting its Web site at **www.aarp.org/hcchoices**.

Outlook

"My generation is the first in which couples have more parents than children. That's a very dramatic change. We've done a good job of helping families care for their children—providing day care and early childhood education, for example. Now we need to shift our attention to the needs of older family members. Society can help by providing tools to enhance the family's ability to care for its elders and by celebrating the importance of families looking after one another.

"What I hope is happening is an awakening in America, if not in the world, that we've entered a new era with respect to aging and caretaking. Families need tools, resources, and support. There is no magic bullet. We need to develop a whole tool kit—a complete line of assistance for caregivers."

—**ALAN SOLOMONT,** founder of HouseWorks, a Newton, Massachusetts–based organization that helps seniors stay independent

What's more, among many older couples, taking care of the finances is considered the "man's job." If anything happens to the husband, the wife may not be able to manage financially.

For their 63 years of marriage, Martha Perkins, of Lantana, Florida, always relied on her husband, Carl, to deal with the family's financial matters. So when he died suddenly in a car accident, Martha, then 84, found herself trying to balance a checkbook and keep pace with the monthly utility bills for the first time. Frustrated and confused, she knew she needed help. She telephoned her son, John, who lives just a few miles away. Together, they spent days organizing all the financial records.

"Until my husband died, I didn't realize how little I knew of our family finances and how much I needed to learn," says Martha, a retired nurse. "Thank goodness my son is organized."

You'll be organized, too, if you start locating and filing your loved one's key financial documents now. As suggested earlier in the chapter, your best bet is to create a separate folder for each type of document, then store the folders together in a designated desk drawer or file drawer. Here's what you should look for:

- Tax returns for prior years
- Tax information for the current year
- Savings and/or checking account register
- Social Security information
- Pension accounts
- IRA, Keogh, and other deferred compensation accounts
- Real estate documents
- Credit card accounts
- Life, property, and automobile insurance policies
- Prepaid funeral plans and burial plot agreements

Of course, getting your loved one's financial affairs in order means not just accounting for what he has now but also anticipating what he'll need in the future. We'll talk more about financial planning in chapter 23. For now, you might want to start thinking about the following issues.

- What are the chances your loved one will need long-term care? Does anything in your loved one's family medical history or personal lifestyle indicate that he's likely to require special care?

- What financial assets does your loved one have that he'll want to protect in the event that he needs long-term care?

- What, if any, additional investments or savings does your loved one want to make?

- What, if anything, does your loved one wish to set aside for family members or charities after his death?

- What portion of income and assets do you want safeguarded under survivor benefit laws if your loved one requires government assistance for long-term care expenses?

To help make all of these decisions, you might want to consider hiring a financial advisor. These professionals can evaluate your loved one's financial situation, assist in setting goals, and make recommendations for achieving those goals. From there, they'll develop and implement a comprehensive financial plan. For tips on finding a qualified financial advisor, see chapter 22.

OBTAINING LEGAL DOCUMENTS

In caregiving, legal preparedness is just as important as financial preparedness. And discussing it can feel just as awkward, especially for the caregiver.

"It's relatively easier now than perhaps 10 years ago, when the public wasn't all that aware of end-of-life issues," Dr. Edinberg says. "Still, some adult children are reluctant to talk about legal matters because they fear that somehow they'll be perceived as interfering with their parents' lives, or even wanting their parents dead. I reassure them that they are part of their parents' lives and that they have a responsibility to make legal preparations not only for their parents but for themselves, too."

Which legal documents your loved one requires depends on his needs and wishes. Experts suggest consulting an attorney—ideally, one who specializes in elder law—to review all the op-

FOR MORE INFORMATION

The Financial Planning Association can provide names of qualified financial advisors in your area. For a referral, call **(800) 282-7526.**

FOR MORE INFORMATION

The American Bar Association (ABA) Lawyer Referral and Information Service can help you find a lawyer in your area who's knowledgeable in elder care issues. You can write to the ABA at 750 North Lake Shore Drive, Chicago, IL 60611.

Another helpful resource is the National Academy of Elder Law Attorneys. For a referral, call (520) 881-4005, or visit the organization's Web site at **www.naela.com**.

tions before choosing those that will best protect your loved one's interests. From a record-keeping perspective, the documents you should be thinking about now are power of attorneys and advance directives. (For more information on the legal issues associated with caregiving, see chapter 25.)

With a power of attorney, your loved one appoints another person—usually a relative or a close friend—to take certain actions on his behalf. While the designated party (known as the agent or attorney-in-fact) has legal power, your loved one retains his right to make decisions for himself.

For example, let's suppose your loved one is going to be hospitalized for a period of time. The person with power-of-attorney could deposit checks and pay bills, submit insurance claims, and even sell property, depending on the provisions of the power-of-attorney agreement. Keep in mind that the agreement can be terminated at any time, and that it's automatically revoked if your loved one dies. Remember, too, that a power of attorney does not take the place of a will or trust.

Documents known as advance directives can guide family members and health care professionals in making decisions when a loved one is no longer able to make them for herself. The four main types of advance directives are the durable power of attorney for health care, the durable power of attorney for finances, the living will, and the "do not resuscitate" order.

Durable power of attorney for health care. This particular power-of-attorney agreement allows the named individual to make medical decisions on a loved one's behalf should that person become incapacitated. The document may include special instructions and preferences pertaining to a loved one's care. It remains in effect until that person passes away.

Durable power of attorney for finances. The key distinction between this agreement and the durable power of attorney for health care is that this one assigns decision-making powers for money matters. It helps ensure that your loved one's finances are handled according to his wishes in the event that he becomes incapacitated. Instructions in a durable power of attorney for finances may pertain to paying bills, making bank deposits, selling property, and managing insurance and other paperwork.

Living wills. Basically, a living will serves as a legal guide—

though not a binding agreement—for doctors in the event a person becomes so sick he can no longer communicate. It outlines the person's wishes as far as whether certain life-sustaining measures should be used. A living will is not the same as a last will and testament; it has nothing to do with the distribution of personal belongings after death.

"Do not resuscitate" order. This document instructs medical professionals not to administer lifesaving procedures should a person's heartbeat or breathing stop. These days, many hospitals ask patients at the time of admission whether they want to be resuscitated from cardiac or pulmonary failure. In addition, a person with a terminal illness may choose to post a special "do not resuscitate" order in his home, directing paramedics and other emergency personnel not to use life-sustaining measures in the event of a medical emergency. A copy of this form is available from your local ambulance service.

In accordance with the provisions of the federal Patient Self-Determination Act, most hospitals and nursing homes must provide information on advance directives at the time of a patient's admission. Be aware that the laws governing the content of these documents vary from state to state. You may be able to obtain the official preprinted forms for your loved one's state through the county or state medical association or bar association, or the Area Agency on Aging. If your loved one splits his time between residences in different states—for example, spending 6 months with you and the rest of the year with your sibling—he'll need identical advance directives using each state's official form.

Be sure to file your loved one's advance directive in a safe but accessible location, where you can get to it when you need it. (AARP reports that 35 percent of advance directives can't be found when the time comes.) You might also want to give backup copies to your loved one's attorney and primary care physician, or to a trusted friend.

A CONSUMER ALERT FOR CAREGIVERS

As the primary keeper of your loved one's medical, financial, and legal records, you're in an excellent position to help protect him from unscrupulous con artists who prey on older people.

FOR MORE
INFORMATION

You can request free state-specific sample forms for the durable power of attorney for health care and the living will from Partnership for Caring, a nonprofit organization dedicated to end-of-life care. Call **(800) 989-9455,** or visit the organization's Web site at **www. partnershipforcaring.org.**

Many seniors have lost their life savings in scams pitched through the mail, over the phone, and even in person.

Be on the lookout for any kind of solicitation that promises something for nothing, produces unbelievable results, guarantees large sums of money, accepts only cash, or claims to be a risk-free or last-chance offer. This sort of language can clue you in to potentially fraudulent activity.

In addition, Rich O'Boyle, publisher of the Web site ElderCare Online, urges caregivers to follow these guidelines before signing any contracts on a loved one's behalf.

- Read and understand a contract before signing it.

- Never sign a contract with blank spaces.

- Keep a copy of the contract, and make sure the other party in the agreement has signed it, too.

- Get any work estimates in writing.

- Check whether you're entitled to a refund if you're dissatisfied with the goods or services provided.

- Ask for references and call them.

- If you still have doubts, call the Better Business Bureau and find out whether anyone has filed a complaint against the company.

If you suspect fraud regarding insurance policies, legal documents, home improvements, or other too-good-to-be-true offers, report it to your local police department as well as your local consumer protection office. (For a phone number, look under "Consumer Services" in the blue pages of your telephone directory.) You can also contact the National Fraud Information Center toll-free at (800) 876-7060. If you or your loved one receives any suspicious mail solicitations—for questionable contests, work-at-home schemes, dubious charitable organizations, and the like—notify the U.S. Postal Service.

CHAPTER 11

RELATIONSHIPS REDEFINED

What You Need to Know

- Both you and your loved one will need to make psychological and logistical adjustments as you assume a caregiving role.

- In general, psychological adjustments are greatly influenced by individual personality traits. The better your and your loved one's personalities mesh, the easier the adjustments may be.

- Logistically, perhaps the greatest challenge in caregiving is getting used to another person's lifestyle and habits. One way to make the transition easier is to work on preserving as much of each person's daily routine as possible.

- Plan for as many of the adjustments caregiving will bring as you can. This creates a foundation for managing your situation, even if it changes suddenly.

As a caregiving situation unfolds, everyone involved tends to focus on logistical issues—what needs to be done when, and by whom. Perhaps these matters come to mind first because they seem to affect the status quo most. Each new task has the potential to shake up lifestyles and daily routines—especially for the caregiver and the care recipient, but also for their immediate family (including spouses, siblings, and children) and anyone else on the caregiving team.

The best way to minimize the sometimes detrimental impact of caregiving on day-to-day life is to approach it in an organized manner right from the start. That might be obvious advice, but it's easily overlooked, particularly by caregivers who are overwhelmed at the prospect of taking on new responsibilities when they already feel stretched thin.

Outlook

"Chances are you were stressed even before your loved one needed care," observes Gail Hunt, executive director of the Bethesda, Maryland–based National Alliance for Caregiving. "Now you may wonder whether you'll have time for anything other than caregiving. You will, but you need to make every minute count. That means getting organized."

Lois Escobar, M.S.W., agrees. Through her job with the Family Caregiver Alliance, a caregiving support organization based in San Francisco, Escobar works closely with families in distress because of caregiving's demands. "They call us because they feel overwhelmed. They're at their wits' end," she says. "Many factors can contribute to such feelings, but a big one is disorganization. To stay sane as a caregiver, you have to get organized—perhaps more organized than you've ever been."

Establishing a caregiving relationship isn't just a logistical matter, however. It's a psychological one, too. Caregiving requires you to interact with your loved one as you haven't before. Your respective roles are shifting, as are the issues you need to discuss. That takes some getting used to, especially if you're caring for a parent.

"Studies have shown that adult children tend to be less distressed by caregiving's logistical challenges than by its emotional demands," notes Claire Berman, author of *Caring for Yourself While Caring for Your Aging Parents*. The ability to manage emotions can have just as great an impact as the ability to manage tasks in terms of providing care.

The information in this chapter can help ease you into your caregiving role by identifying the sorts of psychological and logistical adjustments you may need to make, and giving you advice on how to plan for them. You can't anticipate everything, of course; that's not the nature of caregiving. But when surprises do arise, you'll be ready to deal with them without undue stress. That's one of the perks of getting organized: You feel better able to manage your situation, even through all the inevitable changes.

Take Action... ANTICIPATE EMOTIONAL CHALLENGES

The ability to adjust psychologically to a caregiving relationship depends on a host of factors, including family history, personal belief systems and behavior patterns, and expectations and desires. But all of these things are filtered through an individual's personality. Both you and your loved one have attributes that affect how you perceive those around you and how you express yourself. These attributes can influence your relationship for better or for worse.

Even when two people get along exceptionally well, caregiving can introduce issues into the relationship that evoke complex and often unexpected emotional responses. To help manage these emotions through the transition both you and your loved one are making, experts offer these tips.

✗ Be careful not to "parent your parent." This phrase comes up often these days, as a growing number of adult children find themselves looking after Mom and Dad. If you're in this situation, you need to remember that your parents are still adults. Their sense of dignity and self-worth very much depends on their being treated as adults. "People want to be as independent as possible, even if they're being cared for," Hunt observes. "It's important to recognize what care recipients can't do, to respect what they can do, and to encourage them to keep doing what they can. Don't over-intervene. It hurts your loved one's self-esteem—and it may make that person resent you."

✗ Turn feelings of guilt to your advantage. "For caregivers, guilt is inevitable," explains Percil Stanford, Ph.D., professor of gerontology and director of the Center on Aging at San Diego State University. "It can be paralyzing, or it can serve as motivation to examine an issue more closely and make a change for the better." For example, suppose your father enjoys getting together with his buddies for a weekly poker game, but because of your schedule at work, you can't take him. He says he understands, but you know he misses going, and you feel bad about it. Instead of letting guilt get the best of you, look for a solution to the situation. Perhaps one of his buddies can pick him up. Or he can host the game at your house, so he doesn't need to travel. Either way, he'd get to play poker and see his friends—and you'd both feel better.

✗ Encourage your loved one to express herself openly. Perhaps you've heard the joke making its way around caregiving circles:

> Q. How many aging parents do you need to change a lightbulb?
> A. You don't have to change it. They'll sit in the dark.

It may be a weak attempt at humor, but it raises a serious issue: Most care recipients—especially the elderly—don't want to feel they're a burden, so they're reluctant to ask for help. And that can be dangerous, especially if they're experiencing a medical problem of some kind. Talk with your loved one often. By conveying your concern about her well-being, she may feel more comfortable speaking up when she requires assistance.

✗ Find ways to maintain your loved one's social ties. If your mom moves in with you, she may be forced to leave behind friends and neighbors whom she has known for years, and a community where she has firmly planted roots. This loss of a social network can come as a major psychological blow. Do what you can to help her stay in touch with the people in her life. Suggest that she write letters, make phone calls, and send e-mails. Invite those to whom she's especially close for a visit, or take her to see them. She'll enjoy the company, and you may get some welcome respite from your caregiving duties. Also, check whether her hometown newspaper has a Web site. Most papers do.

✗ Try to accommodate your loved one's spiritual practice. People who consider themselves religious often experience a deepening of their faith in later life. Even those who haven't been particularly devout sometimes feel spiritual stirrings. If your loved one isn't able to attend church, perhaps a member of the clergy can visit her on a regular basis. Many churches and synagogues offer outreach services for shut-ins.

✗ Establish priorities and stick with them. You can't take on all the caregiving responsibilities while juggling a marriage, a family, friendships, and a career. No one can do all that—

and no one needs to. You must decide what you can handle and what you can let go, or at least delegate to someone else. Once you've identified your priorities, discuss them with your loved one and with other family members. Allow yourself to be flexible, but stand firm when the situation warrants. Let's say your sibling informs you that she's no longer able to do your father's housecleaning. You may consider taking on the responsibility yourself, but then you realize you'd be away from your family for several hours a week. Already you feel you're not seeing them nearly enough. So work on making other arrangements, such as hiring a housekeeping service.

✗ Be sure to block out time for your spouse and children. This lets them know they're still top priorities in your life, even though you're busier because of your caregiving responsibilities. If you ask them to pitch in with your work, be careful not to treat that as your "quality time" together. They want and deserve your undivided attention. So schedule plans in advance: Order tickets to a baseball game, concert, or movie; make reservations for dinner; or book a room at a bed-and-breakfast for a weekend getaway. If you need to, arrange for someone else to look after your loved one. Then you can truly focus on your family.

✗ Remember that life isn't perfect. Especially in caregiving, striving for perfection can be a one-way ticket to depression and burnout. Still, it's a habit that's tough to break. If you consider yourself a perfectionist, you may need to make an extra effort to stick with your priorities. And rather than striving for perfection, focus on doing your best as a caregiver. That's certainly a worthy goal.

✗ Find support among your fellow caregivers. No matter how wonderful your family and friends are, you may have times when you need to commiserate with people who truly understand what you're going through emotionally. One way to do that is to join a support group. "These groups really can help people cope with all aspects of caregiving," Hunt says. "I'd urge every primary caregiver to explore the option." If you can't find a group that suits your needs or your schedule,

Point of View

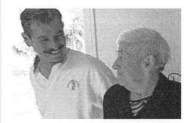

"I've learned a lot from my wife, Alicia, caring for my mother-in-law. I've learned to be more tolerant because of all the stress she's under. I've learned to be more helpful. I began by doing the dishes. Since then, I've learned to cook. When Alicia takes her mother to a late doctor's appointment, I make dinner.

"We've had our tough times, of course. Tempers get a little short. I try to be understanding. I've never spoken with other husbands in my situation. If there were a support group for husbands, maybe I'd go. It would probably be helpful."

—**TONY FRANCO,**
Santa Barbara, California

To find a support group in your area, you can start by looking in the blue pages of your phone directory, under "Self-Help Support Groups." Also check with the Area Agency on Aging that serves your community. The staff there can help you find a group that meets your needs.

If you'd like to launch your own support group, an organization called the Self-Help Clearinghouse has lots of useful resources available. Call **(212) 817-1822** or visit the organization's Web site at **www.selfhelpweb.org**.

you might want to start your own with other caregivers you know. You might even be able to share your caregiving tasks. For example, if several of you have loved ones in adult day care, perhaps you can arrange for carpooling. Or you can take turns looking after your loved ones for an afternoon each week.

Take Action... PLOT OUT THE LOGISTICS

Adapting a "divide and conquer" approach to caregiving—divvying up tasks with other caregivers, or assigning them out to family members—can help ease the psychological as well as the logistical transitions in your relationship with your loved one. Even so, adjusting logistically involves more than just making room for new caregiving responsibilities. It means getting accustomed to another person's lifestyle and habits, especially if that person is moving into your home. It means making sure the living arrangements work for everyone involved.

To avoid some of the logistical hurdles common in caregiving situations, you might want to try these preemptive measures.

✗ Discuss your loved one's daily routine. Older people, in particular, get accustomed to doing things a certain way, explains Ellen Rubenson, M.S.W., a social worker at Providence Medford Medical Center in Medford, Oregon, and author of *When Aging Parents Can't Live Alone*. By learning about your loved one's habits and preferences, and taking steps to preserve them to the extent possible, you may help that person feel more comfortable with any logistical changes she must make. (To familiarize yourself with your loved one's lifestyle, complete the Caregiver's Checklist to the right.)

✗ Assess the kind and level of physical assistance your loved one requires. For this task, you may want to consult with your loved one's caregiving team—her primary care physician, geriatrician, and/or geriatric care manager, plus any other health professional with first-hand knowledge of your loved one's situation. (For a refresher on creating a caregiving team, see chapter 8.) And take time to complete the Caregiver's Checklist on page 30.

Caregiver's Checklist

Is Your Loved One's Lifestyle in Sync with Yours?

The information you collect for this checklist is especially important if your loved one is moving into your home, but it can be helpful for any caregiving situation. Use it to identify those aspects of your loved one's routine that are similar to yours, and those that may require some logistical adjustments for one or both of you.

1. In the spaces provided, note what time your loved one usually does the following:

Awakens _____

Bathes_____

Takes medication _____

Eats breakfast _____

Eats lunch_____

Eats supper _____

Exercises _____

Goes to bed _____

2. In the spaces provided, note which foods your loved one prefers for the following:

Breakfast _____

_____

Lunch _____

_____

Supper _____

_____

Snacks _____

_____

Desserts/treats _____

_____

3. Mark "yes" or "no" to indicate whether your loved one enjoys the following:

Spending time with friends   ☐ yes ☐ no

Reading newspapers   ☐ yes ☐ no

Reading magazines   ☐ yes ☐ no

Watching television   ☐ yes ☐ no

Listening to the radio   ☐ yes ☐ no

Listening to music   ☐ yes ☐ no

Taking walks   ☐ yes ☐ no

Going to museums   ☐ yes ☐ no

Gardening   ☐ yes ☐ no

Other activities   ☐ yes ☐ no

What are they? _____

_____

4. Mark "yes" or "no" to indicate whether your loved one has any of the following:

Food restrictions   ☐ yes ☐ no

If yes, what are they?_____

Allergies   ☐ yes ☐ no

If yes, what are they?_____

Strong likes or dislikes   ☐ yes ☐ no

If yes, what are they?_____

✗ Ensure the safety of your loved one's living environment. Whether your loved one lives alone or moves into your home, you can help protect against falls and other mishaps with a few simple do-it-yourself modifications. Among the changes experts recommend: installing handrails in the bathtub and/or shower, removing throw rugs, replacing oven knobs with disabling switches, and using special door and window locks if your loved one is prone to wander. (For more suggestions, see chapter 9.)

✗ Respect and protect your loved one's privacy. If the person moves into your home, the ideal scenario is for her to have her own bedroom and bathroom. But that may not be possible. In that case, work with your loved one and your family to come up with a living arrangement that everyone feels good about.

✗ Review your loved one's personal expenses. This can become a real issue in a caregiving situation, especially if you bring your loved one into your home. You want to decide

Getting Help When the Family Is Far Apart

If your family is like the majority in caregiving situations, some of your relatives may not live close enough to provide hands-on support. But they can help in other ways, especially in terms of the psychological and logistical adjustments you and your loved one need to make. Some suggestions:

Psychological Adjustments

- Encourage family members to call at pre-arranged times. That way, both you and your loved one can be available for important discussions.

- Ask family members if they'll come visit your loved one so you can get some much-needed respite.

- Recruit family members to help work through specific issues and conflicts. For example, if you

haven't been able to persuade your loved one to divulge an important piece of medical or financial information, perhaps someone else can coax her to do it.

Logistical Adjustments

- Tap into your family members' expertise. For example, if one of your siblings is an accountant, you might want to ask him to manage your parent's financial matters. Or approach the nurse in your family about helping to assess the sorts of physical assistance your parent may require.

- Farm out tasks that can easily be handled from a distance, like preparing income taxes or collecting information on community caregiving services.

Who Picks Up the Tab?

Depending on your loved one's living arrangements and financial situation, you and other family members may need to chip in to cover a portion of the person's expenses. To track who's responsible for what, place an X in the appropriate column(s) for each item listed below. For those items that will be paid by other family members, you may want to write in peoples' names. Then photocopy this form and distribute it to your family for reference.

Expense	Paid by care recipient	Paid by caregiver	Paid by family	Not applicable
Rent/mortgage				
Utilities				
Water				
Garbage				
Phone				
Insurance				
Credit cards				
Medical care				
Medication				
Home health supplies				
Food				
Clothing				
Home maintenance				
Transportation				
Travel				
Gifts				
Incidentals				

up-front who's going to pay for what—and whether other family members should help cover the costs. You can use the Caregiver's Checklist on page 123 to work out a payment plan. (We'll discuss the particulars of managing your loved one's finances in chapter 23.)

Don't hesitate to ask for help. As mentioned earlier, assigning caregiving tasks to willing family members and friends—or sharing the work with other caregivers—can make managing the logistics of the caregiving situation much easier. And don't forget to take advantage of the support services offered by community agencies, from meal delivery and telephone check-in to adult day care and housekeeping assistance. (For more particulars on these services, see chapters 19 and 20.)

A FUTURE IN FLUX

Keep in mind that the logistical and psychological adjustments associated with caregiving are not a once-and-done deal. Whenever your loved one's situation changes, the two of you—and everyone else in the immediate caregiving circle—must regroup accordingly. The most challenging adjustments tend to occur as you assume the caregiving role (and your loved one becomes a care recipient). The rest may feel easier, because you know what to expect and you've gained experience in making decisions and finding resources.

"Try not to become obsessed with future changes—but try not to deny them, either," advises Suzanne Mintz, cofounder and president of the National Family Caregivers Association, based in Kensington, Maryland. "The more organized you are today, psychologically and logistically, the better prepared you'll be for tomorrow—whatever it may bring."

PART FOUR

Giving Care

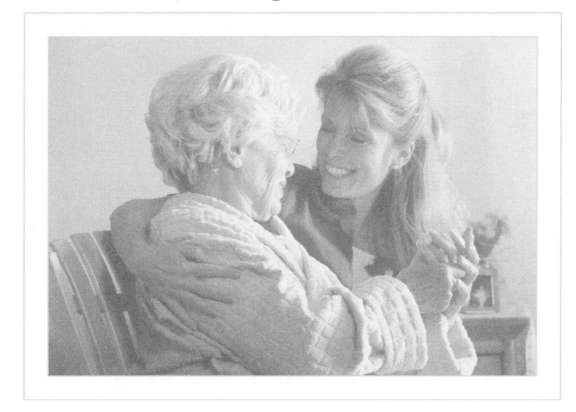

CHAPTER 12

EASING THE TRANSITION

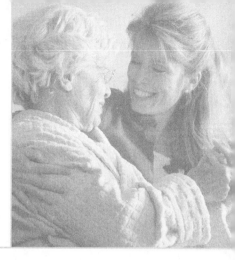

What You Need to Know

- When a person becomes a care recipient, he relinquishes some of his independence. Over time, this can undermine his self-esteem.

- As a caregiver, you can help your loved one cultivate a sense of independence by focusing on what he can do rather than what he can't.

- Once a person can no longer manage a particular task or activity, give him a chance to grieve that loss. With time, he'll be ready to move on.

- Two of the most challenging transitions faced by a care recipient involve relinquishing financial responsibilities and driving privileges.

- As your loved one adapts to the role of care recipient, stay alert for signs of depression. Though quite common in older people, it often goes undiagnosed.

At the outset of a caregiving relationship, you spend a lot of time planning and preparing, with what can seem like a million different details demanding your attention. Somewhere in this process, you need to sit down with your loved one and have a heart-to-heart conversation about the changes that will be affecting his life as well as yours. And you need to ask him one very important question: "How do you feel about all of this?"

You may not get a direct answer right away; the person may not be sure how he feels, or may not be comfortable sharing his thoughts—at least not immediately. Be persistent but gentle in your efforts to draw out a response. Try phrasing your question differently, depending on the situation: "How do you like the housekeeping service that was hired for you?" or "How can I help you feel more at home?"

What you're really trying to find out, of course, is how the person is coping with the transition to care recipient. The fact is, every caregiving task taken on by you or someone else means a little less independence for your loved one. If he perceives the changes taking place as irretrievable losses, his self-confidence and self-esteem can suffer. He may become angry or defiant, or show signs of depression. And that can undermine his physical well-being.

This sort of fallout can be minimized, or possibly transformed, just by talking with the person early on and often. Unfortunately, most caregivers get so caught up in their day-to-day responsibilities that they forget the care recipient is feeling stressed out, too. "The person is likely to be upset about needing care and perhaps not being able to live on his own, but he may not articulate it,"

Caregiving around the World

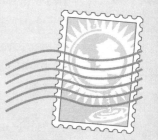

Japanese families have a long tradition of living in three-generation homes, reducing the need for institutional care. But that's changing now, as the elderly are living longer and women are working outside the home in growing numbers. In 2000, Japan unveiled a public, mandatory long-term care insurance program. Known as care insurance, the program shifts much of the caregiving responsibility from families to the nation. It provides for home helpers, adult day care centers, and short-term care facilities—all of which are paid for by the government.

POST CARD

FROM JAPAN

explains Gail Hunt, executive director of the National Alliance for Caregiving, based in Bethesda, Maryland. "Even if your loved one opens up, you may have to listen very carefully to fully understand the emotions he's experiencing."

Yet once you have this information, you can provide the support and encouragement your loved one needs to feel better about himself and his situation. Find ways to reassure him that becoming a care recipient in no way diminishes his worth as a human being. Foster his independence by helping him focus on what he can do, rather than on what he can't. And always keep the lines of communication open, so your loved one knows that his thoughts and feelings matter.

All of this can go a long way toward helping your loved one accept and adapt to his role as care recipient. So can the strategies that follow, which seek to overcome the specific emotional hurdles that are common among people who require care. (As a caregiver, you're likely wrestling with some negative emotions yourself; we'll address those a bit later, in chapter 26.)

Take Action... NURTURE YOUR LOVED ONE'S SELF-ESTEEM

When a person realizes he can no longer perform certain tasks on his own, he may begin to lose his sense of purpose, his reason for being. And that can take a serious toll on his emotional and physical health.

You want to help your loved one feel good about himself, because his attitude weighs heavily on your caregiving relationship. Still, you need to tread carefully, says Suzanne Mintz, cofounder and president of the National Family Caregivers Association, based in Kensington, Maryland. "Helping care recipients preserve their self-esteem is a balancing act," she explains. "They should pursue their own interests, but they may not be able to do that on their own. You want to encourage them but not smother them."

So what's the best way to give a loved one's self-esteem a boost? Try these suggestions.

✗ Refrain from intervening with any task your loved one can handle independently. Perhaps your mother has difficulty

EXPERT OPINION

"I believe that as long as there is breath, there is significance in a senior's life. I may see that they are still vibrant, that they can do many things for themselves. But they don't see it. That's the challenge for caregivers: to help seniors find their significance and help them respond to it and act on it."

—**SUSANA CHAN FONG,** center manager for OnLok, a community elder program in San Francisco

getting dressed on her own, but she's able to choose her clothes without assistance. Encourage her to do that.

✗ When your loved one completes a task without help, offer your praise. This lets the person know you noticed her efforts, which contributes to the sense of accomplishment she's experiencing. Just don't overdo accolades, at the risk of sounding patronizing.

✗ Ask for help around the house. Many care recipients worry about being a burden to their caregivers. Assigning them chores appropriate for their abilities supports their desire to feel like contributing members of the household.

✗ Cultivate your loved one's interest in gardening. Besides being a relaxing pastime, it does wonders for self-esteem, as people can see the fruits—or vegetables, or flowers—of their labors. Your loved one doesn't even need a yard to garden. Planting in containers and window boxes is just as therapeutic.

✗ Consider making a pet part of your family. Many studies have shown that older people, in particular, benefit physically and emotionally from being around animals. Pets depend on their people, which can foster a sense of purpose in care recipients. And if the pet happens to be a dog, he'll need to go for walks—which could mean much-needed exercise for your loved one as well as ample opportunity to socialize.

✗ Introduce activities that provide intellectual stimulation. The options are endless: listening to music and books on tape, assembling puzzles, using computers, attending concerts and lectures, whatever piques your loved one's interest. Gaining knowledge or mastering a skill can be a marvelous elixir for flagging self-esteem.

✗ Commend your loved one for trying something new. Older people, in particular, tend to have set routines. Venturing outside that structure can feel awkward and intimidating; it certainly takes courage. By acknowledging your loved one's efforts, you might encourage him to broaden his horizons even more.

Take Action... HELP EASE LOSS THROUGH ADAPTATION

Whenever your loved one gives up a task or activity, he's left with a void that—no matter how small—can erode his perception of who he is. One of the challenges of caregiving lies in finding ways to fill the voids, so your loved one feels needed and valued.

In some cases, you may be able to modify a task or activity so your loved one can participate in it, even if he can't manage it on his own. "I'm involved in this sort of situation myself," says Percil Stanford, Ph.D., professor of gerontology and director of the Center on Aging at San Diego State University. "A friend of mine developed a rare blood disease several years ago, and he has been declining ever since. Those around him have helped adapt his interests to his abilities. For example, he used to read a great deal. He still can, but he gets tired, so we read to him. He also enjoyed walks on the beach. He had to go on a cane for a while, then a walker. Now that he's in a wheelchair, we push him.

"What's important is to nurture enjoyment and continuity," Dr. Stanford adds. "When people become care recipients, look for ways to adapt their interests to their abilities." Other strategies that can help offset any loss and emptiness your loved one may feel include the following:

- ✗ Respect the person's need to grieve. Coming to terms with a decline in abilities isn't easy; your loved one must be given a chance to accept and let go. Acknowledge and respect his feelings. Then when the time is right, he will feel able to move on.

- ✗ Stay alert for all-or-nothing thinking. As the people around him take over various tasks, your loved one may begin to think, "I can't do anything anymore." The reaction is understandable, but it's most likely a distortion of reality. You can help shift the person's mindset in a positive direction by engaging him in tasks that remind him of all he can do.

- ✗ Suggest activities that complement your loved one's interests but are better suited to his abilities. Suppose your fa-

EXPERT OPINION

"Becoming a care recipient is about loss—loss of independence, loss of a former life. Loss means grieving. And people grieve differently. Your loved one may get angrier than you might like, or remain in denial longer than you think is healthy. It's important for caregivers to give their loved ones the space to be themselves, to work through their grieving in their own way—while at the same time, being alert for signs of depression."

—**SUZANNE MINTZ,** cofounder and president of the National Family Caregivers Association, based in Kensington, Maryland

ther, an avid golfer, had to give up the game. He just might warm up to playing the computer or video version.

✗ Check into groups designed for people with special hobbies or pastimes—such as watching birds or building model trains—that might appeal to your loved one. Often these groups list their events in the lifestyle or entertainment section of the local newspaper. And invariably, they're open to the public. If the person seems hesitant at the prospect of going to a meeting or outing alone, perhaps you or someone else could accompany him. Once he gets acquainted with other members, he'll feel comfortable on his own.

A Matter of Privacy

In becoming a care recipient, your loved one has to contend with not only a loss of independence but also a loss of privacy. The transition can be especially challenging if the person has been living on his own for any length of time and now finds himself in new surroundings amid an unfamiliar family structure. To help your loved one feel more comfortable in his new surroundings, you can try the following strategies.

• Respect the person's lifestyle. If your father prefers to spend time by himself, don't force him to take part in family activities. It will only make him more uncomfortable. Extend the invitation, but then let him decide what he wants to do. This shows respect for his independence—and over time, he may warm up to the idea of joining in. Remember that you are there not to control his life, but to let him live it.

• Provide as much privacy as possible. The ideal scenario is for your loved one to have his own bedroom and bathroom. If he must share sleeping quarters with someone else, you can make temporary walls using freestanding room dividers. In a shared bathroom, designate storage space for your loved one's toiletries, and make sure the bathroom door has a lock.

• Create opportunities for privacy in common areas. Suppose your mother loves to listen to opera, but the stereo is in the family room, where everyone watches television. You may want to buy your mom a set of headphones, so she can play her Pavarotti while the rest of the family tunes in to the tube.

• Invite your loved one to personalize her living space. Family photos, artwork, books, a favorite piece of furniture—familiar items like these can help a person feel more at home in his new surroundings.

• Make a point of talking with your loved one about the living arrangements. This lets the person know that you're concerned about his comfort, and that you welcome his opinions. If specific issues do arise, work with the person to resolve them.

Take Action... PROVIDE COMFORT THROUGH TOUGH TRANSITIONS

Of all the losses a care recipient may face, perhaps the most difficult to accept are also the most threatening to personal independence: relinquishing financial management and giving up driving privileges. For most of us, a driver's license and a checkbook are symbols of our passage into adulthood. When they're taken away, the effects on a person's self-esteem can be devastating. And it isn't just the care recipient who's hurting. Sometimes the caregiver is put in the awkward position of having to intervene on a loved one's behalf.

Not all care recipients become unable to drive or oversee their finances. For those who do, the strategies that follow may help temper the loss and the emotional upheaval that often accompanies it.

Relinquishing Financial Management

At some point in our lives, most of us have inadvertently missed a bill payment or overdrawn a check. In your loved one's case, it's not necessarily a sign that you need to intervene. You should become concerned if the late charges and overdraft notices start piling up, or if questionable financial decisions threaten to wipe out the person's savings. Older people, in particular, are easy targets for unscrupulous businesses and their fraudulent schemes.

Of course, *thinking* about intervening in your loved one's financial affairs may not be nearly as intimidating as actually *doing* it. To make the process less stressful for both of you, try these tips. (We'll get into the specifics of managing personal finances in chapter 23.)

- First and foremost, consult an attorney, preferably one who specializes in elder law. You need to understand your loved one's legal rights before you step in. The fact is, as long as the person is legally competent, he is entitled to make his own financial decisions. The law protects him against loss of financial control, even if well-meaning caregivers believe they're acting in his best interests.

- Tailor your actions to your loved one's point of view. Perhaps the person has a significant emotional investment in being

---

FOR MORE INFORMATION

The National Academy of Elder Law Attorneys can refer you to a lawyer in your area who specializes in the legal aspects of eldercare. For more information, call **(520) 881-4005** or visit the organization's Web site at **www.naela.org**.

Another good resource is the Area Agency on Aging or legal aid society in your loved one's community. Look in the blue pages of your telephone directory, under "Guide to Human Services."

able to handle his own checkbook. In that case, you need to broach the subject of financial management gingerly.

✗ Once you initiate the conversation, make a point of soliciting your loved one's input. You want the person to feel that he's a part of the decision-making process, which gives him a sense of control over the situation.

✗ Assume financial responsibilities gradually. The transition will be much easier for both of you if you zero in on specific tasks that your loved one isn't able to manage. For example, if the person has difficulty organizing his tax information, you might offer to pitch in with that. You can take on other tasks as it becomes necessary.

✗ Find out whether your loved one's financial institution offers automatic bill-paying services. Any bills would go directly to the bank, which would deduct the payments from a specified account. These deductions would show up on your loved one's monthly statements. Automatic bill payment is a good option for people who frequently miss or forget payment due dates but who aren't ready to turn over their checkbooks.

✗ Talk with your loved one about assigning power of attorney. This would give you or anyone else of the person's

Do You Need a Conservatorship?

If your loved one becomes incapacitated and has not executed a durable power of attorney for finances, you will need legal permission to take control of the person's financial affairs. This arrangement is called a conservatorship (or, in some states, a guardianship); you become the conservator, and your loved one, the conservatee.

Anyone—a spouse, a relative, or a friend—may petition a court to appoint a conservator on a person's behalf. In turn, the court will appoint an investigator to assess the competence of the potential conservatee, and to talk with those close to the person. The investigator presents his findings before the judge, who then decides whether to grant the conservatorship. The judge is also responsible for selecting the conservator and specifying that person's powers.

As you might imagine, these legal proceedings are expensive and time-consuming. But once a conservatorship is established, it remains under the court's supervision, which reduces the likelihood for abuse. Your best bet is to consult an attorney, who can help determine whether a conservatorship is appropriate for your situation.

choosing legal authority to act on his behalf in certain matters. With power of attorney, you could pay your loved one's bills by writing checks that draw on his bank account, for example. He would retain all of his legal rights, including the ability to revise or terminate the agreement at any time. Be aware that a regular power of attorney is automatically rescinded in the event your loved one becomes incapacitated. A durable power of attorney for finances, on the other hand, stays in effect until death. (For more information on power of attorney and other legal matters pertaining to caregiving, see chapter 25.)

Giving Up Driving Privileges

Maintaining responsibility for their own finances is a point of pride for many people. Given a choice, though, they'd probably hand over their checkbooks if it meant they could keep their car keys as long as they wanted.

As the creators of TV commercials are acutely aware, few things in life convey freedom like being able to slide behind the wheel of a vehicle and drive just about anywhere. But driving is a skill, and like many skills, it can deteriorate significantly with age or illness. Unfortunately, even hinting to a loved one that he should think about parking his car for good may fuel a hostile response. Then again, not intervening allows the person to stay on the road, where he may do harm to himself and others.

If you feel that your loved one has become a hazard behind the wheel—the Caregiver's Checklist on page 136 can help you assess his skills—please consider stepping in now, before he's involved in a serious accident. The conversation may not be easy, but remember, your loved one's life is at stake. You can temper the sting of the subject matter by using the following strategies.

✗ Talk with your loved one about enrolling in a driver safety program. Perhaps the best known is AARP's 55 Alive program, which provides classroom instruction to improve driving skills in people ages 55 and older. If your loved one seems reluctant to sign up, you may want to mention that some insurance companies offer premium discounts to motorists who complete the course.

FOR MORE INFORMATION

To learn more about AARP's 55 Alive driver safety program, or to find classes in your loved one's area, visit their Web site at www.aarp.org/55alive/.

While online, you might also want to check out the AAA Foundation for Traffic Safety's Web site for senior drivers and their families: www.seniordrivers.org. It features self-assessments, safe driving tips, emergency information, and more.

Is Your Loved One a Hazard behind the Wheel?

Researchers at the Massachusetts Institute of Technology AgeLab recommend keeping a record of incidents that may indicate a decline in your loved one's driving skills. The list below highlights the kinds of incidents you should watch for. You may want to make a copy of the list and distribute it to family members and close friends, so they can jot down their own notes. The more evidence you have, the stronger your case will be for getting your loved one off the road.

Warning Signs	Date(s) Observed	Specifics
Signaling incorrectly	_____	_____
Trouble making turns	_____	_____
Changing lanes improperly	_____	_____
Confusion at highway exits	_____	_____
Difficulty parking	_____	_____
Stopping inappropriately in traffic	_____	_____
Confusing the brake and gas pedals	_____	_____
Driving too fast or slow	_____	_____
Hitting curbs	_____	_____
Failing to notice stop signs or traffic lights	_____	_____
Reacting slowly to traffic situations	_____	_____
Failing to anticipate potential dangers	_____	_____
Getting lost in familiar places	_____	_____
Scrapes or dents on car, house, garage, or mailbox	_____	_____
Traffic violations	_____	_____
Near-misses	_____	_____
Accidents	_____	_____

✗ Advise your loved one to avoid those driving situations that put him at greatest risk. Simply encouraging the person to avoid certain situations—like driving at night, during rush hour, or on freeways—might help ease your concerns about his being behind the wheel.

✗ Offer to make arrangements for alternative transportation. Depending where your loved one lives, he may be able to take advantage of public transit, even getting discounts on his fares. He might also be eligible for the special van services that are provided in many communities for elderly or physically disabled residents. And don't forget to check with the local senior center, churches, and chapters of community organizations such as the American Red Cross. Many have their own transportation programs.

✗ If your loved one brushes aside your concerns about his driving, enlist other family members and close friends to share their observations. You might even want to plan a family meeting, if you think it might help. Just remind all of the participants to remain respectful of your loved one's feelings. You don't want him to feel he's under attack.

✗ Involve your loved one's primary care physician, if necessary. Many states require doctors to report health problems that may compromise a driver's performance, such as Alzheimer's disease and Parkinson's disease. The state then revokes the person's license. Even if your loved one doesn't have a particular condition, he may be willing to heed his physician's advice to turn in his car keys, or at least change his driving habits.

FOR MORE INFORMATION

Every community has a federally funded Area Agency on Aging, which can provide information about public and private transportation services. Try looking in the blue pages of your phone directory, under "Guide to Human Services." You can also call the Eldercare Locator at **(800) 677-1116**, or visit the Web site at **www.eldercare.gov.**

Take Action... MASTER YOUR RESPONSE TO DIFFICULT BEHAVIOR

Even when handled with the greatest tact and respect, common caregiving transitions like cutting back on driving privileges and letting go of financial matters can trigger a host of emotional reactions in your loved one, ranging from occasional crankiness and melancholy to frequent hostility and despair. As

Outlook

"My sense is that one major challenge for the future lies in the shift from an individual model of caregiving to a community or societal model. Currently, individuals are called upon to provide care for a short but consuming and overwhelming time. Then, like a storm, the caregiving episode passes—often because the care recipient passes away—and pre-caregiving life resumes. But the caregivers are changed forever by the experience.

"Caregiving must be re-engineered so that caregivers feel less isolated and can draw upon community resources to reduce their burden. Their response team could include current, past, and future caregivers, all coordinated by public agencies, community-based organizations, or religious groups. In this ideal scenario, when caregiving is needed, the community will respond."

—DAVID B. REUBEN, M.D., professor of medicine and chief of the division of geriatrics at the UCLA School of Medicine

the primary caregiver, you may bear the brunt of the person's mood swings and outbursts. And they can elicit equally emotional reactions from you.

To keep your loved one's behavior in perspective, remember that his sense of self has been shaken. He has grown accustomed to living as he pleases. Now he has to answer to someone else—quite possibly an adult child, whom he may not see as his peer. Keep in mind, too, that a decline in mental function can influence the person's behavior in ways he can't control.

Even so, your loved one's words and actions can hurt. How do you stop them from getting under your skin? These tips can help.

✗ Rather than arguing with the person, tell yourself not to get caught in the heat of the moment. You don't want your emotions to dictate your response. Give yourself time to cool off and collect your thoughts.

✗ Try not to take your loved one's behavior personally. "This isn't easy," Mintz acknowledges. "But more than likely, the person is rebelling against the situation, not against you." If he does make an unkind comment about you specifically, the Alzheimer's Association recommends responding this way: "I know you're upset. You don't deserve what has happened to you." Then change the subject and move on.

✗ Remember that you can't control the other person's behavior, only your own. "It's all about the caregiver's attitude," Dr. Stanford explains. "You can tie yourself in a knot over a particular incident, or you can work at maintaining a healthy perspective on it."

✗ When discussing your loved one's behavior, choose your words carefully, always staying focused on the situation. Being critical of the person only hurts his self-esteem even more.

✗ Encourage the person to share his feelings with someone not directly involved in the caregiving relationship—perhaps a close friend, a member of the clergy, or even a therapist. Having an "outsider" as a sounding board can bring fresh insight to the situation. And that can help your loved one cope with the changes he's experiencing.

✗ If your loved one's behavior is impeding your ability to provide care, consider consulting a social worker or geriatric care manager. This professional can assess the situation and recommend a course of action.

DEPRESSION: A DISEASE IN DISGUISE

Among older people, difficult behavior can be a symptom of depression. In fact, so many in the 65-and-older population suffer from depression that the National Institute of Mental Health describes it as "a serious concern." Unfortunately, a lot of these cases remain undiagnosed.

Part of the problem is that depression affects older people differently. They may not become sad and weepy, or express feelings of helplessness and hopelessness. Instead, says Margaret Norris, Ph.D., a psychologist at Texas A&M University in College Station, they're more likely to experience appetite loss, weight loss, sleep impairment, persistent fatigue, and concentration problems.

These same symptoms can occur with certain chronic conditions or as side effects of medication, however. As a result, says Daniel E. Ford, M.D., M.P.H., associate professor of medicine at Johns Hopkins University in Baltimore, depression is easily overlooked by family members and physicians alike.

Even when depression is suspected, a definitive diagnosis can prove elusive. Without one, patients might not get the treatment they need. Some doctors may prescribe antidepressants just to see if they help, but most physicians will avoid doing this because the medications can have serious side effects.

Left untreated, depression can take a serious toll on physical health. Research shows that elderly people who have depression are less likely to survive heart attack, stroke, and cancer than those who don't. Even more alarming, they're twice as likely to commit suicide as their younger counterparts.

What makes the situation especially tragic is that, according to the National Institute of Mental Health, 70 percent of elderly people who committed suicide had visited their family doctors within a month before their deaths. Thirty-nine percent had a medical encounter within 1 week of taking their lives. Still, their depression remained undiagnosed and untreated.

FOR MORE INFORMATION

Your loved one's primary care physician should be able to recommend a qualified social worker or geriatric care manager. The following organizations can also provide referrals to professionals in your area.

• The National Association of Social Workers. Phone: **(800) 638-8799**; Internet address: **www.socialworkers.org**.

• The National Association of Professional Geriatric Care Managers. Phone: **(520) 881-8008**; Internet address: **www.caremanager.org**.

EXPERT OPINION

"Many people believe that given the losses associated with aging, depression is unavoidable. Not true. While change and loss are an inevitable part of growing older, depression is not. If elderly people exhibit any symptoms of depression, they should be treated. Treatment helps."

—DANIEL E. FORD, M.D., M.P.H.,
associate professor of medicine at
Johns Hopkins University in Baltimore

If your loved one seems to be showing some of the symptoms described above, urge the person to see his primary care physician. If that doesn't work, schedule the appointment yourself. Don't tell yourself that you don't need to worry until the person starts talking about suicide, because that may not happen. Compared with the younger population, the elderly talk about killing themselves less, but take action more.

Your loved one may resist the suggestion that he's depressed; like many older people, he may perceive depression as a moral weakness. It isn't. Try to explain to the person that depression is an illness, not a reflection on his character. And reassure him that in most cases, it's very treatable.

One final thought: As Dr. Ford observes, the leading reason for suicide among older people is loneliness. Caring for your loved one provides not just assistance and support but also companionship. In that sense, caregiving can be a real lifesaver.

CHAPTER 13

GOOD HEALTH MATTERS

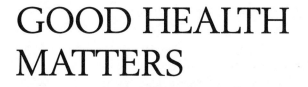

What You Need to Know

- You can help improve your loved one's quality of life through a combination of regular exercise, good nutrition, adequate rest, and controlled stress.

- Physical activity enhances strength and mobility, which can help preserve your loved one's independence.

- While many people worry about taking in too many calories, older care recipients may not be getting enough. Undereating compromises the body's immune system, impairing its ability to fight disease.

- Insomnia and other sleep problems are not a normal part of the aging process.

- Among care recipients, one of the most common sources of stress is the perception that they're losing control of their personal lives.

At its best, caregiving is equal parts proactive and reactive. Even though your loved one may have a particular condition that requires treatment, attending to all aspects of the person's health can significantly improve her quality of life. This may seem like a tall order. In fact, it simply means creating an environment that enables and encourages the person to exercise regularly, eat nutritiously, get adequate rest, and manage stress. Together, these practices make for sound preventive medicine.

If your loved one hasn't followed the most health-conscious lifestyle, that's not to say she can't start now. Experts agree that it's never too late to adopt healthy habits—anything from drinking enough water to lifting light weights.

Of course, you also need to contend with the not-so-small

EXPERT OPINION

"Americans are now living into their eighties and beyond. The fastest growing segment of the population is over 85, and the number of centenarians—people over 100—is exploding. That means the bodies we're taking care of have to last a lot longer than they used to. They have to be fed better, and they have to be exercised better."

—JANE BRODY, personal health columnist for *The New York Times*

matter of persuading your loved one that she would do herself a world of good by, say, increasing her fluid intake or strengthening her muscles. This chapter offers the scientific evidence to help you make your case, as well as many practical tips to help you motivate your loved one to start tweaking her lifestyle. Even the smallest changes can have a big impact, physically and emotionally.

These changes are not without their challenges, however. For example, increasing physical activity is the most direct way to improve health, according to scientific studies. Yet it's a notoriously tough sell, especially since it takes time out of a person's daily routine. By comparison, eating well seems to fit better within the framework of everyday life; after all, food is necessary for survival. Still, a nutritious diet can easily veer off course, sidetracked by too many temptations.

Perhaps the greatest challenge is that as long as your loved one remains mentally competent, she can make her own lifestyle choices—healthy or not. So what's a caregiver to do? Let the person know that you want her to feel good about herself, and to be as vital as possible for as long as possible. Think of stealthy ways to introduce healthy changes, like asking her to walk to the end of the driveway to fetch the mail every day. Perhaps most important, set a good example by taking care of yourself. (We'll talk about lifestyle strategies for the caregiver in chapter 29.)

Even if your loved one embraces the idea of revamping her lifestyle, encourage her to adopt changes gradually, one at a time. Trying to accomplish too much all at once can be overwhelming and increases the likelihood that nothing will stick.

EXERCISE: GETTING FIT FOR LIFE

As mentioned earlier, the biggest boost to your loved one's health will come from a regular exercise program. The research confirming a positive relationship between fitness and vitality has reached critical mass.

"We don't need more studies to prove that people at any stage of life can benefit from increasing their physical activity," says Walter Bortz, M.D., clinical associate professor of medicine at Stanford University and a researcher who specializes in aging populations. "Physical activity is good for everything. It decreases blood pressure and resting pulse. It increases the size of arteries, which is good for the cardiovascular system. It lowers the risk of depression. It raises the odds of staying independent longer."

According to groundbreaking research sponsored by the National Institute on Aging, even the frail elderly can grow stronger and more independent with regular physical activity. The first significant study, performed at Tufts and Harvard universities in 1989, involved residents of a local elder rehabilitation center, all in their late eighties to nineties. For 6 weeks, they engaged in strength training with leg weights. Their muscle strength improved by an average of 180 percent, and their overall walking speed increased by 48 percent. Two participants were able to stop using their canes. These results astounded even the researchers.

Unfortunately, many elderly care recipients see themselves as too old or too weak for exercise. The same is true for those who are chronically ill. Yet experts say this assumption couldn't be far-

Caregiving around the World

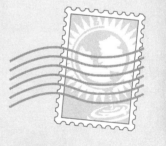

According to German law, children are obligated to support their parents in old age. Seniors can't apply for social assistance until after the family's financial resources have run out. In 1994, Germany enacted a long-term care insurance program that covers everyone, with the exception of a few who opt for private plans. The premiums are 1.7 percent of salary, split equally between employers and employees. Benefits include extensive institutional and home care services. Informal caregivers receive up to 4 weeks of respite care each year as well as pension credit for providing high levels of unpaid services. In 1999, about 600,000 people received pension contributions as caregivers.

POST CARD

FROM GERMANY

EXPERT OPINION

"We believe that through exercise, we can bend the aging curve. Up to this point, everyone has been working with an aging curve that says once people turn 50, they just go downhill. We don't believe that's true. We've already proven it's not true. We are creating the ideal aging curve, more like an aging continuum. Straight across and then leave the Earth. That's it."

—JOE SIGNORILE, senior researcher at the Stein Gerontological Institute of the Miami Jewish Home and Hospital

ther from the truth. If anything, regular physical activity makes people feel younger and stronger, among other important benefits. For example:

- Exercise is an essential component of any weight management plan. It burns calories while increasing muscle mass, helping to shed unwanted pounds that can raise the risk for heart disease and diabetes, among other health problems.

- Activities such as swimming and walking help reduce high blood pressure, a common forerunner to heart disease and stroke.

- Exercise significantly lowers the risk of type 2 (adult-onset) diabetes. For those who've already been diagnosed with diabetes, exercise can help control blood sugar levels more effectively.

- Everyday activities, including walking and gardening, appear to nearly halve the risk of severe intestinal bleeding that's associated with colon cancer and other gastrointestinal illnesses in later life. Scientists theorize that exercise helps move food through the digestive tract, preventing it from becoming trapped and breeding harmful bacteria that cause infections and bleeding.

- Strength training increases muscle mass and power, improves balance, and builds bones. In fact, it even slows the progression of the brittle-bone disease osteoporosis. And some research suggests that it helps relieve arthritis pain by toning muscles and reducing strain. By the way, strength training doesn't necessarily mean lifting weights. Using resistance tubing or performing isometric exercises, in which the body provides resistance, can be just as effective.

- Light exercise has been linked to improved mental health, including a reduced risk of depression. In one study, participants reported that they felt less stress and anxiety after 1 year on an exercise program. Another study found 5 months of strength training to be just as effective as antidepressant drugs and psychological counseling, relieving symptoms in nearly 75 percent of cases.

Note, too, that physical activity can help reduce a person's dependence on medication. Fewer drugs means fewer side effects, plus fewer opportunities for potentially life-threatening interactions. (We'll delve into the problem of drug interactions in chapter 15.)

Function Follows Fitness

For your loved one, perhaps the most compelling reason for getting active is to maintain independence. Regular exercise improves and protects a person's ability to get out of bed, take a bath, climb stairs, and perform assorted tasks of daily living on her own.

That said, the opposite is also true: In the absence of regular exercise, your loved one is likely to lose an even greater percentage of her basic functionality as she gets older. In other words, she'll need help with many aspects of her daily routine.

Surveys have shown that less than one-third of all Americans

Exercising Caution

Everyone, no matter what their age or health status, can reap the rewards of a regular exercise program. But they must make safety a top priority. People who are older or chronically ill may be vulnerable to injury if they try to work beyond their fitness levels and abilities, especially when they're just starting out.

Before your loved one starts exercising, make sure she has her doctor's approval. Then help her get active with these precautions in mind.

- Warm up before working out. Five minutes of gentle activity—such as walking, stationary cycling, or arm-pumping—is sufficient.

- Be careful not to overdo. A little soreness and fatigue can be expected. But if your loved one complains of pain or exhaustion, then she's pushing herself too hard.

- Pay attention to breathing technique. You don't want your loved one to hold her breath while straining. It can cause her blood pressure to spike. The proper technique is to exhale on the muscle exertion—for example, during the rising motion of a push-up—and inhale on the relaxation or release.

- Keep tabs on intensity. The most common method is to check the pulse, but this can be misleading for people on medications that affect their natural heart rates. Instead, many exercise scientists advocate a measure that they call perceived rate of exertion. It's very easy to use: A person just ranks the intensity of her workout on a scale of 1 (easy) to 10 (difficult). Beginning exercisers should aim for an intensity of 5, which means they can carry on a conversation during their workouts without getting winded. A personal trainer can help your loved one find the proper intensity for her age and fitness level.

- Make water a prerequisite. Experts recommend drinking at least eight 8-ounce glasses of water a day. When she's exercising, a person needs even more to stay adequately hydrated.

age 45 and older get some form of regular exercise. That's too bad, because according to the American College of Sports Medicine, a sedentary lifestyle can cause a person to lose about 10 percent of her muscle mass by age 50. The rate climbs even higher after that, leading to a roughly 15 percent decline in muscle strength for someone in her sixties, plus another 15 percent when she's in her seventies.

On the other hand, even light to moderate physical activity can offset many of the health concerns once thought to be an inevitable part of aging, such as bone loss and joint pain. At least one study suggests that exercise might actually turn back the clock. In this study, conducted at the Veterans Administration Medical Center in Salt Lake City, physically fit men in their fifties had higher oxygen uptakes and lower resting heart rates (by 20 beats per minute, on average) during peak workout periods than sedentary men in their mid-twenties. The older men also weighed less—an average of 166 pounds, compared with 192 for the younger men. While the fountain of youth may not exist, physical activity seems like the next best thing!

Take Action... FIND OPPORTUNITIES TO INCREASE PHYSICAL ACTIVITY

As a caregiver, you can help your loved one buck the national trend by developing a fitness habit. Of course, you may have a hard time imagining the person doing anything strenuous if she has difficulty climbing a flight of stairs or getting into and out of the bathtub. That goes double if the person tends to resist any new wrinkle in her usual routine. But the right approach can make all the difference. These tips can help.

✗ Make sure your loved one eases into exercise, so she doesn't become discouraged or, worse, risk injury. For beginners, controlled stretching is an ideal workout, because it improves flexibility and increases bloodflow. It's relaxing, too. You may want to join your loved one in practicing this simple daily routine: neck stretches (slowly tilting the head side-to-side and front-to-back, avoiding full rolls), arm circles, and trunk twists (slowly turning the upper body to

FOR MORE INFORMATION

The National Institute on Aging has developed an exercise guide for older people. To request a copy, call **(800) 222-2225** or visit the NIA Web site at **www.nia.nih.gov**. You can also write to the NIA Information Center, PO Box 8057, Gaithersburg, MD 20892.

The Fifty-Plus Fitness Association, which originated at Stanford University, is dedicated to promoting an active lifestyle among older people. For more information, visit the Web site at **www.50plus.org**.

one side, then the other). Whether the two of you perform these exercises standing up or sitting in a chair, work to maintain good posture. And if your loved one shows any sign of discomfort or shakiness, stop right away.

X Once your loved one has gotten comfortable with stretching, encourage her to add walking to her fitness routine. Many experts recommend walking for 30 minutes a day because it's low-impact, it can be done at any pace, and it requires no equipment other than a good pair of shoes. What's more, it can help strengthen the lower body—an important benefit, if Dr. Bortz's research is any indication. "We've found that leg strength is the best predictor of whether someone ends up in a nursing home," he says. "It reflects a combination of power and speed in the muscles and nerves."

X Introduce your loved one to the gentle, graceful movements of tai chi. In research at Northwestern University in Chicago, elderly people who studied the ancient Chinese martial art showed significant reductions in falls and balance problems after just 12 weeks. Many health clubs and martial arts studios offer tai chi classes, as do some churches and hospital wellness programs.

X Combine exercise with activities your loved one already enjoys. If your mother likes to window-shop, head to the nearest mall for a leisurely stroll. Or take your dad bowling; lifting the ball provides some impromptu strength training.

X Involve your loved one in household chores. If the leaves need raking or the garden needs weeding, ask your loved one to pitch in. Even something as simple as emptying the dishwasher or folding towels counts as physical activity. As an added benefit, it helps your loved one feel like she's contributing to the family.

X If you have young children at home, find opportunities to engage them in active play with your loved one. For example, they could play a gentle game of catch or hide-and-

EXPERT OPINION

"The most wonderful thing about physical activity is that it can begin at any age. Even if you are 80 years old and you have a chronic illness, you can improve your health. You will not only be healthier but also feel better. You'll have a better appetite, and you'll better match your caloric intake with your caloric output. Exercise does not increase people's appetites. It helps them match their appetites to the number of calories they really need."

—**JANE BRODY,** personal health columnist for *The New York Times*

Collage Video is a Minneapolis-based company that specializes in exercise videos. To view their merchandise online, or to request a print catalog, visit **www.collagevideo.com**.

seek. Or they could jump rope, with your loved one helping out as a "turner."

✗ Look around for an exercise video tailored to your loved one's fitness level and ability. Among the titles available: *Smile: So Much Improvement with a Little Exercise*, a low-intensity 35-minute workout for more frail seniors, produced by the University of Michigan School of Public Health (write to Department of HB/HE, 1420 Washington Heights, Ann Arbor, MI 48109); *Armchair Fitness*, a 1-hour gentle exercise session set to big-band music (CC-M Productions, call 800-453-6280); and *Exercising with Dorothy*, a slow-paced routine appropriate for people using walkers or wheelchairs (Stuart Choate, call 800-779-8491).

✗ Recognize even small advances in fitness as big victories. As Dr. Bortz observes, just convincing your loved one to take a walk around the block or to do some simple stretches while watching TV is progress.

Strength Training by the Numbers

Most experts on aging agree that older people can regain function most efficiently through strength training. Before your loved one begins a strength-training program, she must get clearance from her physician. In addition, she should receive some basic instruction from a personal trainer, to learn proper technique and protect against injury. A trainer can also recommend exercises tailored to your loved one's needs and abilities.

In general, though, any strength-training program designed for an older person should follow these guidelines from the National Institute on Aging.

1. Start with a weight your loved one can lift five times without too much effort. Using 1- or 2-pound dumbbells is fine, if that's what the person can handle.

2. Once your loved one is comfortable with five repetitions, increase to two sets of five, with a few minutes of rest in between.

3. When the person can manage two sets, work up to three, with rest in-between.

4. Once your loved one has mastered three sets of five repetitions, aim for 10 repetitions in each set.

5. When the person can easily do three sets of 10 repetitions, try for 15 repetitions per set.

6. Once your loved one reaches five sets of 15 repetitions, move on to a slightly heavier weight.

NUTRITION: GOOD HEALTH IS ON THE MENU

Unlike exercising, which most of us don't do every day (even though we should), eating is a fixture in our daily routines. That gives us plenty of opportunities to change our diets for the better—and just as many opportunities to slip up.

In a caregiving situation, perhaps the best way to approach nutrition is to consider one issue at a time. It's just like preparing a delicious meal: You need to pay attention to each ingredient in turn so that the "recipe"—in this case, for a healthy diet—comes out right.

As a caregiver, your most pressing concern may be whether your loved one is getting enough of the nutrients she needs. But for older care recipients, in particular, an even greater challenge is getting enough calories, period. An inadequate food intake can depress the body's immune defenses so that they're less able to fend off infections. Worse, it can play a role in the downward physical and emotional spiral that some in medical circles refer to as the dwindles.

People in their seventies and eighties are prime candidates for the dwindles, also known as failure to thrive, explains Anne M. Egbert, M.D., a geriatric physician and associate professor at the University of Kansas School of Medicine in Wichita. The most common indicator of the condition is withdrawal—physical, social, or both. But rapid weight loss and mental confusion also occur, and they're often brought on by not eating.

"All of us have seen people who sort of curl up and hide from the world," Dr. Egbert says. "They just don't feel like seeing anybody or eating anything."

If the condition remains unchecked, it can lead to serious illness and death. On the other hand, if the warning signs are spotted early enough, the downward spiral can be stopped and even reversed. Good nutrition supports the recovery process.

The Rules Change with Age

Other factors can challenge the appetites and eating habits of care recipients. Sometimes the sense of taste is compromised as a result of certain medications or a lifetime of smoking or excessive drinking. Often the sense of smell deteriorates with age. Even

EXPERT OPINION

"We want to care for our elders at home, because that's their culture. They have their native foods and their families. If they go into a long-term care facility, everything is different. Even the food is different; they have to be on a diet that they're not used to. They're not accustomed to eating chicken or hot dogs or fish; they want to eat the kinds of foods they had at home. I find that's one of the biggest complaints of people in nursing homes."

—**AURELIA NEHOITEWA,** ombudsman for the Office of Hopi Elderly Services, Kykotsmovi, Arizona

Water Works

Experts advise caregivers to pay close attention to the amount of water and other fluids consumed by a loved one. Much like an inadequate food intake, a lack of fluids can contribute to a host of health problems.

"A person's thirst mechanism becomes less efficient with age," explains Irwin H. Rosenberg, M.D., dean of nutrition sciences at Tufts University in Medford, Massachusetts. "Dehydration or partial dehydration can lead to dizziness, falls, increased blood pressure, and a higher risk of kidney stones." And in older people, poor hydration can be made even worse by medications they're taking, such as diuretics and laxatives, which increase the excretion of fluids from the body.

Dr. Rosenberg notes that in the "70+ pyramid" created by two of his colleagues at Tufts University—a version of the USDA Food Guide Pyramid tailored to the nutritional needs of older people—water sits prominently at the base. The revised pyramid recommends drinking at least eight 8-ounce glasses of water and other fluids a day.

poor-fitting dentures or lack of dental hygiene can interfere with a healthy diet by making chewing painful.

In people who are older or disabled, the stomach can actually shrink, reducing appetite in the process. Usually this problem can be circumnavigated by adjusting meal frequency and size. The rest of the family might get the standard three squares a day, while the care recipient eats smaller meals more often. Irwin H. Rosenberg, M.D., dean of nutrition sciences at Tufts University in Medford, Massachusetts, describes the ideal eating plan for care recipients as "a healthful version of an all-day buffet."

Of course, for some people, the problem lies in eating too much rather than too little. Your loved one's daily calorie requirement will decline as she gets older. If she hasn't adjusted her calorie intake accordingly, and if she isn't as active as she should be, she's a prime candidate for gaining weight. And that has health risks of its own, from heart disease and diabetes to gallstones and joint pain.

While no doctor would discourage a person who's overweight from trying to slim down, many agree that caregivers don't need to worry if their loved ones are carrying 5 to 10 extra pounds. In fact, research has shown that the extra weight can help elderly or disabled people recover from surgery or illness.

Some experts would argue that the American obsession with weight doesn't belong on an older person's plate. "I've seen 80-year-olds who won't eat certain foods because they're concerned about weight gain," Dr. Egbert says. "Sometimes older people need to loosen up with dietary standards that are better targeted to the young."

Take Action... CULTIVATE HEALTHFUL EATING HABITS

Your loved one probably has food preferences and dietary patterns that go back decades. Convincing him to try something new and healthful takes no small amount of patience. But it can be done. You can nudge the odds in your favor by making every dining experience inviting, comfortable, and pleasant. Here's how.

X Offer a variety of nutritious choices at each meal. Let's face it: None of us likes to be told what to eat. The best strategy is to serve more items, only in smaller portions.

✗ Serve up some old-fashioned comfort foods. Depending on the care recipient's age, she may derive the most pleasure from familiar menu items like meat loaf, mashed potatoes, creamed corn, and fruit cocktail. As long as she's eating it, she's reaping the nutritional benefits. Dr. Egbert even endorses the inclusion of milk shakes in eating plans for older people.

✗ If your loved one has difficulty using utensils, build her meal around finger foods—perhaps a sandwich, cherry tomatoes, celery sticks and dip, and a piece of fresh fruit. That way, she can enjoy her meal with the rest of the family, without feeling self-conscious. (Another option is to buy adaptive utensils, available from medical supply stores and catalogs.) Likewise, if your loved one has difficulty chewing, offer her soft food items like soups and smoothies. For swallowing problems, cream soups, nectars, and vegetable juices are good options. (Remember that slightly thick liquids are easier to swallow than thin ones.)

✗ Make water and other fluids available at every meal. The care recipient might try to limit her fluid intake, especially if she is incontinent. She probably doesn't realize that drinking too few fluids actually stimulates the production of urine, which can irritate the bladder and increase the likelihood of a mishap. Besides water, fluid choices include decaffeinated coffee and tea (caffeine is a diuretic), juice, broth, gelatin, sherbet, and ice pops. To further encourage frequent sipping, you might want to place a water bottle on your loved one's nightstand.

✗ Create a relaxed mealtime environment, keeping the pace leisurely and the conversation pleasant. If your loved one refuses to eat, don't dwell on it. You can't make her clean her plate, as you might have done with your kids. So wait until after the meal to find out why she reacted the way she did. You're entitled to enjoy your dining experience, too.

✗ For mid-morning and mid-afternoon snacks, use your imagination. Leftover pancakes, cereal with milk, half a sandwich, rolled meat slices, cut-up vegetables, yogurt, pudding,

Supplemental Insurance for Seniors

Even with the healthiest eating habits, your loved one may need a little extra nutritional support. Research has shown that compared with other age groups, older people eat less and get fewer vital nutrients from their diets. Yet they may need even more of these substances because of illnesses they have or medications they take.

Older people should take daily supplements of vitamins B_{12} and D, recommends Irwin H. Rosenberg, M.D., dean of nutrition sciences at Tufts University in Medford, Massachusetts. The B vitamin helps maintain nervous system function and memory, while the extra D compensates for decreased intestinal processing and absorption of nutrients.

You may be able to find the recommended amounts of both nutrients in a multivitamin. Check labels and choose a product that supplies 6 to 15 micrograms of vitamin B_{12} a day, plus 400 to 800 IU of vitamin D a day.

dried fruit, popcorn, peanut butter and crackers—all of these choices can satisfy.

SLEEP: THE REST OF THE STORY

In the grand scheme of good health, sleeping well doesn't get nearly as much attention as eating nutritiously and exercising regularly. But it should. For care recipients, in particular, getting a good night's sleep every night can transform quality of life.

Unfortunately, many people assume that sleep problems—difficulty falling asleep or staying asleep—come naturally with age. According to the National Institute on Aging, while our sleep patterns do change over time, "disturbed sleep or waking up tired every day is not a normal part of aging."

What researchers do know is that compared with younger people, the elderly get less of the "quiet" sleep known as non-REM. Everyone experiences four or five cycles of REM (rapid eye movement or "dreaming" sleep) and non-REM in a typical 8-hour night. Older people stay in non-REM for shorter periods.

The fact is, care recipients of all ages—not just the elderly—may struggle with sleep problems. The most common is insomnia, which is defined as taking a long time (between 30 and 45 minutes) to fall asleep, waking up too early and being unable to fall back asleep, or waking up tired. Research indicates that about one-third of all people age 65 and older experience insomnia symptoms.

What's behind all those sleepless nights? According to a Stanford University study involving more than 13,000 residents of Italy, Germany, and the United Kingdom, physical inactivity is a common culprit. So is a dissatisfying social life. And medical conditions like arthritis can make even the simple act of lying in bed painful.

When you look at this list, you can see why lack of sleep seems so prevalent among care recipients. But sleeping pills are not the answer, warns Mark S. Lachs, M.D., M.P.H., chief of geriatrics and gerontology at New York Hospital in Manhattan. At most, they're a last resort, to be tried when all other lifestyle approaches have been exhausted.

One reason for Dr. Lachs's concern is that older care recipients are likely to be taking at least one other medication. If they add a sleep aid to the mix, they're at greater risk for a potentially serious drug interaction. Another issue is that older people tend to eliminate drugs from their bodies more slowly. With sleep medications, they may experience a sort of morning-after hangover, or even mental confusion. Other common side effects include dry mouth, constipation, blurred vision, and ringing in the ears.

If your loved one is having trouble sleeping, first try the strategies described below—and give them a chance to work. If they don't seem to help, a sleep medication may be your only option. Dr. Lachs recommends that it be used as briefly as possible. In some cases, just one night of treatment is enough to break the cycle of sleeplessness. In other cases, longer treatment is necessary. Stay alert for side effects, too. They should be listed on the product label.

Take Action... SET THE STAGE FOR SLUMBER

Ideally, your loved one will experience truly restful, rejuvenating sleep without any assistance. If not, the following self-care strategies could provide the relief she needs. All are supported by research from the country's leading sleep laboratories.

- Make consistency a priority. This means your loved one should go to bed at the same time every night and get up at the same time every morning, even on weekends. Awakening at a regular hour is especially important, scientists say, because it sets the body's biological clock. In fact, they recommend that people arise on schedule even when they've had a rough night, sleep-wise. It helps keep that inner clock running as it should.

- Allow time for a 20-minute nap during the day. By knowing that she'll have a chance to rest during the day, your loved one may feel a little less anxious about getting to sleep at night. Just be sure to set the alarm for 20 minutes, since longer naps can disrupt the body's sleep/wake cycle. Some people may need to avoid napping altogether for this reason.

✗ If worries seem to be keeping your loved one awake at night, encourage her to put pen to paper and make note of them, along with any possible solutions that she thinks of. This exercise can help clear her mind so she doesn't toss and turn so much. It's best done in the early evening, to allow adequate downtime before she retires.

✗ Limit strenuous physical activity within 5 hours of bedtime. While exercising is important for your loved one, doing it too late at night can disrupt sleep.

✗ Have your loved one refrain from drinking coffee, tea, cola, and other caffeinated beverages after lunchtime. Caffeine, which lingers in the body for a full 8 hours, only worsens a sleep problem. The same is true for alcohol.

✗ Encourage your loved one to get some natural light in the afternoon hours, whether by going outside or by sitting near a sunny window inside. Exposure to natural light helps regulate the body's sleep/wake cycle.

✗ Put two drops of lavender essential oil on your loved one's pillowcase to induce sleep. Lavender is an ancient folk remedy known for helping people nod off. You can buy essential oils in many health food stores and bath-and-body shops.

STRESS MANAGEMENT:
THE HEALING POWER OF CALM

Of the four cornerstones of good health—regular exercise, good nutrition, adequate rest, and controlled stress—the last one may seem most elusive in a caregiving relationship. After all, caregiving is stressful business. For the caregiver, it means shouldering extra responsibilities and extra worries. For the care recipient, it means coping with change and loss.

The renowned Holmes-Rahe scale, developed nearly 40 years ago, quantifies the stress levels associated with a variety of life events. Personal illness, retirement, change in financial status, and moving into a new home all rank among the top 10 stressors. And all may factor into a care recipient's situation.

Helping your loved one manage any stress she may be feeling is important. Research over the past 15 years has identified some of the more serious health consequences of letting stress fester. It can increase cholesterol levels as much as poor dietary habits can. It can raise blood pressure, which in turn elevates the risk of stroke. In one in five healthy people, it triggers responses that can harm the cardiovascular system. (The ratio climbs to one in two among people with high blood pressure.)

That's not all. A recent report implicates stress as a factor in delayed healing of the skin. Stress has also been linked to depression, and the incidence of depression has tripled since World War II.

While the physical effects of stress on a care recipient may not be readily apparent, the behavioral effects usually are. Many a caregiver has seen a loved one turn anxious, resistant, or demanding—or even all three within the span of a few minutes. Often these behaviors result from the care recipient's perception that she's losing control of her personal life.

Research proves that perceived lack of control can be a major stressor. In one landmark study of British civil workers, the people under the most stress were those in low-level positions with no say in their work assignments. Even middle managers with more responsibility (but only slightly higher salaries) reported less stress, presumably because they had the ability to make decisions.

Of course, many events in a caregiving relationship can trigger a stress response. To help your loved one cope, you need to figure out what's behind any uncharacteristic behavior. Notice whether it follows a pattern. For example, she may become agitated when she has to go to the doctor or when she's asked about financial matters. She may get upset because *you're* having a bad day, and she's feeding off of your mood.

When stress threatens to turn a caregiving interaction into a confrontation, the best advice is to remove yourself from the situation, if only for 10 minutes. This gives you and your loved one a chance to cool off, so neither of you says or does something that you might regret. If the time-out doesn't defuse your loved one's mood, your calm demeanor and voice just might.

Another easy and effective way to neutralize stress, for the care recipient and caregiver alike, is to practice deep breathing. Researchers at the University of Missouri–Kansas City developed

Outlook

"A significant challenge for the caregiving community, and for all of us, is to recognize that we need to help each other, especially as we age. The American spirit prizes independence, and asking for and accepting help is very difficult for many people. It's not easy to change a culture, yet unless we allow the true spirit of community to be part of our lives, we may well make matters worse for our loved ones and ourselves.

"My hope for the future is that family caregivers will be considered an integral part of the care system and be given the training, support, remuneration, and benefits that are their just due. We can't continue to marginalize the millions of family caregivers in this country, upon whom not only aging or disabled loved ones but also the entire health care system depends."

—**SUZANNE MINTZ,** cofounder and president of the National Family Caregivers Association, based in Kensington, Maryland the following breathing exercise especially for the elderly. It's intended to counteract stiffness in the rib cage, which constricts full oxygen flow. But it also evokes a sense of relaxation and inner peace.

1. Sit up as straight as possible, with your shoulders relaxed. Exhale.

2. Inhale. At the same time, relax your abdominal muscles. Feel as though your belly is filling with air.

3. Continue inhaling, letting the middle of your chest fill up with air. Feel your chest and rib cage expand.

4. Hold in your breath for just a moment, then begin to exhale as slowly as possible.

5. While exhaling, relax your chest and rib cage. Begin to contract your abdominal muscles to force out the remaining air.

6. Close your eyes, and concentrate on your breathing. Allow your face to relax and your mind to clear. Let everything go.

7. Continue the exercise for about 5 minutes, staying focused on your breathing the entire time.

Encourage your loved one to practice this exercise whenever she's feeling distressed, as well as before she goes to bed. You can take advantage of it, too. It's an effective antidote for the body's stress response.

Finally, keep in mind that moodiness or behavioral problems exhibited by your loved one may have nothing to do with stress. Be sure to consider other causes, such as undereating, lack of sleep, or even medication.

CHAPTER 14

MANAGING ILLNESS

What You Need to Know

- When a caregiving situation involves a specific health problem, the foremost goal of care is to maintain—or even improve—quality of life.

- You can best support your loved one by learning as much as you can about his health problem. Then the two of you can work together to make informed decisions about treatment and care.

- Finding a physician whom you and your loved one like and trust is critical to managing a health problem effectively.

For most families, a caregiving relationship evolves from concern about a loved one's health. Perhaps the person has experienced a sudden medical crisis, such as a heart attack or stroke. Or she's dealing with a chronic condition such as arthritis that's beginning to affect her ability to perform routine tasks.

No matter what the circumstances driving the need for care, the goal for the caregiver remains the same: to maintain or improve the loved one's quality of life. Above all else, this means managing any health issue in a way that enables the care recipient to function well on her own for as long as possible, says Donna Wagner, Ph.D., director of the gerontology department at Towson University in Maryland. "A person doesn't have to go straight into a nursing home or care facility because of an illness," she observes. "Home care might be enough."

Ideally, a plan for home care is in place *before* a loved one actually needs it. Even in the early stages of a disease, the person can work with her physicians and family to make decisions about her future care and treatment.

Is Your Loved One's Doctor Good Enough?

When you're deciding the best means of managing your loved one's illness, it's helpful to have guidance from someone who understands the situation but isn't as emotionally attached to it as you are. The best person for the job is your loved one's primary care physician. That's why having a doctor whom both you and your loved one like and trust is so critical.

The following list of questions, based on a checklist developed by the National Institute on Aging, can come in handy whether you're looking for a new physician or reevaluating your loved one's current doctor. Some of the questions are easily answered, while others may require some research.

☐ yes ☐ no   Is the doctor board-certified in a specialty, such as geriatric medicine?

☐ yes ☐ no   Is the doctor a participant in your loved one's health insurance plan?

☐ yes ☐ no   If not, can your loved one afford to pay for treatments and services that are not covered?

☐ yes ☐ no   Is the doctor affiliated with the hospital of your loved one's choice?

☐ yes ☐ no   Is the doctor's office close by?

☐ yes ☐ no   Are the doctor's hours convenient?

☐ yes ☐ no   Does the doctor have a plan in place for handling patient calls after hours or while she's on vacation?

☐ yes ☐ no   Are the doctor's age, gender, and/or language skills relevant?

☐ yes ☐ no   Does the doctor show genuine interest in and concern for your loved one's well-being?

☐ yes ☐ no   Does the doctor welcome your questions?

☐ yes ☐ no   Is the doctor open to treatment options other than conventional medicines and surgery?

Once a health issue makes care necessary, your most important task as the caregiver is to become informed. Learn everything you can about your loved one's condition—and when you think you've exhausted your resources, keep digging. Talk with doctors, nurses, and other health practitioners, as well as with support organizations and other patients. Check out Internet sites and search bookstores for useful references.

In the face of illness, knowledge is power. It can turn up new and promising treatments that a doctor may not yet be aware of. It can provide leads to assistive devices that a loved one might use to continue living independently, with minimal help. It can deliver the reasoned perspective that a loved one may need to consider other housing options when home care is no longer enough.

This chapter can help in your search for knowledge. It's intended as a primer on the health concerns that most often require care or otherwise factor into caregiving relationships. You'll learn about the latest treatment options, as well as self-care strategies that can minimize symptoms and maximize quality of life.

ARTHRITIS

Forty-three million Americans have some form of arthritis, which translates to unquantifiable pain and discomfort. Depending on its severity, the condition can turn the most ordinary action—like getting out of bed—into an exercise in agony. That can have a significant impact on a caregiving situation.

The most common form of arthritis is osteoarthritis. It involves a degenerative breakdown of cartilage in the joints, especially in the hands, back, hips, knees, and feet. Without cartilage to provide cushioning, the bones in the joint rub together. That's what causes pain and impedes movement. Osteoarthritis most often affects older people, though obesity and overuse of joints—as in certain sports—can increase risk in anyone of any age.

Second to osteoarthritis is rheumatoid arthritis, a condition in which the linings of joints become inflamed. It tends to affect many joints in the body, causing pain, stiffness (especially in the morning), redness, swelling, and possibly fever. Over time, the compromised linings in the joints lose their ability to protect the bones and cartilage, setting the stage for deformities.

These are just two of the more than 100 forms of arthritis known to doctors. That's why getting an accurate diagnosis is so important. The more detailed the diagnosis, the more targeted and effective the treatment.

Invariably, that treatment includes exercise—which may seem counterintuitive, considering that all forms of arthritis impair movement. But exercise helps keep joints flexible and their supporting muscles strong. The type of workout regimen that's prescribed will vary from one patient to the next. The goal is always the same: to decrease pain and increase range of motion.

Medicines That Manage Pain

Besides exercise, your loved one's arthritis treatment plan may include some sort of pain-relieving medication. The first choice among physicians is a category of drugs known as nonsteroidal anti-inflammatory drugs (NSAIDs). This group includes over-the-counter ibuprofen and naproxen as well as the prescription COX-2 inhibitors. If your loved one's doctor recommends one of these medicines, be sure to get clear dosage instructions and follow them to the letter. The side effects of NSAIDs tend to become more serious as the dosage increases. Even over-the-counter ibuprofen can cause gastrointestinal problems in some patients when taken daily for a long time.

If an NSAID doesn't provide relief, your loved one may be given oral steroid medications or periodic steroid injections in the affected joint. The side effects of steroids can be serious, ranging from weight gain and hormonal disturbances to hair loss and bone loss. Your loved one's doctor should order regular blood tests to monitor the effects of steroid treatment on the liver and kidneys.

For rheumatoid arthritis, a number of promising new treatments—including both oral and intravenous medications—are in development. A rheumatologist will be up-to-date on the latest research. One caveat is that the new medicines won't help in cases where the disease has already reached an advanced stage. It needs to be caught early on.

For osteoarthritis, some doctors and many natural health practitioners recommend trying a glucosamine and chondroitin supplement to alleviate pain. A study funded by the National

Institutes of Health found that the supplement may indeed provide modest relief. Equally intriguing is the theory that glucosamine might help restore lost cartilage to arthritic joints. If your loved one decides to try this or any other kind of nutritional supplement, be sure that his doctor knows about it. That's the best way to avoid a potentially serious supplement-drug interaction. (For more on these kinds of interactions, see chapter 15.)

Take Action... ESTABLISH A JOINT-FRIENDLY LIFESTYLE

If your loved one is living with arthritis pain, he'll appreciate the following self-care strategies, adapted from the Arthritis Foundation. They pamper hurting joints—and in the process, they just might reduce the need for medication.

- Be careful not to overtax the affected joint. Using assistive devices can take the pain out of various routine tasks, like getting out of a chair or buttoning a shirt. In addition, maintaining a healthy weight can ease pressure on arthritic hips and knees.

- When a joint is inflamed, apply something cold. Ice is best, but a frozen gel pack or even a frozen bag of peas will work. (Be sure the cold source is wrapped in a towel to prevent direct contact with the skin.) The coldness reduces pain and swelling by constricting blood vessels and preventing fluids from leaking into surrounding tissues.

- Schedule a walking date at least once a week. Walking is the ideal exercise for most people with arthritis. It strengthens muscles and builds bones without jarring fragile joints. Your loved one might be reluctant to engage in any physical activity, so as motivation, do your walking at one of his favorite spots—perhaps in a nearby park or even on a golf course.

- Suggest a swimming class. Exercising in water effectively works the joints with minimal impact. Many YMCAs and community pools offer fitness swimming and aqua aerobics classes, some especially for older people.

Preparing for a Medical Emergency

Suppose your loved one experienced a sudden illness or injury—perhaps a heart attack or a broken hip. What would you do?

Now is the time to prepare for just such a possibility. Together, you and your loved one can come up with a plan of action, such as which hospital to go to (if more than one is close by) and who should be called—physicians, family members, and the like.

You might also want to make arrangements for your loved one's care in case you'd become sick or incapacitated. Perhaps a family member or friend would look after your loved one for the time being. Other options include home care or short-term respite care at an assisted living facility or nursing home.

✗ Ask your loved one's physician or physical therapist to recommend a stretching routine. Stretches promote flexibility in joints and muscles, which helps preserve range of motion. Yoga has the same benefits, though it may require more strength and agility.

✗ Make audiotapes of your loved one's favorite music. Listening to music can lift the spirits and take the mind off pain.

✗ Keep oranges and orange juice in the house. Recent research has confirmed the importance of vitamin C and other antioxidants in reducing the risk of osteoarthritis as well as slowing progression of the disease.

✗ Find ways to tickle your loved one's funny bone. Laughter has many proven health benefits. It helps relax muscles and relieve pain, and it boosts the immune system.

✗ Make sure your loved one wears sunscreen, as well as a hat and protective clothing, when out in the sun. Some forms of arthritis are hypersensitive to sunlight. In addition, some medications increase the likelihood of skin damage from the sun's ultraviolet rays.

CANCER

Every case of cancer is unique in its treatment and prognosis. But it's universal in its need for some kind of care, whether that entails a promise of unconditional love and support or full-time assistance with routine tasks.

Cancer can strike many different organs and glands in the body. When its multiple forms are taken into account, it ranks as the second-leading cause of death in the United States, trailing only heart disease. These days, some cancers—like colon cancer—have very impressive cure rates when they're caught early. Others, like pancreatic cancer, remain extremely difficult to slow down.

Often the conventional wisdom about cancer is misleading, if not plainly wrong. For example, among women, breast cancer is perceived as the deadliest form of the disease. While it does take an estimated 40,000 lives every year, the number of long-term survivors has reached the hundreds of thousands. Statistically, women are more likely to die from lung cancer than breast cancer.

Among men, prostate cancer is the most worrisome. While some cases do spread quickly, others are contained relatively easily and without surgery.

Misinformation only fuels the anxiety and dread that invariably accompany a cancer diagnosis. One of a caregiver's most important jobs is to find out the facts about a loved one's particular kind of cancer. Along with that comes the responsibility of acting as gatekeeper, deciding how much of this knowledge should be shared with the care recipient.

It's an issue that apparently even physicians wrestle with. According to a study conducted by researchers at the University of Chicago, more than half of all doctors choose to withhold vital information about the severity of symptoms or the length of life expectancy in the interest of protecting their patients. Other doctors are inclined to be straightforward, even blunt, about a poor prognosis. But neither approach is appropriate for every patient.

Cancer Coping Techniques

The American Cancer Society offers the following list of do's and don'ts to help caregivers and care recipients come to terms with a cancer diagnosis.

Do . . .

- Pay attention to verbal and nonverbal expressions of fear, such as anger, denial, excitability, headaches, muscle tension, and trembling.

- Listen carefully to each other. Try waiting a few seconds before responding, to allow comments to register.

- Talk candidly about feelings. Discovering that the other person is experiencing the same emotions can be reassuring.

- Seek help through counseling and support groups.

- Turn to prayer and other forms of spiritual expression, if desired.

- Practice a relaxation technique to calm down during times of stress. One example: Close your eyes and breathe deeply. Concentrate on relaxing a single body part at a time, working your way from your toes to your head. While breathing, imagine yourself in a relaxing setting, like on a beach at sunrise.

Don't . . .

- Keep feelings inside.

- Force your loved one to talk if she isn't ready.

- Blame yourself for being fearful or anxious. Instead, identify the source of your emotions and talk about it. The same goes for your loved one.

- Try to reason with your loved one if fear or anxiety is extreme. Instead, talk with her physician about medications, counseling, and other kinds of assistance.

EXPERT OPINION

"I think that an important piece of caregiving is empowering patients to make their own decisions. That's something that I do personally. I see my responsibility as educating people, regardless of their backgrounds, in a way that enables them to understand their situation well enough to make their own decisions for themselves. That way, patients are more likely to adhere to whatever treatment outline the two of us have decided upon."

—**JEFF MEYERS, M.D.**, medical director of the AIDS Healthcare Foundation in Sherman Oaks, California

To figure out what's best for your loved one, you need to talk directly with him. Ask how he feels about all of the information that can bombard a cancer patient. Find out if he has concerns that haven't been addressed by his physician.

Likewise, you need to speak frankly with the doctor about her manner of communicating with your loved one. Encourage your loved one to express his thoughts about the sorts of information he wants to know. And be careful about consulting the doctor in private conferences. Your loved one may feel left out, even though he is the patient.

Interestingly, many cancer patients say their most distressing interactions involve not their physicians but their family and friends. Some people try too hard to make a connection and inadvertently belittle the situation ("I know how you feel . . . my son just had chicken pox, and it was scary"). Others avoid mentioning the C word altogether. As a caregiver, you can subtly coach well-meaning relatives and friends in their conversations, remaining respectful of their good intentions while shielding your loved one from unintended distress.

After the Diagnosis

For most newly diagnosed cancer patients, the most urgent issue is choosing an appropriate course of treatment. Understandably, they want to rid their bodies of the disease as quickly as possible. Yet many experts recommend taking time to explore all the available treatment options before making any decisions. Cancer patients who do this frequently report that they feel greater peace of mind with their chosen treatment plans.

Some patients want to try every drug and procedure possible. Others prefer to use less invasive holistic measures. As a caregiver, you can help your loved one sort through the options and settle on an approach that feels right for him.

That's only the beginning of your involvement in your loved one's treatment. If he is using chemotherapy, for example, you can keep tabs on side effects to make sure they're being managed as well as possible. The same is true for pain. Actually, you and your loved one might want to establish a sort of rating system in which the person assesses his pain on a scale of 0 (no pain) to 10 (intolerable pain). Based on this information, the two of you can work with a doctor to set up a medication schedule that provides maximum relief.

Besides pain, many cancer patients struggle with fatigue. And often it goes untreated, perhaps because it's perceived as tolerable when compared with other side effects. But it shouldn't be ignored, especially since it compromises a person's ability to enjoy life. Being a caregiver puts you in the position to monitor your loved one's energy level and to raise any concerns about it during doctor visits.

Also be aware that many cancer patients become depressed after completing their course of treatment, even when it's successful. Experts attribute this phenomenon to a sense of loss, as the patients are no longer preoccupied with beating a disease. Depression can affect care recipients and caregivers alike. Both you and your loved one may need additional support or counseling to get through this difficult time. (You'll find more strategies for treating depression in chapters 12 and 26.)

Take Action... LIVE WELL WITH CANCER

Self-care is a critical component of any cancer treatment plan. It keeps the body and mind strong, so they're better able to tolerate powerful cancer medicines and withstand the effects of the disease. Among the lifestyle strategies recommended for cancer patients:

✗ Get as much exercise as possible. Even if your loved one is confined to bed, he can sit up in a chair for meals or walk to the bathroom (with assistance, if necessary). One man with colon cancer did leg stretches and other exercises while standing up to read his e-mails. Any physical movement is beneficial. Keep in mind, though, that no exercise should cause pain.

✗ Stick with a regular meal schedule. Nutritious foods are best, but ice cream and other favorite snacks are okay, too—as long as they're enjoyed in moderation. The goal is to ensure that your loved one is getting enough calories and nutrients.

✗ Drink plenty of fluids. This helps prevent dehydration and improve energy levels.

✗ Maintain a record of bowel habits to detect any unusual

FOR MORE INFORMATION

The American Cancer Society sponsors support groups for cancer patients and their families. For more information, check with your local chapter or visit the American Cancer Society Web site at **www.cancer.org**. The site features message boards and live chats, for those who feel more comfortable with online support.

Another good resource is the National Cancer Institute Web site, **www.cancer.gov**. It provides general information about cancer resources, including support groups and services, along with the latest news in cancer research. Its toll-free hot line is **(800) 422-6237**.

and persistent changes. They can provide valuable clues in some cancers.

✗ Keep up with grooming and hygiene, including dental care. You want your loved one to feel good about himself; it's vital to his well-being. If he is confined to bed, perhaps someone can come to give him a shave or a haircut.

✗ Indulge in some pampering. Your loved one might enjoy a manicure or pedicure, or even a massage. Any "treat" that's relaxing and rejuvenating can lift the person's spirits.

DIGESTIVE PROBLEMS

The digestive system doesn't change with age. But older people do experience more digestive problems, most likely because food doesn't pass through the body as quickly as it used to. This slowdown can result from taking certain medications, getting less physical activity, eating more processed, low-fiber foods—or a combination of all three.

Among the most common digestive conditions—especially in older people—are constipation, heartburn, irritable bowel syndrome, and ulcers. At the very least, an untreated digestive ailment can affect quality of life. At worst, it can set the stage for a serious medical crisis, including infection or inflammation of the liver, gallbladder, or pancreas. That's why caregivers should closely monitor their loved ones for signs of digestive distress. Any of the following is reason to see a doctor as soon as possible.

- Stomach pains that are severe, long lasting, recurring, or accompanied by chills and clammy skin

- Recurrent vomiting and/or blood in the vomit

- A change in stool or bowel habits that lasts for more than 3 days, including constipation and diarrhea

- Diarrhea that keeps the person awake at night

- Dark, tea-colored urine

- Yellowing of the eyes or skin

- Painful or difficult swallowing of food

- Loss of appetite or unexplained weight loss

FOR MORE INFORMATION

Among the best sources of information about digestive disorders is the National Digestive Diseases Information Clearinghouse. Call **(301) 654-3810** or write to 2 Information Way, Bethesda, MD 20892-3570.

Online, visit the American College of Gastroenterology Web site, **www.acg.gi.org**, and the federal government site, **www.healthfinder.gov**. Both can direct you to research and resources for specific digestive ailments.

Beyond watching for these symptoms, you can help your loved one make lifestyle adjustments to delay the development or progression of digestive problems. As might be expected, many of the recommended changes target a person's eating habits. Let's look at each condition in turn.

Constipation

Although constipation is quite common, it remains a source of confusion. For starters, it's not a disease but rather a symptom. Of course, the distinction probably won't matter much to someone who is experiencing difficult and painful bowel movements.

Furthermore, a person isn't necessarily constipated just because she doesn't pass stool every day. According to geriatrics experts, many older people believe they should be having bowel movements like clockwork. In fact, the digestive tract may empty less frequently with age.

To add to the confusion, doctors cannot always pinpoint why a person has constipation. Not eating enough fiber or drinking enough water can cause a problem. So can misusing or overusing laxatives, which sometimes creates a dependency that prevents the body from stimulating bowel movements on its own. Other drugs that could cause constipation include antidepressants, antihistamines, antacids, diuretics, and medicines for Parkinson's disease.

Depending on the severity of a person's constipation, treatment options range from simple lifestyle changes to surgical procedures that eliminate intestinal blockages. In your loved one's case, the following measures may do the trick.

- Don't ignore the urge to have a bowel movement. Some people put off going to the bathroom for hours, especially if they're away from home. In the long run, this practice can worsen constipation.

- Eat plenty of fiber-rich foods. The best sources include fresh fruits and vegetables (served raw or cooked), as well as whole grains. Dried fruits such as apricots, prunes, and figs also supply lots of fiber.

- Add small amounts of unprocessed miller's bran to baked goods and cereals. Experiment to figure out how much your loved one can tolerate. Some people experience significant bloating and gas when they add bran to their diets.

Is It Really Constipation?

To help determine whether your loved one is truly constipated, answer these four questions. Even one "yes" response suggests a possible problem.

- Does the person have fewer than three bowel movements in a week?
- Does the person struggle to pass stool?
- Does the person experience pain during bowel movements?
- Does the person have any other problems, such as bleeding during bowel movements?

Outlook

"In the first half of the 21st century, demography and technology will radically change the landscape of caregiving in the United States. Healthier and more engaged baby boomers, and their children, will be reluctant to withdraw from the workforce to assume the full burden of family caregiving. Their demands will reshape the ways in which care is provided to elders, in the same way the baby boomers reshaped aspects of society in the 1960s and 1970s.

"Aided by technologies that we are just beginning to glimpse, caregivers will be empowered to find the resources they need to continue to be active members of society while providing for the needs of their loved ones. These same forces—boomers' demands and technological advances—will drive a redesign of the formal care system so that it's much more responsive to consumer needs."

—**GLORIA CAVANAUGH,** president and chief executive officer of the American Society on Aging, based in San Francisco

Note: If your loved one has heart or kidney problems, check with his doctor before trying miller's bran.

- Drink lots of water, at least eight 8-ounce glasses per day. But go easy on milk; in some people, drinking large quantities contributes to constipation.

- Engage in regular exercise. Walking is an excellent choice, because it's convenient and very low impact. But any physical activity helps.

Heartburn

Chronic heartburn, also known as gastroesophageal reflux disease (GERD), occurs when stomach acid flows backward into the esophagus. This produces a burning sensation behind the breastbone and, in some people, a sour or bitter taste at the back of the throat. A flare-up of heartburn can last for up to 2 hours and is made worse by eating food.

More than 60 million Americans say they experience heartburn at least once a month. For another 15 million, it occurs daily. The condition seems to affect a disproportionate number of elderly people (though pregnant women are also very vulnerable).

As chronic heartburn worsens, so can its symptoms. People with GERD have reported a sensation of food being trapped behind the breastbone, bloody vomit, tarry or black bowel movements, and a sensation of choking that may cause shortness of breath, coughing, or a hoarse voice. The condition also has serious complications, including narrowing of the esophagus and the onset of Barrett's esophagus (a premalignant disorder).

To treat chronic heartburn, many doctors recommend a combination of lifestyle changes and over-the-counter remedies. Among their suggested strategies:

- Avoid foods and beverages that could trigger a flare-up. They include alcoholic beverages, coffee, chocolate, peppermint, tomato products, and anything spicy or greasy.

- Refrain from eating within 2 or 3 hours of lying down or going to bed.

- Maintain a healthy weight.

- Give up smoking.

For short-term relief, your loved one may want to try antacids or H2 blockers (such as Pepcid AC or Zantac 75), some of which are available without a prescription. If the person must use these medications more than twice a week, she needs to see a doctor.

Ulcers

An ulcer is an area of the stomach or small intestine that has been damaged by stomach acid and digestive juices. Even though most ulcers get no bigger than a pencil eraser, they still cause significant pain.

Ulcers come in two basic forms. Duodenal ulcers, located in the small intestine, most often occur in people ages 30 to 50. Stomach ulcers are more common in the over-60 population.

In many cases, the primary symptom of an ulcer is a gnawing or burning pain somewhere between the bottom of the breastbone and the navel. The pain tends to occur between meals and can disturb nighttime sleep as well. A flare-up can last for min-

---

Health Care Timetable

Regular doctor visits are vital to your loved one's well-being, especially as he gets older. Many of the chronic conditions commonly associated with aging can be caught early, and even prevented, through routine screenings and immunization. As part of your medical record-keeping, you'll want to schedule appointments with your loved one's primary care physician for the following:

Frequency	Immunization/Screening
Monthly	Blood pressure screening. Readings consistently above 140/90 are considered a risk factor for heart disease and stroke.
	Skin exam, checking for any suspicious-looking moles or sores that may be signs of skin cancer
Yearly	Complete physical exam with a head-to-toe skin cancer screening and colon cancer screening, including stool tests
	Flu shot in the fall
Every 5 years	Examination of the rectum and lower colon for colon cancer
Every 10 years	Tetanus-diphtheria booster shot
By age 65	One-time immunization to prevent pneumonia

utes or hours. Other, less frequent symptoms include nausea, vomiting, diminished appetite, and weight loss.

Complications from ulcers can cause bleeding, which over time may lead to fatigue and anemia. A person with an ulcer may vomit blood or pass black or tarry stools. Sometimes bleeding, not pain, is an ulcer's primary symptom.

Left untreated, an ulcer can cause perforations in the intestinal or stomach lining. This allows bacteria, food, and digestive juices to spill into the abdominal cavity, prompting sudden, intense pain that may require hospitalization or surgery. Another possible outcome of an untreated ulcer is chronic inflammation and scarring. The scar tissue can prevent food from leaving the stomach and passing into the intestinal tract, leading to vomiting and weight loss.

The good news is, the majority of ulcers are highly treatable. Among the most significant medical breakthroughs in recent years was the discovery that most ulcers result from a type of bacteria called *Helicobacter pylori*. Between 80 and 90 percent of these ulcers can be healed permanently with antibiotics.

Caregivers should be aware that some ulcers are caused by long-term use of nonsteroidal anti-inflammatory drugs (NSAIDs) such as aspirin, ibuprofen, and naproxen. Your loved one may be taking one of these medicines to treat arthritis or another type of chronic pain. If so, you may want to ask the person's doctor about switching to acetaminophen or a low-dose corticosteroid.

In decades past, physicians told patients that they could avoid ulcers by steering clear of spicy, fatty, or acidic foods. Now doctors know that developing an ulcer has little to do with diet. Still, some foods may aggravate pain and should be avoided. Quitting smoking can also help.

HEART ATTACK

A heart attack occurs when one of the heart's arteries suddenly becomes blocked by a tiny blood clot. Usually, the clot forms inside an artery that has been narrowed by plaque buildup.

Perhaps the best-known sign of a heart attack (also known as a myocardial infarction) is intense, crushing chest pain. The pain tends to concentrate in the center of the chest or just below the center of the rib cage, though it may spread to the arms, neck, lower jaw, or abdomen. Other symptoms may include sudden weakness, sweating, nausea, vomiting, breathlessness, loss of consciousness, palpitations, and confusion. Sometimes the combination of "burning" chest pain, nausea, and vomiting is mistaken for indigestion.

The severity of a heart attack, and the chances of survival, depend primarily on the extent of the blockage and the part of the heart muscle that's affected. Sadly, 15 percent of heart attack patients die before leaving for the hospital. Another 15 percent die before they even get there.

Of course, modern medicine offers greatly advanced technology for identifying people who are at risk for heart attacks. Imaging equipment can detect problems even years in advance, allowing ample time to take preventive action.

The trouble is, relatively few people have shown an interest in getting screened. That's too bad, because for one in four American adults, the first sign of cardiovascular disease is a sudden heart attack resulting in death. An estimated 1.5 million heart attacks occur in the United States every year, taking more than 450,000 lives.

You can help change these statistics—and protect your loved one against a first heart attack—by being aware of the risk factors. Among those identified by the American Heart Association are high total cholesterol, low HDL cholesterol (the beneficial kind), high blood pressure, diabetes, obesity, lack of physical activity, smoking, and family medical history. The presence of even one of these factors means your loved one should be making lifestyle changes to reduce his risk.

Mending a Broken Heart

If your loved one has already experienced a heart attack, your focus as a caregiver is on preventing a recurrence. The person may need some convincing that she can improve her heart health, even though it has taken a beating. If she won't listen to you, she may heed her cardiologist. Most have seen their fair share of repeat patients, and they would love to reverse the trend.

Any good cardiac rehabilitation program will include strategies for controlling heart disease risk factors such as high cholesterol, high blood pressure, diabetes, and obesity. All of these risk factors can be reduced with regular exercise and a proper diet. Random-

Surviving a Heart Attack

With heart attacks, as with so many health matters, prevention is the best medicine. But aspirin might run a close second. It can greatly improve a person's odds of survival by preventing further clotting.

The next time your loved one sees his doctor, you may want to ask whether an aspirin would help in the event of a heart attack. Then you're prepared in case the need arises. One caveat: The aspirin must be chewed slowly, not swallowed whole.

You can also plan ahead by making a list of all the medications your loved one is taking. This information is vital to emergency room physicians, who need to make a fast decision on the best course of treatment.

If your loved one ever experiences chest pain, take it seriously—even if he says it's no big deal. Drive him to the emergency room, or better yet, call for an ambulance.

FOR MORE INFORMATION

The American Heart Association provides a wealth of resources and support services for people with heart disease and their families. Your best bet is to contact the chapter that serves your area. You can also call the organization's national offices at **(800) 242-8721** or visit the Web site at **www. americanheart.org**.

ized clinical trials show that physical activity, in particular, significantly increases the rate of heart attack survival. Quitting smoking also boosts the odds of surviving a heart attack, as well as avoiding a recurrence.

An increasing number of cardiac rehabilitation programs are putting greater emphasis on emotional support for participants. Pioneering cardiologist Dean Ornish, M.D., believes the support segment of his holistic program to reverse heart disease is vital to the successful outcomes that have been published in major medical journals.

But as Dr. Ornish and other heart experts point out, the effectiveness of any cardiac rehabilitation program is in direct proportion to the willingness of a participant to stick with it. Caregivers must embrace this principle and find ways to help their loved ones feel "ownership" for the outcomes they experience.

Another important task for the caregiver is to keep tabs on any medicines that may have been prescribed to reduce the risk of another heart attack. Make sure they're taken as directed, and watch for any serious side effects. As your loved one's heart health improves, ask her doctor whether she needs to change medications or adjust her dosage.

HIV AND AIDS

Perhaps the best place to begin any discussion of HIV and AIDS is with a translation of the abbreviations. HIV stands for human immunodeficiency virus; infection with the virus can lead to AIDS, or acquired immunodeficiency syndrome.

When a person has AIDS, the body's immune system breaks down and becomes unable to fight off other infections and illnesses. Some people infected with HIV develop full-blown AIDS rather quickly. Others don't have symptoms for 10 to 12 years, or even longer.

Scientists have yet to find a cure for AIDS, or a vaccine to prevent it. New drug protocols are helping many people with HIV and AIDS live longer. But the medications are not problem-free. In fact, they can be highly toxic, causing osteoporosis, heart damage, and kidney failure.

The unpleasant, sometimes serious side effects, along with the complex daily dose regimens, often convince patients to skip their medicines. But this can seriously undermine treatment. In the absence of the necessary dose, HIV cells seize the opportunity to produce new strains of the virus that are resistant to medications.

In fact, even if a person follows his daily dose regimen, HIV can rapidly mutate into new drug-resistant strains. Still, doctors and researchers are more optimistic than ever about finding effective treatments that enable people with HIV and AIDS to live longer and better.

The past 10 years have produced a number of medications that effectively slow down HIV and treat the opportunistic infections associated with AIDS. You and your loved one must work with a physician to figure out which drug regimen makes the most sense for your loved one's circumstances. Here's a rundown of the leading treatments for preventing HIV from reproducing and destroying the body's immune system.

Reverse transcriptase inhibitors. These drugs work by attacking an HIV enzyme called reverse transcriptase. The category includes abacavir, delavirdine, didanosine (ddI), efavirenz, lamivudine (3TC), nevirapine, stavudine (d4T), zalcitabine (ddC), and zidovudine.

Protease inhibitors. These medicines target another HIV enzyme, called protease. Examples of protease inhibitors include amprenavir, indinavir, nelfinavir, ritonavir, and saquinavir. The dosage and side effects of each drug vary from one person to the next.

Highly active antiretroviral therapy (HAART). Many people with HIV take inhibitor-type drugs in combination with this medicinal "cocktail." When successful, HAART can drop HIV cells to practically undetectable levels while elevating the body's CD4 immune cells to normal levels. (In healthy people, CD4 counts range from 450 to 1,200 per cubic millimeter. In a person with AIDS, the count drops below 200.)

Take Action... ANTICIPATE SPECIAL NEEDS

Coordinating multiple medications and dose schedules is one of the many challenging tasks facing caregivers whose loved ones have HIV or full-blown AIDS. Indeed, these conditions present

EXPERT OPINION

"There is a mentality that [an HIV diagnosis] is a death sentence, which is no longer the case with adequate health care. In fact, people who are HIV positive can effectively manage it as a treatable chronic disease, which allows them to leave behind the role of care recipient. It's difficult, though, for people who have begun to prepare themselves for chronic care-receiving to return to being more active members of society. It's a new challenge that we're facing in HIV treatment."

—**JEFF MEYERS, M.D.,** medical director of the AIDS Healthcare Foundation in Sherman Oaks, California

FOR MORE INFORMATION

The federal government provides information and assistance to people with HIV/AIDS and their families through the National AIDS Clearinghouse. You can visit the organization's Web site at **www.cdcnpin.org**.

such a unique set of care requirements that many experts advise prospective caregivers to take a course in home care. To find one in your area, check with the state health department or the local chapters of HIV/AIDS support organizations.

In addition, the U.S. Department of Health and Human Services offers these helpful guidelines for HIV/AIDS care.

- Talk with your loved one constantly. This is the best way to understand his needs.

- Work with your loved one and his team of health professionals to develop and implement a plan for care.

- Request written instructions for medications and other treatments. Make sure you're clear on dosages and possible side effects. Pharmacists can help with this information.

- Keep a written record of your loved one's symptoms and health status. Ask the person to provide input, if he's able.

- Bring any changes in your loved one's health or behavior to his physician's attention. Symptoms such as coughing, fever, diarrhea, and confusion may require immediate care.

MEMORY LOSS, ALZHEIMER'S DISEASE, AND DEMENTIA

Anyone who is caring for a parent or elderly relative harbors some concerns about Alzheimer's disease. It's easy to understand why. After all, many older people show signs of memory loss, which can be an early indicator of Alzheimer's. And the statistics seem to support the belief that the longer a person lives, the more likely he is to develop the disease. In fact, the number of Alzheimer's cases is expected to triple in the next 50 years if no effective cure or preventive is found.

While the prospect of Alzheimer's may worry caregivers, it's downright frightening to care recipients. That's why they may be reluctant to get tested for the disease, or to tell anyone that they're struggling with certain tasks.

Alzheimer's is a progressive, degenerative disease that attacks the brain and impairs memory, thinking, and behavior. It is the most common form of dementia, which physicians define as a loss of intellectual function so severe that it interferes with a person's day-to-day routine.

In the United States, Alzheimer's is the fourth leading cause of death, after heart disease, cancer, and stroke. The time from onset of symptoms until death can range from 3 to 20 years, though the average is 8 years. Age and family history are the most documented risk factors.

The majority of people diagnosed with Alzheimer's are in the 65-and-over population; by some estimates, almost half of all people age 85 and older have the disease. It affects roughly equal numbers of men and women. Symptoms include gradual memory loss, reduced ability to perform daily tasks, disorientation, difficulty learning, loss of language skills, impaired judgment, and personality changes. Over time, a person with Alzheimer's becomes completely unable to care for herself.

The problem with many of these symptoms is that they could indicate something else gone awry, such as an underactive or overactive thyroid, a nutrient deficiency, or depression. As a result, caregivers and care recipients alike may worry more than necessary—or may not catch on soon enough. Many physicians who specialize in geriatrics contend that even when family members suspect a loved one has Alzheimer's, they allow too much time to pass between observing symptoms and seeking professional help.

Part of the problem may be that symptoms such as forgetfulness and poor judgment develop slowly. Gradual but progressive damage to the brain may not become evident until a highly stressful event, such as the death of a relative or the onset of another health problem.

Then, too, family members may mistakenly attribute a loved one's behavioral changes to old age. But an automobile mishap caused by disorientation behind the wheel, or repeated late notices on unpaid utility bills, should never be ignored.

Early Detection Is Key

While a diagnosis of Alzheimer's disease is never welcomed, the sooner the condition is caught, the more effective treatment will be. Just 15 years ago, doctors might have acquiesced to a caregiver's wishes not to inform a loved one of his condition. But

Outlook

"Studies suggest that between 35 and 45 percent of people age 85 and older are likely to have dementia. If that's true, and if most people can live past 85, we're talking about a huge potential burden in the future. Until scientists find a preventive or cure for dementia, the kind of four-part support proven effective here at NYU—which includes individual counseling, family counseling, support groups, and the availability of a counselor as needed—can be extremely helpful to family caregivers and their relatives with dementia. How these services would be paid for under the current medical system isn't clear, however."

—MARY MITTELMAN, DR.P.H.,
director of the caregiver research program of the Silberstein Institute for Aging and Dementia of the New York University School of Medicine

that was when Alzheimer's was hardly understood, and no viable treatment options existed.

These days, certain therapies can slow the progress of Alzheimer's and help sustain mental function for longer periods. But these treatments aren't as effective in advanced cases, observes Mark S. Lachs, M.D., M.P.H., chief of geriatrics and gerontology at New York Hospital in Manhattan and faculty scholar for the American Federation for Aging Research. For example, donepezil and vitamin E therapy work best in the early stages of the disease, before too many brain cells have been destroyed. Other govern-

Is It Alzheimer's?

Many of the symptoms of Alzheimer's disease can mimic those of other health problems. To assess whether your loved one has Alzheimer's or something else, the Alzheimer's Association recommends paying attention for these 10 warning signs.

Memory loss. Forgetting appointments, names, and telephone numbers is normal. People with Alzheimer's forget such things more often—and they can't recall them later.

Difficulty performing familiar tasks. Someone with Alzheimer's will struggle to complete a once-easy task, such as cooking dinner or playing a favorite game.

Problems with language. A person with Alzheimer's forgets simple words or substitutes unusual ones. His speech and writing can be hard to understand.

Disorientation in time and place. People with Alzheimer's can become lost in their own neighborhoods, or forget where they are and how they got there.

Poor judgment. Someone with Alzheimer's might wear three layers of clothing on a hot summer day, or a sleeveless shirt in the middle of winter. Worse, the person can lose perspective on money, paying large sums to telemarketers or home care contractors.

Problems with abstract thinking. Everyone struggles to balance a checkbook now and then. People with Alzheimer's completely forget what the numbers mean and how they're calculated.

Misplacing things. While anyone might misplace car keys or a wallet, a person with Alzheimer's stores household items in bizarre places—an iron in the freezer, a sandwich under the sofa, a wristwatch in the fruit bowl.

Changes in mood or behavior. Someone with Alzheimer's experiences rapid mood swings, going from calm to tears to anger within a matter of minutes, and for no apparent reason.

Changes in personality. People with Alzheimer's can become confused, suspicious, fearful, or completely dependent on another family member.

Loss of initiative. A person with Alzheimer's can become extremely passive, sitting in front of the television for hours or sleeping more than usual. He may not want to engage in activities he once found pleasurable.

ment-approved Alzheimer's medications include tacrine, rivastig-mine, and galantamine.

Besides providing a jump start on treatment and support, early detection of Alzheimer's allows your loved one to make his own decisions about end-of-life care. Once the disease is in its advanced stages, this sort of decision-making becomes virtually impossible. What's more, your loved one may have an opportunity to participate in studies of experimental Alzheimer's treatments. This field of research is booming. And of course, a screening may show that your loved one's symptoms are caused by something other than Alzheimer's.

Taking the early detection argument one step further, some researchers have suggested that the best preventive measure for Alzheimer's is genetic testing, followed by treatment for anyone who gets a positive result, regardless of whether the person displays symptoms.

Right now, no single clinical test exists for diagnosing Alzheimer's. The best a doctor can do is a comprehensive medical exam, consisting of a complete health history, a physical evaluation, blood and urine tests, and neurological and mental status assessments. The mental health testing can last for hours; it might need to be done over the course of several doctor visits. Some newer technology does allow for more sophisticated tracking of brain cells.

After going through the exam, your loved one may get a diagnosis of "probable" or "possible" Alzheimer's. (Only an autopsy can prove "definite" Alzheimer's.) "Probable" means the physician has ruled out all other conditions that might be causing dementia. "Possible" means Alzheimer's is the primary cause, but another health problem may be influencing the disease's progression.

Take Action... AIM FOR CLEAR COMMUNICATION

In caring for a loved one with Alzheimer's, perhaps one of the greatest challenges is adjusting to the person's level of function. You may become frustrated when he doesn't listen or follow instructions. In fact, he probably wants to do those things, but he's just not able. His brain's communication centers won't allow it.

EXPERT OPINION

"In dementia, changes happen continuously over time as the person declines. So first the caregiver must come to terms with the disease, and the fact that it's really happening. Then she can begin to learn about it—understand the symptoms, identify the support she and other family members can provide, find out about available resources. As changes occur and more problems arise, the caregiver is always adjusting, always learning."

—**MELITTA MADDOX,** clinical nurse specialist at the Veterans Administration Geriatric Research, Education, and Clinical Center in Minneapolis

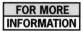

FOR MORE INFORMATION

The Alzheimer's Association has a 24-hour "hotline" for Alzheimer's information, services, and support. Call **(800) 272-3900**. The organization's Web site, **www.alz.org**, is also an excellent resource.

Of course, effective communication is critical to a caregiving relationship. These tips might help improve the process, even as Alzheimer's progresses.

X When talking with your loved one, turn down the radio or television and eliminate any other distracting background noise.

X Be concise. If your message is long-winded or filled with too many details, your loved one might zero in on one minor point rather than hearing the important information.

X Listen for and address the person's feelings. Don't argue over small details (which may seem big to your loved one) or make light of insecurities. Keep the exchange positive.

X Avoid information overload. Even a long restaurant menu can seem overwhelming to your loved one.

X Use written notes. Some people who have trouble with short-term memory retain good writing and reading skills.

X Communicate through touch. A gentle hug or hand squeeze can say more than words ever could. Besides, research shows that stimulating the senses helps keep the brain active.

Putting the Day on Paper

We tend to take our daily routines for granted. But for a person with Alzheimer's, even the most ordinary tasks can present a challenge. Creating a daily to-do list provides a sense of structure, which helps your loved one function at his best. Ideally, the items in the list should focus on enjoyment rather than achievement. Here's a sample suggested by the Alzheimer's Association.

Morning

- Bathe, brush teeth, and get dressed
- Prepare and eat breakfast
- Discuss the newspaper or reminisce about old photos

Afternoon

- Prepare and eat lunch; clear and wash the dishes
- Read the mail
- Listen to music or do a crossword puzzle

Evening

- Prepare and eat dinner; allow time for meaningful conversation
- Play cards or watch a movie
- Read a book or magazine

✗ Try not to take your loved one's words and actions personally. Extremes in emotion reflect your loved one's disease, not his heart or mind.

✗ If you're feeling frustrated, count to 10. Showing your anger can agitate your loved one even more.

OSTEOPOROSIS

The word *osteoporosis* means "porous bone." True to this translation, the disease is characterized by accelerated bone loss.

The human body builds bone up to about age 35. Then it begins losing bone mass at the rate of about 1 percent each year, though regular exercise and proper diet can help offset the decline. Women who've gone through menopause and men age 65 and older experience even more rapid bone loss.

If not detected and treated, osteoporosis can make bones increasingly fragile. Eventually, a person with the disease may suffer a fracture—typically in the wrist, hip, or spine. Hip and spinal fractures are particularly worrisome because they may require hospitalization, surgery, and a long recovery process with a little too much pain mixed in. Even with treatment, these kinds of fractures can lead to prolonged or permanent disability or, in the worst case, death.

The trouble with osteoporosis is that it produces no outward symptoms, so unless a person undergoes bone density testing or suffers a fracture, the disease can remain undetected. A woman might go to the doctor with severe back pain that she thinks was caused by overzealous housecleaning, only to find out that one of her vertebrae has collapsed.

An estimated 10 million Americans have osteoporosis. Another 18 million have low bone mass, which makes them more vulnerable to complications from the disease. In terms of risk factors, gender ranks near the top of the list; women account for about 80 percent of osteoporosis cases. Other indicators of increased risk include a petite or thin frame, advanced age, family history, smoking, excessive alcohol use, long-term corticosteroid therapy, and a low-calcium diet.

The National Osteoporosis Foundation recommends bone density testing for every woman age 65 and older, as well as

FOR MORE INFORMATION

The National Osteoporosis Foundation specializes in osteoporosis research and outreach. To learn more about the organization's services, call **(202) 223-2226** or visit the Web site at **www.nof.org**.

for women under 65 who've suffered bone fractures. Among men, anyone who has had a fracture should get tested, regardless of age.

If your loved one fits into one of these categories but has yet to undergo testing, you definitely should try to persuade her to consult her doctor. At the very least, the test results provide a baseline for monitoring the person's future bone health. And if they do show signs of osteoporosis, catching the disease early means your loved one could begin treatment now, before she experiences a fracture.

The preferred method of bone density testing uses technology called DEXA, or dual energy x-ray absorptiometry. It is relatively fast and harmless. Newer handheld devices—one is a sort of wand that's waved over the person's heel—produce even faster results, but their accuracy compared with DEXA is still under evaluation.

Caregiving around the World

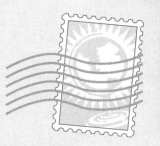

In some Finnish municipalities, children's day care and short-term care for older people are provided on the same premises. In addition to traditional service centers and day care centers, municipalities and parishes run interest clubs, called granny chambers, which keep seniors active and reinforce their social networks.

POST CARD

FROM FINLAND

Pills That Protect Bones

While researchers have yet to find a cure for osteoporosis, the U.S. Food and Drug Administration has approved certain medications to treat and even prevent the disease. Hormone replacement therapy is a common if controversial treatment for women, while a drug called alendronate is available for both women and men. Another medicine, teriparatide (sold under the brand name Forteo), just recently went on the market. It's administered via injection, similar to the insulin prescribed for people with diabetes.

Other new and promising therapies are in the works as well. One study, published in the *New England Journal of Medicine*, made a case for injections of parathyroid hormone, which significantly reduced the risk of fracture. Other treatments under investigation include sodium fluoride, vitamin D metabolites, and a group of drugs known as selective estrogen receptor modulators (SERMs).

Take Action... SUPPORT GOOD BONE HEALTH

Beyond medical treatments, a number of lifestyle strategies can help preserve bone mass, even if your loved one has already been diagnosed with osteoporosis. Here's what experts recommend.

✗ Eat a balanced diet rich in calcium. If your loved one doesn't like milk, try low-fat cheese and yogurt. You can also add powdered milk to gravies, shakes, puddings, and other recipes. Nondairy sources of calcium include broccoli, canned salmon, and kale. Remember that the vitamin C and magnesium in orange juice enhance calcium absorption.

✗ Consider a calcium supplement to make up for any dietary shortfall. Nutritionists recommend that women and men over age 65—the age group most vulnerable to osteoporosis—get a total of 1,500 milligrams of calcium a day.

✗ Spend 5 to 15 minutes in bright sunshine every day. This enables the body to manufacture a sufficient supply of vitamin D, which also enhances calcium absorption.

Strike Back against Stroke

To increase your loved one's chances of surviving a stroke, the American Stroke Association recommends following its four-step Chain of Survival.

- Recognize the warning signs and note the time they first occur. Call 911 immediately. Tell the operator that your loved one is experiencing stroke symptoms and that you need an ambulance.

- Obtain early assessments and prehospital care from ambulance personnel.

- Have ambulance personnel transport your loved one to the hospital. They can notify the emergency room that they're on their way.

- Make sure the emergency room personnel provide rapid diagnosis and treatment. A properly staffed and equipped hospital can evaluate medical data promptly and begin treatment to restore bloodflow to the brain.

✗ Engage in weight-bearing exercise such as walking or strength training with light dumbbells. Even pushing up out of a chair is helpful.

✗ Steer clear of bone-harming habits like smoking and excessive alcohol intake.

✗ Avoid consuming large quantities of cola and salt. The former increases calcium excretion in the urine, while the latter can block calcium recovery in the kidneys.

STROKE

Some experts believe that if strokes were referred to as brain attacks, which they feel is a more accurate description, people would better understand the devastating effects of these catastrophic medical events. In the United States, stroke is a leading cause of long-term disability and the third most common cause of death, behind heart disease and cancer. About 600,000 Americans have strokes each year.

The word *stroke* refers to a loss or impairment of body function caused by insufficient bloodflow to the brain. To operate at peak efficiency, the brain needs an adequate blood supply. If the supply is obstructed in any part of the brain—even for a few minutes—the nearby cells are damaged, and the tissue dies.

The region of the brain that is "attacked" determines the type and extent of disability that results. For example, a stroke on the right side of the brain can lead to paralysis on the left side of the body (especially the limbs), as well as vision problems, memory loss, and a change in behavior to a quick, inquisitive style. A stroke on the left side of the brain may paralyze the right side of the body and cause speech and language problems, in addition to memory loss and a change in behavior to a slow, cautious style. Speech problems can range from trouble finding the right words to a total inability to speak. Some stroke victims have difficulty understanding what others are saying. Others lose their reading, writing, and math skills.

Once in progress, a stroke can't be stopped. Still, in terms of medical treatment, time is of the essence. New clot-busting drugs can successfully minimize or even prevent a stroke's damaging effects if they're administered within the first 3 hours. So every second counts.

The American Stroke Association recommends paying attention for the following warning signs in your loved one. They're your cue to call for an ambulance and get to the hospital as quickly as possible.

- Sudden numbness or weakness in the face, arm, or leg, especially on one side of the body
- Sudden vision trouble affecting one or both eyes
- Sudden difficulty walking
- Sudden dizziness or loss of balance or coordination
- Sudden severe headache with no known cause

Don't wait to see if these symptoms subside. One tragically common mistake is allowing a loved one to try to "sleep them off" when they occur in the middle of the night. Remember, treatment must begin within that critical 3-hour window—and the sooner, the better.

About 10 percent of all strokes are preceded by what are known as transient ischemic attacks (TIAs). They're also known as ministrokes—though in reality, they don't have much in common with full-blown strokes. Their symptoms can be vague; a person who is having a TIA may seem disoriented, confused, or "spaced out."

If your loved one experiences a TIA, it doesn't automatically make him a candidate for a stroke. But it may increase his risk for one. Some statistics indicate that a person who has had at least one TIA is 9½ times more likely to be affected by a stroke than someone of the same age and gender who hasn't had a TIA.

Even though a TIA may not seem as serious as a stroke, it still warrants a visit to the emergency room. Doctors can determine whether your loved one is predisposed to a full-blown stroke and recommend an appropriate plan of care.

Relearning to Live

After a stroke occurs, proper rehabilitation becomes the top priority. Your loved one may need retraining in the most basic tasks, such walking, talking, and eating a meal.

The long-term goal of rehabilitation is to help a stroke survivor

FOR MORE INFORMATION

To learn more about stroke symptoms and recovery, visit the American Stroke Association Web site at **www. strokeassociation.org.**

live independently. The short-term goal is to boost the person's confidence in a full recovery. Skilled physical and occupational therapists specialize in teaching the daily functions; caregivers play a major role in the confidence-building. They can help their loved ones feel less self-conscious about the recovery process.

Rehabilitation begins when a doctor deems a stroke patient medically stable. It can take place in an inpatient or outpatient setting, or even at home, through a home health agency. Caregivers should not shy away from asking their loved ones' doctors, nurses, and therapists—as well as other caregivers and informed friends—for their opinions on what works best.

Keep in mind that every stroke patient is unique. Your loved one may require treatment and support that's beyond the scope of certain rehabilitation programs. Finding care that matches your loved one's needs is absolutely critical to his recovery.

Among the services that may benefit stroke patients are rehabilitation nursing, physical therapy, occupational therapy, recreational therapy, speech-language pathology, audiology, nutritional care, rehabilitation counseling, social work, psychiatry/psychology, chaplaincy, and patient/family education. Some of these services are included in rehabilitation programs, while others are available only through community organizations.

URINARY INCONTINENCE

The loss of bladder control is a sensitive issue for care recipient and caregiver alike. The care recipient may be embarrassed about living at the mercy of a bodily function, while the caregiver may be reluctant to discuss it. But with incontinence more so than with any other condition, open communication can lay the groundwork for improvement in a person's quality of life.

For example, caregivers may be able to convince their loved ones to seek medical care. Roughly 80 percent of people who receive treatment for incontinence report better bladder control. Unfortunately, only about one in five people with the condition actually tell their doctors about it. According to the National Institute on Aging, some patients—as well as some caregivers—may not realize that incontinence is treatable.

At least one in every 10 people age 65 and older has some de-

FOR MORE INFORMATION

The Stroke Family Support Network offers support services to those caring for stroke patients. Call **(888) 478-7653** and ask for the Stroke Family Support Network.

FOR MORE INFORMATION

To learn more about incontinence treatments, contact the National Association for Continence at **(800) 252-3337** or the Simon Foundation for Continence at **(800) 237-4666**.

gree of incontinence, ranging from occasional leakage to regular wetting. Doctors have identified four forms of the condition.

- In *stress incontinence*, urine leakage is triggered by exercise, coughing, sneezing, lifting—any physical movement that puts pressure on the bladder.

- *Urge incontinence* means a person cannot hold urine long enough to reach the toilet. This form often affects people with diabetes, stroke, dementia, Parkinson's disease, or multiple sclerosis. It can also be a warning sign for bladder cancer.

- In *overflow incontinence*, small amounts of urine leak from a bladder that is always full. It's common in older men, who may have blocked urine flow. People with diabetes are also at risk.

- *Functional incontinence* is diagnosed when a person has relatively normal urine flow but can't get to the toilet in time because of arthritis or another disabling condition.

While stress incontinence is considered the most treatable, all four forms can benefit from a doctor's care. Perhaps the most frequently prescribed therapy is Kegels (pronounced KAY-gulls). These exercises involve strengthening the pelvic muscles by contracting and holding them, as if to stop urine flow. Kegels can be performed anywhere, while standing, sitting, or lying down. A 5-minute session two or three times a day can enhance bladder control.

Some doctors recommend biofeedback, which can help a person get a better sense of when her bladder is filling. Another therapy, bladder training, gradually prolongs the time between toilet visits.

Some medications help treat incontinence by relaxing the bladder (if it's overactive) or by tightening the sphincter muscle (if the bladder is underactive). But these drugs can produce side effects such as dry mouth, vision problems, and urine buildup. Surgery may be recommended if a person has a physical problem such as an abnormally positioned bladder or an enlarged prostate.

If treatment for incontinence isn't successful, a caregiver can still help a loved one retain dignity and function. Special absorbent underclothing is no more bulky than underwear and can

The Other Kind of Incontinence

The loss of bowel control, or fecal incontinence, presents a significant challenge in a caregiving situation. A caregiver may get angry or frustrated when a loved one soils himself, but scolding the person will only add to his embarrassment.

If your loved one has fecal incontinence, try to remember that he's not soiling himself intentionally. Sometimes eating a healthful diet—lots of fresh produce and whole grains, plenty of water—can improve bowel habits. Another option is glycerin suppositories, which can stimulate bowel movements 15 to 20 minutes after insertion. To help decide on a course of treatment, keep a written record of your loved one's bowel habits to share with his physician.

be worn comfortably in social settings. Perhaps a less appealing option is a flexible tube known as an indwelling catheter, which collects urine in a container. This technology surely will improve in the years ahead.

In addition, the FDA has approved an injectable collagen implant that adds "bulk" to the tissues around the urethra, helping improve urinary control. To learn more about this treatment, check with a knowledgeable physician.

VISION AND HEARING LOSS

Few things make a person feel older more quickly than a decline in vision or hearing. That may be why so many care recipients are reluctant to admit to any impairment. Then again, they may be worried about losing whatever independence they have left. Either way, their quality of life may suffer needlessly.

As a caregiver, you can help your loved one make lifestyle adjustments to accommodate any vision or hearing loss. But first, you need to figure out that the person is having a problem seeing or hearing. That's where your own sharp senses come into play.

For instance, you may notice that your loved one squints when reading or bumps into objects when walking. She may complain about poor lighting or start wearing mismatched clothes. All of these are clues that your loved one may not be seeing as well as she used to.

A person's vision can deteriorate for various reasons, from ordinary aging of the eye to eye diseases such as cataracts, glaucoma, and macular degeneration. Treatment can help restore vision, or at least slow vision loss. But it must start in the early stages of the disease, which is why getting a diagnosis is so critical.

For hearing loss, the most familiar treatment is a hearing aid— a device your loved one may balk at wearing. But new hearing aid technology can greatly improve hearing without causing too much self-consciousness on your loved one's part. Implants and surgery may also be options, depending on your loved one's situation.

How can you tell if your loved one is becoming hard of hearing? She may complain about people mumbling or about hearing hissing or ringing sounds. She might also respond inap-

FOR MORE INFORMATION

The National Center for Vision and Aging, operated by The Lighthouse International, provides information and support for those with vision loss. Call **(800) 334-5497** or visit the Web site at **www.lighthouse.org.**

FOR MORE INFORMATION

You can find out more about treatments and support services for hearing loss by contacting the International Hearing Society. Call **(800) 521-5247** or visit the Web site at **www. pitt.edu/~uclid/ihs.htm.**

propriately to questions or have difficulty following a conversation.

Take Action... ACCOMMODATE CHANGES IN YOUR LOVED ONE'S VISION

For a person with vision loss, the goal of care is twofold: first, to maintain a comfortable and familiar living environment; and second, to promote independence. The following strategies can help on both counts.

✗ Refrain from assisting with daily tasks your loved one can manage alone.

✗ Stand directly in front of your loved one when speaking to him.

✗ Keep your voice at a normal level, unless your loved one also has a hearing problem.

✗ Always announce your entrance or exit from a room.

✗ Decide together if you plan to move furniture or other household items.

✗ Keep furniture away from main traffic paths around the house.

✗ Decorate with contrasting colors, especially around doors, stairways, light switches, and electrical outlets.

✗ Adjust the blinds to allow for a maximum amount of natural light.

✗ Install enough indoor lighting to provide even and bright distribution.

✗ Remove any loose or uneven walking surfaces, as well as any wiring that stretches across the floor.

✗ Be consistent about keeping doors open or closed.

✗ Encourage your loved one to ask for help when necessary.

✗ Schedule regular checkups with an optometrist or ophthalmologist.

✗ Scout around for rehabilitation programs that target vision loss.

Take Action... HELP YOUR LOVED ONE HEAR BETTER

Hearing loss can impede your ability to communicate effectively with your loved one. To overcome any potential problems, try these tips.

✗ Stand in a spot that has good lighting, so the person can see your face.

✗ Face the person and speak clearly.

✗ Minimize background noise. Turn off the TV or radio, if necessary.

✗ Don't talk too fast or too slow.

✗ Do not cover your mouth, eat, or chew gum while talking.

✗ If the person doesn't understand a statement, try rewording it.

✗ If the person has a hearing aid, encourage her to wear it regularly. And remind her to make adjustments—for example, when she's in a restaurant with a lot of background noise.

✗ Be patient and positive in your conversations. It always pays off.

CHAPTER 15

WHEN DRUGS DON'T MIX

What You Need to Know

- A leading reason for nursing-home placement is improper management of medicines. When people confuse or miss doses, they may experience adverse reactions that their families may misinterpret as symptoms of illness.

- The elderly are especially vulnerable to interactions and side effects. As the body ages, it stores medicines more readily but doesn't break them down as efficiently.

- Medications can interact with each other as well as with herbs, vitamin and mineral supplements, and other dietary supplements. Maintaining a master list of all your loved one's remedies—pharmaceutical and natural—is essential to managing them effectively.

When people become caregivers, they usually have no idea how many medications their loved ones are taking. And they're astounded when they find out.

Then they face the daunting task of trying to coordinate all the dose schedules. Some drugs must be taken in the morning, others at night; some must be taken with food, others on an empty stomach. It's no wonder care recipients might confuse or miss doses. Anyone could.

Studies indicate that about one-quarter of all residents of nursing homes ended up there because they couldn't manage their drugs. Not that they didn't try; they did. More than likely, they made mistakes that adversely affected their health, and possibly endangered their lives.

"These people can cook, drive, and manage their money," says

Jack Fincham, Ph.D., dean and professor at the University of Kansas School of Pharmacy in Lawrence. "But they get in trouble because they're unable to juggle six, eight, even 10 medications. And so their conditions deteriorate from good to bad."

Then, too, their families—the ones who decide on nursing-home placement—may not recognize the difference between symptoms of a disease and side effects of a medication. Nor are they familiar with drug interactions, when one pill can block or overboost the effects of another.

But the family members are no more at fault than the care recipients themselves are. If anything, the times they live in are to blame. People are living longer than ever, which is wonderful. But as they get older, they're more vulnerable to health problems like high cholesterol, high blood pressure, adult-onset (type 2) diabetes, and osteoarthritis. Doctors attempt to manage these conditions with prescription and over-the-counter drugs. And so medicine cabinets are brimming.

Caregiving around the World

Largely because of China's "one family / one child" rule, the country's fertility rates are declining. The population of China will age faster than any population in history. At the same time, rapid economic growth may weaken traditional caregiving institutions and increase the demand for leisure activities and high-tech health care. In response, one of the many benefits Chinese employers are offering to their valued employees is eldercare.

POST CARD

FROM CHINA

FOR SENIORS, A SERIOUS HEALTH CONCERN

Among all age groups, older people are at highest risk for adverse drug interactions and side effects. One reason is that they take more medications than anyone else. Another is that they see more doctors than anyone else—and all those physicians can write out prescriptions. Unfortunately, those in the medical community don't always communicate with each other to make sure the therapies they're recommending won't have adverse interactions with other therapies the patient has been prescribed. That's why the patient and the caregiver should feel free to ask questions themselves.

Still, the situation is more complicated than monitoring the quantity of pills and coordinating prescriptions between doctors. For starters, older people lose lean muscle mass and gain fat cells over time. Many drugs are designed to be stored in fat tissue. The presence of more fat means the accumulation of more medicine, creating side effects.

What's more, as a person ages, the liver and kidneys become less efficient at breaking down medicine. In other words, the people taking the highest proportion of medications have bodies that can't fully process the drugs' ingredients.

As a caregiver, you can help manage your loved one's medications to maximize their effectiveness while minimizing their side effects and potential for interactions. But first, you must get a handle on the person's pills and dosages. A proactive approach is best. You may need to employ your most savvy skills of persuasion to get as many details as possible. For instance, you might bring up the topic this way: "Mom, I'm planning to see my doctor next week to make sure my blood pressure is okay. I was wondering what kind of blood pressure medicine you're taking." Then gently nudge her to talk about other medications and treatments she's using.

And when your mom goes to the doctor, don't be afraid to ask whether any of her dosages should be adjusted because her body might be storing too much medicine. For her, these sorts of questions might make the difference between independent living and an assisted living facility.

If your loved one eventually requires the level of care provided

Outlook

"Compared with previous generations, baby boomers have fewer children per person, but children are so critical in the provision of support. As a result, the adult children of disabled older people are going to need a lot of help. Already we see older wives caring for their aging husbands; sisters caring for each other; and nephews and nieces, and children of cousins, caring for their families' elders. Sometimes these people don't even identify themselves as caregivers, so helping the general public define who a caregiver is, what the caregiving role is, and where the caregiver can find help would all be big steps."

—ROSE DOBROF, D.S.W., Brookdale professor of gerontology at the Brookdale Center on Aging at Hunter College in New York City by such a facility, you must remain vigilant about her medication regimen even after she's placed. A study in the December 2001 issue of the *Journal of the American Medical Association* reports that 10 percent of residents in assisted living facilities were being given medicines that are rarely prescribed for the elderly—or should never be used by them. This finding reinforces the fact that caregivers need to be proactive in making sure treatments are helping and not harming their loved ones.

Take Action... ROUND UP YOUR LOVED ONE'S REMEDIES

Of all that you'll be asked to do in this chapter, your most important task by far is to put together a comprehensive list of remedies that your loved one is currently using. These tips can help you do the job quickly and easily.

✗ Contact your loved one's doctors and pharmacist for complete records of the prescription drugs your loved one is taking. You might need her written permission to get these records. Once you have them, they should provide a comprehensive picture of your loved one's current prescription program.

✗ With assistance from your loved one and other family members, write down all the over-the-counter drugs the person is using, as well as herbs, vitamin and mineral supplements, and any other dietary supplements.

✗ Ask your loved one whether she has experienced an allergy or bad reaction to any drug. Also find out whether she has been told by a health professional to avoid a particular drug. Knowing what a loved one shouldn't take is just as important as knowing what she is taking.

✗ Check your loved one's medicine cabinet to make sure you've documented everything. Look any place else she might store remedies, too—like in the kitchen.

✗ Compile all the information you've gathered into one "master list." Be sure to update it regularly, as your loved one's treatments change.

Take Action... STAY ON TOP OF THE TREATMENT REGIMEN

Now that you've identified what your loved one is taking, you can turn your attention to "how much," "when," and "how." Coordinating this information can help ensure proper dosing and safeguard against problems. Just follow these guidelines, developed with input from the National Professional Society of Pharmacists.

✗ Identify those health professionals who can answer questions and provide information about the various treatments your loved one is using. Primary care physicians, specialists, and nurses are excellent resources. And of course, don't forget your loved one's pharmacist. He might be the most accessible, though you may need to make an appointment to see him. "And honestly, if he isn't willing to help out, you should find another pharmacist," Dr. Fincham says. If you live near a pharmacy college, that can be a good resource, too.

✗ Schedule a 15-minute consultation with one of these health professionals to go through all of the treatments your loved one is using. Be sure to take your master list—or even better for this appointment, throw all the pill bottles into one big bag. Having one expert scrutinize the entire regimen at once might help zero in on any potential problems right off the bat.

✗ Whenever you talk with a health professional about a particular treatment, be an active listener. Take notes (or, even better, tape record the conversation—with the person's permission, of course). Ask whether he has printed materials he can provide. Repeat any instructions you're given so he knows you've understood.

✗ Ask your loved one's doctor to write the purpose of any medicine on the prescription slip. It can say something simple, like "for high blood pressure" or "for rash." As long as it's on the slip, it will be put on the label. Then the bottle is clearly marked for anyone who helps your loved one with her medications.

✗ Ask your pharmacist to include both the generic and brand names on pill bottles. According to Lana Witt, Pharm.D., a

FOR MORE INFORMATION

The Mayo Clinic maintains an impressive collection of information about prescription and over-the-counter drugs, as well as herbal remedies and nutritional supplements. You can explore their resources online at **www.mayoclinic.com.**

Do You Know Enough about Your Loved One's Meds?

To be truly well-informed about your loved one's treatment regimen, you need to ask the following questions about each prescription and over-the-counter drug, advises Lana Witt, Pharm.D., a pharmacist at Stanford University Hospital. You may want to make extra copies of this checklist, so you can take them with you to the doctor or pharmacist.

Question	Notes	Answer
What is the name of the medication?	Get both the generic and brand names, to avoid confusion.	
How much should be taken?	The doctor determines the proper dose based on your loved one's condition. You need to know the strength of each pill (often in milligrams), the number of pills to be taken at each time, and the frequency with which to take them. If a dosage changes, make sure the doctor informs the pharmacist.	
Why is this medication being prescribed?	This information allows you to monitor whether the drug is serving its purpose, its dose needs to be adjusted, or it's no longer necessary.	
What benefits should be observed?	Knowing what to expect and when helps a great deal. For instance, if the doctor says your loved one's pain should subside over several days, you can follow up if that doesn't happen.	
What side effects may occur?	By finding out what they are, you can take appropriate precautions. For example, if a drug might cause drowsiness, you can make sure your loved one doesn't drive or consume alcohol after taking it.	
How will this medication interact with others?	Asking this question reminds the doctor that your loved one might be taking more than one medicine. A pharmacist can help most in determining whether any over-the-counter drugs, herbs, and supplements might inadvertently affect the medication.	

pharmacist at Stanford University Hospital, using the generic name ensures clear communication between doctors, pharmacists, and other health professionals.

✗ When picking up a prescription for your loved one, read the label before you leave the pharmacy. Also, look at the medicine in the container. Question any changes in size, color, markings, quantity, or dosage. If you are uncertain about the medicine, check with the pharmacist or your loved one's doctor.

✗ Make sure your loved one takes prescription and over-the-counter medications according to their instructions. Ask the pharmacist or doctor what to do in the event of a missed dose.

✗ Throw out any of your loved one's medicines that have become outdated. The expiration date applies only if a drug has been stored properly. Humidity, temperature, light, and even air can negatively affect shelf life and potency.

✗ Keep a written record of each drug's effects, based on your loved one's feedback as well as your own observations. A few notes each day or week is sufficient feedback for an informed next trip to the doctor or pharmacist.

✗ If your loved one experiences any unexpected symptoms or changes, contact the doctor or pharmacist right away. Make sure this information goes in your loved one's medical records, as well as on your own master list.

✗ Purchase a pill organizer that is marked for the purpose of managing medications. Several styles and sizes are available at pharmacies and medical supply stores.

✗ Get a calendar that's big enough for you or your loved one to mark each time she takes each of her medicines. This can help prevent missed doses or "double dosing."

MIXING AND NOT MATCHING

One of the lesser-known dangers of taking multiple medicines is that one pill can inhibit or exaggerate the effects of another. The best way to avoid this problem is to ask questions. Your loved

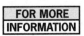

FOR MORE INFORMATION

The American Pharmaceutical Association maintains a Web site with up-to-date information on medication use, including adverse reactions. You can check out the site at **www.pharmacyandyou.org.**

Herbal Alert

With the rise in popularity of alternative therapies, many care recipients are experimenting with herbs and other natural remedies. Sometimes well-meaning family members and friends recommend these treatments. But caregivers need to remember that herbs are plant *medicines*. Like conventional medicines, they can cause interactions and side effects.

Doctors and especially pharmacists are learning more about the hazards of taking certain herbs in combination with prescription drugs. In one landmark study, published in the *Archives of Internal Medicine* in 1998, researchers identified a number of herb-drug pairings that can cause adverse reactions. They're shown in the chart below.

If Your Loved One Takes . . .	Then Avoid . . .
Antianxiety medications	Kava, valerian root
Antiseizure medications	Evening primrose oil
Blood thinners	Chamomile, dong quai, feverfew, garlic, ginger, ginkgo, ginseng
Diuretics (for high blood pressure)	Licorice
Hypoglycemics (for diabetes)	Ephedra, garlic, ginger, ginseng, licorice
Heart failure medications	Hawthorn, licorice, Siberian ginseng
Immunosuppressive drugs, including corticosteroids used for autoimmune disorders	Alfalfa, echinacea, licorice
Iron	Black cohosh, chamomile, feverfew, hawthorn, St. John's wort, saw palmetto, valerian

Since the publication of that study, other researchers have added to the list of dangerous herb-drug combinations. For example, experts at the Mayo Clinic caution against using St. John's wort with any prescription medicines—particularly antidepressants—since the herb appears to stimulate drug metabolism. And taking aspirin in conjunction with a number of herbs, including feverfew, garlic, ginger, and ginkgo, can lead to excessive bleeding.

The efforts to identify other potential herb-drug interactions continue, with some research funded by federal grants. In the meantime, if your loved one is interested in trying an herbal remedy, run it past her doctor or pharmacist first. And stay alert for suspicious symptoms, which may indicate an adverse reaction.

one's doctor or pharmacist should be able to identify potential interactions between prescription and over-the-counter drugs, as well as herbal remedies, vitamin and mineral supplements, and other dietary supplements. And they should be willing to check their references for you if they're unsure.

To recognize all the interactions and adverse reactions that can occur, you'd probably need a degree in medicine or pharmacy yourself. But even with a little bit of knowledge, you can zero in on possible "hot spots" in your loved one's treatment regimen. For instance, did you know that certain conditions can make a person more vulnerable to an adverse reaction? Experts have observed this phenomenon in those with asthma, cardiac arrhythmia, diabetes, epilepsy, hypothyroidism, autoimmune disorders, gastrointestinal diseases, and respiratory problems. Being in intensive care or battling an infection also raises a person's risk.

Beyond the presence of a particular health problem, the use of certain medications can increase the likelihood of an adverse reaction. These drugs have what's known as a narrow therapeutic index. In other words, increasing their effects even slightly can be toxic, while decreasing their effects even slightly wipes out their healing benefits. Among the medicines with a narrow therapeutic index are aspirin, anticoagulants (also known as blood thinners), and some antidepressants.

Doctors and pharmacists readily acknowledge that the elderly population has its own set of risks for drug interactions, as well as for side effects. If you're caring for an older person, don't shy away from asking pointed questions about the medications your loved one is prescribed—for example, whether a particular drug is necessary or, at least, whether the dose can be lowered.

Some prescription medications are designated "best avoided" or "use in reduced doses until full effect is determined" because they're known to trigger adverse reactions in older people. Among the drugs that carry these cautions are antidepressants, antihistamines (prescribed for colds or allergies), anti-inflammatories, beta-blockers (used to reduce blood pressure and slow the heartbeat), diuretics (sometimes called water pills), sleep aids, sildenafil (Viagra), and thyroid preparations. These medicines can also cause confusion and behavioral disturbances. So before you jump to conclusions about any symptoms your loved one is experiencing, consider the possibility that the person might be having an adverse reaction to something she's taking.

Keep in mind that over-the-counter products can cause problems, too. For example, medications containing aspirin are not recommended for people being treated for asthma, high blood pressure, liver or kidney disease, or stomach disorders. And even over-the-counter antihistamines—like their prescription-strength counterparts—can have adverse effects when taken long-term. Whenever you have doubts about a nonprescription medicine, consult your loved one's doctor or pharmacist.

FRONT AND CENTER ON SIDE EFFECTS

The line between interactions, adverse reactions, and side effects can blur. But for a caregiver, being able to make the distinction matters less than being able to recognize when a loved one is being harmed by a medicine that is supposed to be helping.

"Sometimes side effects are subtle," Dr. Fincham says. "The caregiver and care recipient won't notice them. Other times, side effects might be incorrectly associated with the illness. I have seen people become highly disoriented, dizzy, and unable to concentrate just from using over-the-counter antihistamine products."

Side effects are stated on the labels and package inserts of every prescription and over-the-counter medication. It might seem like fine print, but by taking the time to read the information, you'll know what to watch for. For example, you'll learn that nonsteroidal anti-inflammatory drugs such as ibuprofen and naproxen can contribute to various kinds of gastrointestinal problems.

In addition, doctors and pharmacists maintain lists of drugs that cause certain side effects in older people, such as sluggishness, unsteadiness, falling, constipation, and incontinence. These lists exist for a good reason: The elderly population is three times more likely than everyone else to experience side effects, as well as interactions.

If you suspect a drug of causing persistent side effects in your loved one (sometimes they dissipate after a few days), you might ask whether the dosage can be decreased. Discontinuing the medicine completely may not be necessary. Remember that in older people especially, the body just may not process a full dose efficiently.

CHAPTER 16

ADAPTATIONS FOR DAILY LIVING

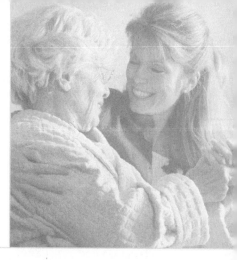

What You Need to Know

- Encourage your loved one to do as much as she can for herself to maintain as much independence as possible, physically and emotionally.

- Recognize your own physical limitations when deciding whether to ask for help with certain caregiving tasks.

- Practice good hygiene to reduce the transmission of viruses, bacteria, and other germs between yourself and your loved one.

- Explore the wide range of adaptive tools and equipment that enable people with physical limitations and disabilities to perform many tasks of daily living without assistance.

If you were to walk into Ethelinn Block's home in Mesa, Arizona, and head for her father's bedroom closet, you would see neat rows of easy-to-match shirts, shorts, and slacks. But you wouldn't find any shoes. Not a single pair. They're stashed in a big box in the garage.

You see, Ethelinn's father has Alzheimer's disease. Keeping his shoes out of sight prevents him from leaving the house and wandering off.

"We also installed an alarm system and double-locked our doors inside and out," Ethelinn says. "In his bathroom, we place everything in clear view so he doesn't open up cabinets to look for things. I store only one extra roll of toilet paper there, because if he finds more, he flushes them down the toilet."

Point of View

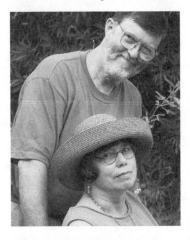

"When you require personal care, it's easy to fall into a pattern of thinking, well, that person is an extension of me and should know what I want, what I need, when I want it, when I need it. I do it regularly, and I must stop and remind myself that . . . I have a responsibility to clearly tell my husband what I need. Otherwise, I get impatient with him: 'Well, why doesn't he just know?' So, I suppose that my honoring him means backing up and looking at him as a person—not as me, or as a part of me, but as a wonderful, separate being."

—NANCY MAIRS,
Tucson

Like many caregivers, Ethelinn continuously adds new safeguards to keep her father out of harm's way both inside and outside the home. She has to make the upgrades to stay apace of the changes in her father's physical and emotional health.

TEAMWORK PAYS OFF

Ethelinn's proactive approach to her father's care illustrates the importance of being able to anticipate and adapt to a loved one's evolving needs. In providing support, caregivers must be careful not to intrude on the care recipients' personal space. Finding the line between the two isn't always easy, especially when a loved one remains mentally competent and capable of managing many tasks himself.

If this scenario sounds familiar, perhaps your best bet is to ask your loved one to help you help him. Letting him handle what he can on his own preserves his sense of independence and self-worth, so he doesn't feel like a burden. And by stepping in only when your loved one requests assistance, you're able to focus your caregiving efforts on what's truly necessary.

Karl Smith, of Newark, Delaware, can vouch for the benefits of caregiver and care recipient working together as a team. That's how he and his 93-year-old father, Luther, manage household chores. For example, after meals, Luther rinses the dishes and sets them in the strainer in the sink. Then Karl transfers them to the dishwasher, fills the soap bin, and turns on the machine. Similarly, on laundry days, Karl runs the washer and dryer, while Luther does the folding.

"When my father moved in, he kept wanting to do something so he'd feel like he's contributing," Karl says. "The chores take longer than if I did them myself, but they get my father moving. They're good exercise for him."

The key to this sort of teamwork is constant communication between the caregiver and the care recipient. This even applies to the execution of a specific task. As an example, let's walk through the process of helping your loved one stand up from a chair. (You wouldn't want to actually attempt this unless you're sure you're strong enough and you have no back problems.)

1. Announce clearly, "I'm going to help you stand up now."

2. Ask the person to move to the front of the chair and slide his feet back under his center of gravity. Check to be sure that he has both feet firmly on the floor.

3. Block his knees with your knees.

4. Place your arms around the person's waist. Don't let him pull on your neck.

5. Ask him to lean forward by saying, "Bring your nose over your toes."

6. If the person has the physical strength and coordination, ask him to use the arms of the chair to push himself up. If not, tell him that you'll lift him on the count of three.

You can see how communicating supports each step so that you and your loved one are working together, not at cross-purposes. In much the same way, it can synchronize your efforts with his needs across all caregiving tasks.

Take Action... ASSIST WITH SAFETY IN MIND

In helping your loved one get out of a chair or perform other basic functions of daily living, you will quickly discover that caregiving is very physical work. And unless you possess the powers of Superman or the boundless energy of an Energizer Bunny, you have physical limits. That's okay. It's what makes you human.

Before you try too many of the really demanding tasks, like getting your loved one out of bed or transferring him from a chair to a wheelchair, consider seeking professional advice. A physical therapist, occupational therapist, or nurse can help assess your capabilities.

Beyond that, you can take precautions to reduce your risk of injury and illness in a caregiving situation. Your best bet is to get training in basic skills from a home care professional. It's worth the effort. After all, if you get knocked out of commission, you may not be able to help anyone—not even yourself.

Protecting Your Back

Dale L. Anderson, M.D., an urgent care physician in St. Paul, Minnesota, reminds caregivers to be especially kind to their backs.

Walk This Way

If your loved one needs some assistance walking, medical experts recommend that you let her take your arm as you walk side by side. Holding on to her arm can actually interfere with her balance.

To provide more support, try walking behind your loved one, placing one hand on her shoulder and using the other to hold her belt or waistband. Be sure to stand close and walk in step behind her to help guide her.

Rather than getting assistance from you, your loved one might be able to get around with a cane or walker. Whichever she chooses, be sure she receives training in proper walking technique from a physician or physical therapist.

Outlook

"In the future, I hope technology becomes more of an aid to caregivers. Right now, for example, the Grotta Foundation sponsors Caregiver Connections, which offers teleconferenced workshops and support programs for caregivers. This enables a home-bound caregiver or a working family member to participate in a range of programming from the home or office.

"Also, because dual-career families are the economic future, we must find low-cost alternatives for caregivers who need to work. In many cases, people won't be able to just leave their jobs.

"Most of all, I would love to see caregiver resource centers, similar to those in California, throughout every county in the United States. Caregivers would have one place where they could go to access services, benefits, and information, such as caregiver education, support groups, and respite care."

—**SUSAN FRIEDMAN,** executive director of the Grotta Foundation in South Orange, New Jersey

"I've had to provide medical treatment to caregivers who, despite their best intentions, did not use proper technique to lift or move a loved one, or to help the person stand up," he says. "The caregiver may be confined to bed temporarily because of back injuries. That makes the person feel guilty, because he's not able to help the care recipient."

Caregiving involves a lot of lifting, reaching, and bending—movements that can hurt your back if done improperly. According to Marion Karpinski, R.N., creator of the *Home Care Companion* video series and author of *Quick Tips for Caregivers*, you can reduce your risk of injury just by practicing good posture whenever you move. "Proper posture maintains the natural curves of the spine, helping to conserve energy and prevent muscle strain," she explains.

To protect your back when doing any kind of lifting, Karpinski and other experts offer these tips.

- Wear a back brace and nonskid shoes for support and safety.

- Before you even begin to lift, think about your posture and body position. Keep your back and neck straight.

- Stand as close as possible to the object, without leaning forward or bending at your waist. This minimizes strain on your back and leg muscles and improves leverage.

- Position your feet about shoulder-width apart, with one foot slightly in front of the other for the broadest base of support. If necessary, get down on one knee or squat so you're on the same level as the object.

- As you lift, tighten your abdominal muscles to protect your back.

- Never try to lift someone heavier than you or to pull the person by his arms or legs. Always hold him at his trunk and hips.

Holding Germs at Bay

Another consideration for the caregiver is potential exposure to infectious diseases. Any time you have contact with your loved one—whether directly (through bathing or changing dressings) or indirectly (by handling laundry and dishes)—you risk picking up germs. You can stop the spread of viruses, bacteria, and other bugs with these precautionary measures.

- Consider using protective barriers whenever you're going to be in direct contact with your loved one. You can buy gloves, gowns, aprons, masks, and protective eyeglasses in medical supply stores and some pharmacies.

- Wash the fronts and backs of your hands in warm soapy water before and after having contact with your loved one, as well as after using the bathroom, after handling medical equipment, and before preparing food. Use a mild antiseptic soap dispensed from a pump bottle rather than bar soap.

- Always wash dishes in soap and hot water. Add a small amount of chlorine bleach to a sink or basin full of water, then soak the dishes in this solution for about a minute before rinsing them in hot running water. Allow the dishes to air-dry.

Caregiving around the World

Australian caregivers, or carers, save their country's economy an estimated $16 billion each year. Carer Respite Centers, with a national toll-free hotline, provide single contact points for caregivers seeking information and advice. The centers also offer free Carer Support Kits, which include materials on financial assistance, legal issues, medication management, home care, respite care, and more.

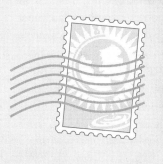

POST CARD

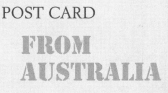

FROM AUSTRALIA

Outlook

"Innovations in technology, improved design and engineering, and new service models for care recipients and caregivers are laying the groundwork for a number of changes that will affect the future of caregiving. For example, many patients with congestive heart failure, diabetes, and other chronic conditions are using in-home devices to monitor and report their health status to medical providers. A wide range of biomeasurements, such as weight and oxygen saturation, can be transmitted by phone (and increasingly over the Internet) to a physician, nurse, or care manager. Many firms are testing and commercializing this technology to meet the needs of the aging population."

—JOSEPH F. COUGHLIN, PH.D.,
founding director of the AgeLab at the Massachusetts Institute of Technology in Cambridge

✗ To sanitize the kitchen and bathroom countertops, wipe them with a clean sponge that has been soaked in a bleach-and-water solution. Be sure to wear latex gloves when you do this.

✗ Use a bleach solution to clean bedpans and commodes. This calls for latex gloves, too.

✗ Wash laundry that has been soiled with bodily fluids as separate loads. Use hot water and add a cup of Lysol or bleach to each load. If you're washing colors, select a color-safe bleach. For hand-washing, use 2 tablespoons of bleach per gallon of water, and wear rubber gloves.

Take Action... PRESERVE DIGNITY IN PERSONAL CARE

Now that you know the basics of safe caregiving, let's turn our attention to the most fundamental of caregiving tasks: hygiene and grooming. They tend to be the most uncomfortable for both the caregiver and the care recipient because of the level of intimacy they require. But with practice, they become almost second nature. Mutual respect and trust are key.

Bathing

Taking a bath is one of life's simplest pleasures. As a caregiver, you can help keep the experience pleasant and relaxing for your loved one. But first, you may need to work through some self-consciousness on her part.

"A person may feel embarrassed about being bathed. She might also perceive a loss of privacy," says Su Bonnet, a professional caregiver from San Marcos, California. "When someone needs bathing, I try to put some kind of compassionate humor into it so the person is more comfortable."

One of Bonnet's clients, an 85-year-old woman named Lillian, gets a bath every other afternoon. Lil's rheumatoid arthritis and macular degeneration, coupled with recent spinal fusion surgery, make her unsteady on her feet.

"Lil felt embarrassed the first time I gave her a bath. She said to me, 'I look like a POW. I'm too thin,'" Bonnet recalls. "I told her that I have pounds to spare and that I'd give her some. She laughed at that. Then she said, 'Oh well, we're both girls.' I made sure she had her balance, then I closed the shower curtain a bit to give her some privacy."

Caregiving experts like the idea of encouraging a care recipient to bathe herself as much as she's able. It helps maintain and possibly improve her level of function. If necessary, you can wash the hard-to-reach places, like the back and the feet.

These strategies can also make for a better bathtime.

✗ Keep the bathroom at a comfortable temperature.

✗ Get out all the necessary bathing supplies and put them where they're easy to reach.

✗ When you're ready to begin, ask your loved one to sit on the edge of the tub. Then have her put both legs into the tub before standing up. This provides balance and stability. Have her follow the same steps when she gets out of the tub.

✗ If your loved one can't sit down in the tub, consider purchasing a tub bench and a handheld shower attachment. You can find this equipment in medical supply stores and some pharmacies.

While a lot of people like to bathe every day, your loved one may not want or need to. At the very least, she should wash her face, hands, and genital area on a daily basis. For this, an old-fashioned basin bath may suffice.

Skin Care

Without proper skin care, your loved one is susceptible to dryness, allergic rashes, and sores. To reduce the risk of these problems, experts recommend applying a moisturizing lotion or emollient cream after every bath. Look for a product that contains aloe, which replenishes and nourishes skin cells while preventing dryness and scaling. Let your loved one rub in the lotion where she can; then offer to help with the hard-to-reach spots.

This is a wonderful opportunity to introduce your loved one to the healing power of therapeutic touch. Using your fingertips (never your fingernails), gently massage lotion into her neck, shoulders, and back. Apply firm, steady pressure to increase bloodflow and ease minor aches. You may want to play soft meditative music to maximize the relaxing effects.

If your loved one requires assistance with facial shaving, choose an electric razor over a blade. It's easier to use, with less chance for nicks and cuts.

Hair Care

Even more so than bathing, hair care has an impact on a person's self-image. But your loved one may have a hard time managing her mane on her own. Here's how you can help.

✗ Urge your loved one to consider a new hairstyle. Something short and low-maintenance is best.

✗ If the person has difficulty navigating the tub or shower, wash her hair in the kitchen sink. It's probably equipped with a handheld sprayer, which you can use to rinse.

✗ If your loved one is bedridden, roll a towel into a U-shape and put it in a large plastic bag. Then place the towel, open end up, on the edge of the bed to cradle your loved one's head. Use a bucket to catch the soap and water as it runs off.

✗ Buy a dry shampoo product for those occasions when your loved one isn't able to wet her hair.

✗ Every 4 to 8 weeks, take your loved one to a beauty salon or barbershop for a professional shampoo and cut. Even better, look for a hairstylist who makes house calls. Many do, although they usually charge more for the service.

Dressing

If your loved one is able to dress herself, give her as much time as she needs to complete the task on her own. You can help her decide what to wear by placing two outfits on the bed and letting her choose one. Stay within shouting distance in case she asks for help with closing buttons or zippers or tying shoes.

When you and your loved one go clothes-shopping, steer her toward easy-to-wear items that feature large front fasteners (zippers or Velcro) and elastic waistbands. Women should seriously

FOR MORE INFORMATION

A number of mail-order catalogs sell clothing that's designed especially for people who cannot dress themselves. One is the Sears Home Health Care Catalog, available by calling **(800) 377-5508**. Another is published by the Buffalo State College Center for Clothing for Individuals with Physical Disabilities. To request a copy, call **(716) 878-5813**.

consider giving up constricting garments like panty hose and bras that fasten in the back. Make sure the person has a pair of non-skid shoes that can be slipped on rather than laced.

HELPER GADGETS FOR THE CARE RECIPIENT

For dressing, and for many other tasks of daily living, companies are constantly introducing products designed especially for people with physical limitations and disabilities. The gadgets currently on the market range from shoe lacers and hands-free beverage dispensers to elevated toilet seats and portable seat lifts. These and similar assistive devices enable care recipients to manage routine functions on their own and, possibly, to remain independent longer.

Your loved one's physician can probably tell you where such products are sold in your area. You can also look in the Yellow Pages under "Medical Equipment and Supplies," or search the Internet using the keywords "assistive devices," "disability-related products," or "medical equipment and supplies."

Let's take a closer look at some of the gadgets that may make life easier for your loved one—and, indirectly, for you as well.

Calendar clock. The display on this clock shows the month, the day, and the time of day, and also indicates A.M. or P.M. It's great for anyone who has trouble remembering this sort of information.

Reacher. This device acts like an arm extension, enabling a person to retrieve objects from high shelves and other hard-to-get-to locations. Some reachers extend nearly 3 feet. Look for one that features an easy-to-use gripper handle and a rubberized gripping end, which can snag objects without slipping.

Wall-mounted jar opener. For people who have arthritis and similar conditions, opening a jar with a vacuum seal can be next to impossible. But not with this gadget, which features a screw cap remover, a bottle hook, and edges for prying.

Dinnerware. Dinner plates with "lips" allow people with poor dexterity to scoop up food without spilling. Also look for molded flatware and beverage glasses that conform to the shape of the hand.

Button hook. The cushioned grip and flexible ribbing on this

FOR MORE INFORMATION

A company called Abledata has information about thousands of assistive devices for home care. Call **(800) 227-0216**, or visit **www.abledata.com**.

device make opening and closing buttons easy. It's ideal for anyone with impaired fine motor skills in the hands.

Cervical support pillow. This specially designed pillow conforms to the natural curvature of a person's neck, cradling the neck and head. It reduces muscle stress and tension by providing proper anatomical support to the neck vertebrae. As an added benefit, it helps open obstructed airways, which often contribute to snoring and sleep apnea. Look for a pillow that is hypoallergenic and machine washable.

Adaptable walker basket. This vinyl-coated steel wire basket attaches easily to most regular and folding walkers, allowing a person with limited mobility to carry small items from one place to another. Look for a model that requires no tools for assembly.

Portable seat lift. Placed on top of a chair seat, this device uses gentle hydraulic action to raise someone off a chair. It safely lowers a person to a sitting position, too.

Elevated toilet seat. Being perched higher on the "throne" is helpful for people with limited mobility. The seat, usually made from durable polyethylene for easy cleaning, firmly fits on top of an oval-shaped toilet bowl. Most models add about 5 inches of height to the existing seat. No tools are needed for assembly.

Personal emergency response system (PERS). This electronic gadget contains a tiny radio transmitter that connects a person's home telephone to a response center. Think of it as a lifeline for your loved one, who may have a medical emergency in your absence. He just has to press a button to activate the transmitter, which then sends a signal to the response center. The staff there will put out the call for emergency personnel. The transmitter can be worn as a necklace or bracelet.

HOME MODIFICATIONS: DO IT YOURSELF, OR LET SOMEONE ELSE?

Depending on the extent of a loved one's physical limitations or disabilities, you may need to do some remodeling to make her living space safer and easier to navigate. The required upgrades can be as simple as rearranging the furniture or as complex (and costly) as adding a bedroom or bathroom.

To determine the extent of the job, first survey the home's in-

---

FOR MORE INFORMATION

In the book *Do-Able Renewable Home*, caregivers can learn about making various kinds of home modifications. The book can be ordered by visiting **www.usc.edu/dept/gero/hmap/library/drhome**, the Web site for the Andrus Gerontology Center at the University of Southern California.

Another excellent resource for home modifications, especially for people with dementia, is Ageless Design. You can visit the Web site at **www.agelessdesign.com**.

terior by going from room to room and making note of any possible hazards. Then head outside and assess the exterior. Depending on what you find, you may be able to achieve peace of mind just by making a few minor adaptations to reduce the risk of falls, burns, and other injuries. (To learn more about these basic home improvements, see chapter 9.)

Next, you need to evaluate your loved one's physical and mental condition. Aging and illness can bring about declines in memory, vision, hearing, strength, flexibility, and dexterity, among other changes. These can compromise a person's function, making home modifications necessary.

Depending on your handiness, you may be able to do much of the work yourself. For example, household lighting can be made brighter simply by switching to bulbs with a higher wattage or using different lamps. Conventional doorknobs and cabinet and faucet handles can be replaced with larger lever-type handles.

Other home improvements that may benefit your loved one include the following:

Countertops. These may need to be raised or lowered. Ideally, they should be at a height that's comfortable for someone who is seated in a wheelchair or standing—usually between 30 and 34 inches.

Kitchen sink. If your loved one uses a wheelchair, she may get back strain from leaning forward to reach items in the bottom of a deep sink. Install a wooden, wire, or plastic rack to raise the working level of the sink to a more comfortable height.

Stove. A person in a wheelchair or with limited mobility could easily burn herself when reaching for a pot on the back burner. Consider mounting a mirror above the stove, so your loved one can safely keep tabs on her cooking.

Refrigerator. Side-by-side refrigerator/freezer units are accessible to everyone in the household, including those who have trouble bending down or reaching up.

Shelves. Consider putting lazy Susans in kitchen and bath cabinets so your loved one doesn't have to reach all the way to the back to retrieve something. Another option for the kitchen is to install wall and ceiling hooks for hanging up frequently used pots and pans.

FOR MORE INFORMATION

Many states and municipalities fund grants and loans for caregivers who need to remodel their homes to accommodate their loved ones. Contact state and local housing authorities to determine the availability of such programs in your area.

EXPERT OPINION

"I encourage caregivers to 'think outside the box' and be creative when rearranging their homes to accommodate an aging parent. In some cases, people have converted their living rooms into bedrooms for loved ones with limited mobility and trouble climbing stairs. Living rooms make nice bedrooms because they are larger in size, with ample space for photos, books, and comfortable chairs. With the care recipient in the living room, a caregiver doesn't need to constantly run up and down stairs. Watch a television show together. Let the aromas from the kitchen waft into the living room. All these sights, sounds, and smells provide comfort for the care recipient and reduce stress for everyone in the household."

—**ANNIE GLASGOW**, a psychotherapist from St. Paul, Minnesota, who works with caregivers

Grab bars. Position these bars near the toilet, tub, and shower. They should be able to withstand a 250-pound load, which means they must be screwed directly into wall studs. If they're fastened to drywall, they won't support the weight.

Doorways. A standard wheelchair is 24 to 27 inches wide. You may need to remove the door of your loved one's bathroom so she can maneuver her chair in and out.

Kickplates. Adding these to doors can protect against excessive wear, especially if your loved one uses a wheelchair. Look for plates made from a durable material such as metal or plastic laminate. The top of the kickplate should be positioned about 10 inches above the floor.

Floors. To reduce the risk of falls, affix nonskid adhesive strips to potentially slippery walking surfaces, especially in bathrooms. For high-traffic areas, consider replacing existing flooring with nonskid ceramic tile or indoor/outdoor carpeting.

Lighting. Put night-lights in all bedrooms, bathrooms, and hallways. If possible, install lighting or illuminating adhesive strips on stairs.

Stairs. For safety, handrails should run along both sides of a stairway. Mount them about 1½ inches from the wall to allow adequate room for grasping fingers and to support up to 250 pounds of weight. Secure the rails with molly bolts through wallboard or with screws into upright studs.

Ramps. These may be necessary for a loved one who uses a wheelchair or has limited mobility. Interior ramps should have a maximum slope of 1 inch of rise for every 12 inches of length. For exterior ramps, the ratio is 1 inch to 20 inches. Portable ramps are available from surgical supply houses and direct from manufacturers.

CHAPTER 17

CARING FOR THE BEDRIDDEN

What You Need to Know

- If you're caring for someone who's bedridden, consider getting training in home health care. It's the best way to learn the proper techniques for assisting the person with the tasks of daily living.

- Experts recommend that a person who's bedridden change positions at least once every 2 hours to protect against bedsores. Good posture and skin care also help reduce risk.

- If your loved one develops a bedsore, you may be able to treat it at home. But stay alert for signs of infection, which can spread to other parts of the body and cause serious complications.

Arlene Garcia remembers when she would greet each sunrise by sharing a 2-mile walk with her mother, Alice Fritz. Out in the crisp desert air near their homes in Moenkopi, Arizona (Hopi Nation), they'd chat about anything and everything as they matched each other stride for stride.

The pair also enjoyed shopping trips into town. A couple of years ago, as they drove the downtown streets in Arlene's car, they were struck nearly head-on by a pickup truck. Though dazed, Arlene instinctively turned toward the passenger seat, where she saw her mother slumped over, unconscious. Alice's neck had been broken.

"It just happened so fast," Arlene recalls. "My mother's spinal cord was crushed between the fourth and fifth vertebrae, leaving her permanently paralyzed from the chest down. Since then, we've been taking care of her."

Arlene and her siblings sought training from home health care experts to learn the right way to tend to their mother's personal needs—how to feed her, how to exercise her, how to transfer her from a bed to a wheelchair and from a wheelchair to a car. They also worked out a schedule so between them, they could provide round-the-clock care.

"My mother always looked after my grandmother, and my grandfather and uncle, too," Arlene says. "She was a caregiver all those years. She was always doing things for me, too. And of course, I just adore her. So I thought, 'Well, now it's my turn.'"

A HIGHER LEVEL OF CARE

Loss of mobility happens for many reasons. In Alice Fritz's case, it was caused by a car crash. It can also result from a fall or a chronic illness. Sometimes it's temporary, as after surgery; other times it's permanent. Invariably, it leaves a person confined to bed.

When caring for a loved one who is bedridden, you'll be faced with responsibilities beyond the usual cooking, housekeeping, and bill-paying. Depending on the person's condition, you may need to perform a lot of physically demanding tasks, like helping him sit up in bed or change positions to prevent bedsores. And you might be challenged to provide him with stimulating activities that can fend off feelings of isolation and boredom.

In this sort of situation, you will benefit tremendously from the expertise and assistance of your loved one's caregiving team—the doctors, nurses, social workers, physical therapists, and other health professionals involved in the person's care. Don't hesitate to consult them. When you do, remember to be very specific with your questions and concerns. You might want to jot down issues as they arise and use your notes as a "script" when talking with members of the caregiving team. Together, you can come up with an approach to care that is tailored to your loved one's needs.

You can also follow Arlene Garcia's lead and obtain training in home health care. According to Trina Tomlinson, a home health care nurse from Vista, California, she and her colleagues understand their role in teaching caregivers as well as tending to care

FOR MORE INFORMATION

The National Pressure Ulcer Advisory Panel (NPUAP) offers booklets and other resources to families caring for loved ones at home. You can contact them by phone at (716) 881-3558, or by writing to NPUAP, SUNY at Buffalo, Beck Hall, 3435 Main Street, Buffalo, NY 14214.

recipients. "It is very rare for clients to have 24-hour, round-the-clock professional care in their homes," Tomlinson observes. "When we aren't there, family members and friends must know how to move the person, change bedding, prevent bedsores, and recognize symptoms that may require medical attention."

At the same time, you need to remember that you're human, not superhuman. Don't expect more of yourself than you can reasonably deliver. One of the smartest decisions you can make is to seek outside assistance in caring for a loved one who is bedridden and in steadily declining health. Likewise, if you're having difficulty following through on a prescribed plan of care, ask for help.

In-home caregiving support takes many forms, from homemaker services to skilled nursing care. We'll discuss all of the options in chapter 20. For now, just be aware that resources are available, and that you shouldn't hesitate to take advantage of them.

ENVIRONMENT MATTERS

Caring for a loved one who's bedridden begins with creating a pleasant yet practical living space. Do you remember those times in your childhood when you were home sick? Just snuggling in bed surrounded by your favorite toys and games, with your mom providing an extra dose of TLC, made you feel better. And you want your loved one to feel the best he can, too.

Start by personalizing his room as much as possible. Hang family photos on the walls, stack favorite books on the shelves, set a familiar chair in the corner. To battle boredom, provide a radio and television as well as a supply of games and puzzles to pass the time. Store these items so they're within easy reach, if at all possible.

Don't overlook the benefits of having a room with a view. While your loved one may not be able to go outside, he still can enjoy the great outdoors from his window. If his room is on the first floor (which is ideal), you might want to install a bird feeder or birdbath so he can do some bird-watching. Depending on his health and abilities, you also might want to buy binoculars and a field guide, so he can identify the various species that fly in. It's great mental stimulation.

FOR MORE INFORMATION

To learn more about training in home care skills, call your local Area Agency on Aging. It's listed in the blue pages of your phone directory, under "Guide to Human Services." In addition, Healing Arts Communications has produced *The Home Care Companion Video Collection* to instruct professionals and laypeople in basic caregiving skills like managing medications, controlling infections, and preventing falls. Log on to **w w w. h o m e c a r e c o m p a n i o n . c o m**.

EXPERT OPINION

"If your mother's health has reached the point that she's bedridden, you can't pretend the bed is not there. But you can improve the situation by dressing your mom in a nice bed jacket, fixing her hair, and putting on her lipstick. And pay attention to the aromas. Air fresheners, perfumed sachets, and potpourri can be wonderful, therapeutic smells. If the weather is nice, open a window and let the fresh air in. For someone who is bedridden, the feel of the outdoors can be a psychological boost."

—**ANNIE GLASGOW**, a psychotherapist in St. Paul, Minnesota, who works with caregivers

Point of View

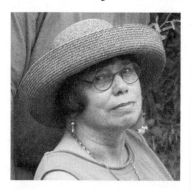

"Confinement is a curse; confinement is a blessing. Nothing about it is straightforward. Oh, I hate the limitations. I was always a walker, and I miss just being able to get up and walk somewhere. On the other hand, by having to sit, I can watch my grandchildren and perhaps see them in a way that nobody else does."

—NANCY MAIRS,
Tucson

BEDDING BASICS

Of course, for someone who is bedridden, the key to comfort may be the bed itself. Unless a member of his caregiving team advises otherwise, your loved one would probably feel best in his own bed. The type of bedclothes he uses is a matter of personal preference. What's important is changing the sheets regularly.

As a rule, health experts recommend changing unsoiled bed sheets every 4 days. But as caregivers know, bathroom accidents can and will happen. Soiled sheets should be removed immediately and washed in hot water with a cup of Lysol or bleach per load. Always keep a clean set of bedding handy, just in case.

In addition, you might want to protect the mattress from stains and odors by placing an absorbent bed pad between the mattress and the fitted sheet. You can find these pads in medical supply stores and some department stores. A heavy towel would work, too.

Incidentally, while we're on the subject of linens, you may want to pick up some extra washcloths whenever you buy towel sets. You'll find yourself using lots of washcloths in caring for your loved one. Because they're used hard, they tend to wear out fast. A good rule of thumb is to buy three washcloths for every pair of hand and bath towels.

No Pressure Here

If you've ever sat in a wooden chair for more than an hour without shifting around or standing up, you know how the no-give design can tax your muscles, especially those in your lower back. A mattress is more accommodating, but still, sitting or lying on one for long periods can be painful. It also increases the risk of bedsores (which we'll discuss next).

This is why health experts recommend taking precautions to protect sensitive body parts from excessive pressure. Your best bet is to provide extra support surfaces between the mattress and your loved one—for example, by sliding pillows underneath her head, neck, and back. Special pillows and seat cushions are available from medical supply stores and some chiropractic offices. Sheepskin and foam "egg carton" mattress pads can help, too.

What sort of support works best? That depends on the person's health, physical build, skin condition, and range of motion. You can do what's known as a hand check to determine if a support surface is indeed reducing pressure. Just slide your open hand underneath the support surface, with your fingers parallel and your palm facing up. At least 1 inch of support surface should separate your hand from your loved one's body. This shows adequate protection.

Be sure to tell your loved one when you're going to do a hand check. And be gentle—remember, you're working around a sensitive spot.

Take Action... DEFEND AGAINST BEDSORES

One reason to provide extra padding for your loved one's body is to prevent bedsores, which can occur on any body part that's under constant long-term pressure (hence their other names: pressure sores or ulcers). They tend to be most common on bony parts not adequately cushioned by surrounding muscle and fat, such as the heels, ankles, hips, base of the spine, elbows, and head. No matter what the affected area, the continuous pressure disrupts bloodflow, causing the skin to break down and form painful ulcers.

Perhaps the easiest way to reduce the risk of bedsores is to make sure your loved one moves her body regularly. Experts recommend changing positions at least once every 2 hours while in bed, and at least once every hour while sitting. These intervals may need adjusting based on a person's skin condition and comfort level.

Beyond regular movement, good posture and skin care on your loved one's part can help stop bedsores from forming. That's why incorporating the following strategies into your caregiving routine is so important.

Maintaining Good Posture

We seldom think about our posture when we're standing up, let alone sitting or lying down. Yet for a person who is bedridden, the position of the body can be a deciding factor in whether bedsores develop.

To help your loved one maintain good posture while in bed, experts offer these suggestions.

EXPERT OPINION

"The first time I went to provide hospice care for a client named Judy, who was dying of cancer, her hair was made up, and she was wearing a beautiful gown, with earrings and a little angel pin. I knew immediately that her family cared for her deeply. I would turn her every 2 hours and prop up pillows for her, moving carefully to avoid bruising her thinning skin. Judy was in a lot of pain—she was taking morphine—but she was a very strong lady who never complained. She maintained her dignity until she died, and I will always respect and admire her."

—**TRINA TOMLINSON,** a home health care nurse from Vista, California

FOR MORE INFORMATION

The National Institutes of Health offers a consumer booklet on reducing the risk of bedsores. You can request *Preventing Pressure Ulcers: Patient Guide* (AHCPR publication number 92-0048) by calling **(800) 358-9295** or writing to Publication Clearinghouse, PO Box 8547, Silver Spring, MD 20907.

The Medicinal Value of Motion

Just because your loved one is bedridden, that doesn't mean he can't take advantage of the therapeutic powers of movement. Slow but deliberate range-of-motion exercises, practiced for even 5 minutes a day, promote good health by improving posture, circulation, heart and lung function, and mental alertness. They also reduce the risk of serious health problems such as heart disease, diabetes, and osteoporosis.

Here's a simple exercise that can help improve bloodflow in someone who's bedridden. Have the person lie on her back and slowly raise her left leg as high as she's able. You can assist by gently lifting her leg, if necessary. Hold for a few seconds, then return to the starting position. Repeat with the right leg, then with each arm in turn.

✗ Use pillows and foam pads to keep the person from applying full body weight to pressure points.

✗ When he wants to lie on his side, have him lean forward at about a 30-degree angle to the bed so that he's not directly on his hipbone. Place a small pillow or foam pad between his knees or ankles, as needed, to keep them from touching.

✗ When the person wants to lie on his back, raise his heels by placing a pillow or thin foam pad underneath his lower legs, from mid-calf to ankle. Avoid putting a cushion directly under the knees when a person is lying on his back, since it can restrict bloodflow to the lower legs and feet.

✗ Avoid using cushions shaped like doughnuts. They impede bloodflow to skin tissues, causing circulation problems and raising the risk of sores.

✗ Elevate the head of the bed to no more than a 30-degree angle. If the person has a respiratory ailment, talk with his doctor about the best positions for lying in bed.

Just like lying down, sitting in a chair or wheelchair can put pressure on sensitive body parts. You can help your loved one hold his body upright, and keep bedsores at bay, with these tips.

✗ Choose a chair with arm supports, on which he can rest his elbows, forearms, and wrists.

✗ Place a cushion on the chair seat to keep the person from sitting directly on any pressure points.

✗ Have him keep his thighs horizontal and parallel to the floor, with his ankles in a neutral position and his feet on the floor or a footrest.

✗ Encourage the person to shift his body weight every 15 minutes or so. Even wiggling his toes and flexing his arms and legs will promote circulation.

Protecting the Skin

Besides being the body's largest organ, the skin might be the one most vulnerable to injury, especially in someone who is bedridden. It's easily irritated by the rubbing of clothes and bedding, as well as by the pulling and tugging of body movement. And this irritation can contribute to bedsores.

The best way to protect the skin from harm is to practice good hygiene, says Dale L. Anderson, M.D., an urgent care physician in St. Paul, Minnesota, who frequently advises caregivers on skin care. Here's what he recommends.

- Above all else, keep the skin clean and dry. Change moisture-absorbing briefs and pads frequently.

- Use soaps sparingly, and when you do, choose an emollient or superfatted bar over an alkaline bar.

- Regularly apply a moisturizing lotion made with vitamin E and/or aloe vera, using a gentle massage motion to increase healthy bloodflow. Avoid rubbing reddened skin or areas with cuts or blisters.

- Place a disposable absorbent pad between the person and his mattress to soak up urine from any accidents, so the skin stays dry. The pads are sold in medical supply stores. Avoid using plastic sheets, which retain urine and body heat. This can irritate the skin.

- Try to keep bed sheets free of wrinkles, as they can put unnecessary pressure on the skin.

- To remove urine or feces from the skin, wash the area with warm soapy water and dry thoroughly with thick, absorbent towels. Be sure to wear disposable latex gloves for this task.

- When helping the person change positions, take care not to pull or drag him across the bed. This creates friction, which can irritate the skin.

Warning Signs to Watch For

If, despite your best efforts, your loved one develops a bedsore, you'll want to begin treatment immediately. Follow the procedures outlined in the Caregiver's Checklist on page 219. In its early stages, a sore will appear red or raw. Over time, it might open and start draining fluid. If that happens, you'll want to monitor the sore for the following signs of infection.

Outlook

"Caring for a loved one can be a demanding job, and a rewarding one, too. Health care professionals could reduce the strain and boost the rewards by supporting the efforts of informal caregivers. Nurses, in particular, could teach straight-forward technical caregiving skills to family members, and they could answer questions, facilitate the use of health services, and provide emotional support to individuals and groups of caregivers. So much could be gained by integrating professional and informal caregiving."

—CHAD BOULT, M.D., M.P.H., M.B.A., professor and director of the Lipitz Center for Integrated Health Care at Johns Hopkins University in Baltimore

Localized (at the Site of the Sore)

- Thick, yellow or green drainage
- Foul odor
- Redness, warmth
- Tenderness
- Swelling, inflammation

Generalized (Elsewhere in the Body)

- Weakness, fatigue
- Fever, chills
- Confusion, difficulty concentrating
- Rapid heartbeat

If you notice any of these symptoms, consult your loved one's doctor as soon as possible. Untreated, an infection from a bedsore can spread. The person may develop cellulitis (infection of the surrounding skin), osteomyelitis (infection of the underlying bone), or sepsis (infection throughout the body).

For a bedsore that doesn't heal with home care, your loved one's doctor may recommend electrotherapy, which uses a mild electrical current to promote healing. Other surgery can repair the damaged skin tissue.

Take Action... MOVE FROM BED TO CHAIR WITH CARE

In the past, bed rest was the treatment of choice for just about every ailment imaginable. These days, physicians like to see their patients get out of bed as often as possible, even if only to sit in a chair. It reduces the risk of bedsores, for one. It's better for circulation and digestion, too.

Unless your loved one's doctor advises otherwise, you may be helping your loved one out of bed several times a day. Here's how to do it safely. (Don't try this without assistance unless you're sure you're strong enough and you have no back problems. Even better, get training in proper lifting technique from a home care professional.)

Do You Practice Proper Bedsore Care?

Medical experts at the National Institutes of Health have developed the following procedure to promote the healing of bedsores and reduce the risk of infection. You may want to make a copy of the checklist and keep it near your loved one's bed, so it's available for easy reference.

This procedure calls for a saline solution, which you can make yourself. You'll need 1 gallon of distilled water and 8 teaspoons of table salt. (You can also use tap water, but be sure to boil it for 5 minutes.) Put the water in a clean container and add the salt. Stir until the salt dissolves completely. If you use boiled tap water, allow the solution to cool to room temperature to avoid accidental burns. You can store any unused solution in a sealed plastic or glass container for up to a week.

Task #1: Preparation

☐ In an easy-to-tote container, gather the necessary supplies: saline solution, irrigation equipment (syringe, portable basin, and large plastic bag), dressings, first aid tape, disposable plastic gloves, small plastic bag, soft clean towel, glasses or goggles, and a plastic apron (optional).

☐ Wash your hands with warm soapy water and rinse thoroughly.

☐ Place the person in a comfortable position.

☐ Place the large plastic bag on the bed to protect the bed linens.

Task #2: Removing Old Dressing

☐ Slide the small plastic bag over your hand.

☐ With your protected hand, grasp the old dressing and pull it off.

☐ Turn the plastic bag inside out to encase the old dressing.

☐ Seal the bag tightly before disposing of it.

Task #3: Irrigating the Bedsore

☐ Put on the disposable plastic gloves, the glasses or goggles, and the plastic apron, if using, to prevent contact with any drainage that may splash.

☐ Fill the syringe with the saline solution.

☐ Place the basin under the sore to catch any drainage.

☐ Hold the saline-filled syringe 1 to 6 inches from the sore and spray it. Use enough force to remove dead tissue and old drainage, but not enough to damage new tissue underneath.

☐ Carefully remove the basin so the fluid doesn't spill on you, your loved one, or the bed.

☐ Dry the skin surrounding the sore by dabbing it with the towel.

☐ Remove the gloves by pulling them inside out and disposing of them promptly in a lidded container.

Task #4: Assessing the Bedsore

☐ Examine the sore. As it heals, it will shrink and drain less. The new tissue underneath should be light red or pink and a little lumpy. Don't disturb this new tissue.

☐ Contact your health care provider if the sore grows in size, drainage increases, or the sore shows no signs of healing within a couple of weeks.

Task #5: Applying a New Dressing

☐ Always wash your hands with warm soapy water before touching a clean dressing.

☐ Follow the instructions provided by your loved one's doctor or nurse to apply a new dressing. Never reuse a dressing.

☐ Store unused dressings in their original packages or sealed plastic bags to protect them from airborne germs. Keep them in a clean, dry place.

☐ Throw away the entire dressing package if it becomes wet, dirty, or contaminated.

✗ Pull back the blankets and top sheet completely, so they're out of the way.

✗ Ask the person to move toward the edge of the bed that's on his strongest side. If he isn't able, try grasping the fitted sheet and slowly pulling the person toward you. Be sure to bend at your knees and not at your waist.

✗ Assist the person in rolling onto his side, so he's facing you. Remember to bend at the knees, not at the waist, to get more leverage and avoid throwing out your back.

✗ Have the person lean on his elbow and push himself to an upright position, lowering his feet over the edge of the bed. If he needs help sitting up, stand as close as possible, making sure your feet are square to his body. Then crouch with your back straight and your knees and hips bent, and raise the person to an upright position. Avoid yanking or pulling his arms.

Once the person is sitting up, you can help him stand up or move to a chair—again, taking care to protect your back. If you find yourself needing a helping hand with this process, check out some of the mobility aids designed to make moving someone easier. They include sliding sheets, hoists, rope ladders, trapeze bars, bed blocks, and adjustable beds. You may be able to rent or borrow these aids from a medical supply store or the local chapter of an organization like the American Cancer Society.

CHAPTER 18

THE FAMILY THAT PLAYS TOGETHER . . .

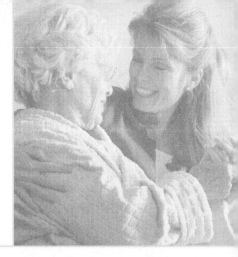

What You Need to Know

- Taking time to relax and have fun can be therapeutic for the care recipient and caregiver alike.

- Activities that focus on family provide an opportunity for interaction outside the caregiving situation itself. By socializing and sharing interests, family members may come to communicate better and feel closer to one another.

- In families affected by a caregiving situation, holiday traditions can take on new significance. They create a sense of continuity and stability, especially for the care recipient.

- Birthdays and other special celebrations present a wonderful opportunity to honor a loved one. The best gifts you can give are time and togetherness.

Play. Do you remember the word? Too often it disappears from the vocabulary of dedicated caregivers, as they devote their time and attention to paying bills, preparing meals, driving to doctor appointments, and handling assorted other caregiving tasks.

No matter how hectic your schedule, you must make time for recreation and relaxation. That goes for your loved one, too.

"Play is absolutely vital. Without it, the whole caregiving/caregetting relationship can become so one-dimensional," says Annie Glasgow, a psychotherapist in St. Paul, Minnesota, who works with caregivers. "I remind my clients that providing and receiving care isn't easy. Through play, family members have an opportunity to lighten up and step out of roles that can be hurtful or stressful."

What's the payoff for you, the caregiver, of including some fun

Outlook

activities in your daily routine? For starters, you'll be less prone to fatigue and irritability, and less vulnerable to burnout. What's more, you may smile a bit more. Studies show that laughter, like exercise, can elevate levels of serotonin and other feel-good hormones produced by the body, Glasgow explains. That's good for you, physically and emotionally.

So give yourself permission to take a break from the day's responsibilities. Even a few minutes of playtime each day can work wonders, Glasgow says. As much as you can, continue to take part in activities that give you pleasure. If you stopped playing golf or practicing yoga when you became a caregiver, start again now. And at least once a month (and ideally more often), arrange for someone else to look after your loved one, so you can enjoy a night out.

While making time for play might squeeze your schedule a bit, the effects of neglecting your own needs can be far worse. "You may start to feel overwhelmed, angry, or resentful," Glasgow says. "Often these emotions are depression turned inward."

Just as you can benefit from embracing play in your life, so can your loved one. It engages him mentally and physically, which can boost his self-confidence and sense of independence. As a bonus, it helps relieve some of the stress that goes with being thrust into the care recipient role.

The best kind of play involves others in the caregiving household, because it allows family members to interact with one another outside their respective caregiving roles. Doing fun things

Fun Defined

In a national poll of senior citizens conducted by the marketing agency Belden, Russonell, and Stewart, respondents identified the following as key areas of enjoyment.

Spending time with family and friends	81%
Having leisure time	65%
Pursuing hobbies	61%
Traveling	51%

together helps break down communication barriers and reinforces familial bonds. It might even forge new ties.

The big question is, what sorts of activities can your loved one do that you and others in the family might also enjoy? As you'll see, the options are as boundless as your creativity and imagination.

Take Action... MAKE HOME LIFE LIVELIER

In its simplest form, play involves finding ways to take some of the "routineness" out of the daily routine. That's especially important in a caregiving situation, where boredom can sap the spirits of both the care recipient and the caregiver. You don't need to do anything extravagant to change the pace and enjoy the moment. Some ideas:

✗ Start with something as simple as adorning the kitchen table with flowers in a vase. Create a different bouquet each week, using blooms from your own garden or the supermarket. The sight and scent of fresh-cut flowers can elevate your loved one's mood, Glasgow says.

✗ Plan a week of "TV appointments." Older care recipients, in particular, may play the television for hours on end—not for entertainment but as background noise. To make TV watching more of an event, you and your loved one can choose programs that you'd like to watch together. Read through the weekly listings—usually they're published as inserts in the Sunday newspaper—and circle the shows you'd both enjoy. Then mark the viewing times on your schedule, and have your loved one do the same.

✗ Rent videos of your loved one's favorite movies, or classic films featuring acting greats like Humphrey Bogart, Katherine Hepburn, and Jimmy Stewart. Show them at in-home matinees—complete with popcorn!—on weekend afternoons. Afterward, the two of you can spend time chatting about the plot and your favorite scenes.

✗ Talk with your loved one about upcoming events, like birthday parties and visits from family members. It might stir a sense of joyful anticipation.

Point of View

"My mother, Judy, simply loved her rose garden. When she was diagnosed with terminal cancer, I just prayed that she would live through the spring, so she could watch the buds bloom. One Sunday afternoon, I helped her out of her recliner and took her for a walk around the garden. Her legs were a little wobbly, but we walked arm-in-arm. We talked about the bushes and about gardening. Eventually, we came upon a peach tree; it was breathtaking, with its hot pink blossoms in full bloom.

"Two days later, her cancer took a turn for the worse. She was in a wheelchair and could no longer walk on her own. She died at age 73, but I will always cherish that spring afternoon we spent together in the rose garden."

—SU BONNET,
Lake San Marcos, California

EXPERT OPINION

"I tell caregivers to never underestimate the healing power of humor. Families need to create time and opportunity for laughter. People who laugh seem to be healthier, more creative, more productive, and better at problem solving."

—**PATTY WOOTEN, R.N.,** a registered nurse, therapeutic humorist, and author from Santa Cruz, California

- Spice up mealtimes with special guests. On a regular basis, invite a few of your loved one's close friends for lunch or dinner, or even afternoon tea. Ask each of them to bring a dish or beverage, so everyone can share in the preparation and fun. Be sure your loved one is involved in putting together the guest list and choosing the date, plus other preparations as she's able.

- Whenever your loved one has guests, take plenty of photos of their visit. Your loved one will appreciate the mementos. If you want, you can assemble a photo album as a birthday or holiday gift.

- Arrange for "play dates" with your loved one's grandchildren. Caregiving experts say that while older people may enjoy reminiscing with their peers, their interactions with youngsters may be just as mentally stimulating. Perhaps all of you can get together for an afternoon of intergenerational card games and board games. If the kids are highly active, keep an eye on your loved one for signs of fatigue.

- Spend 5 minutes a day relaxing with your loved one. Both of you need the break! Play calming music and practice deep breathing, focusing on slow, full breaths.

- Emphasize humor in your household. You've heard the saying about laughter being the best medicine. You and your loved one can get your daily dose by reading the newspaper comics out loud. Somehow, jokes seem better when they're brought to life by the human voice.

Take Action... GO OUT ON THE TOWN

You can overcome the cooped-up feeling that can strain any caregiving relationship by treating your loved one to regular outings. These excursions don't need to be extravagant, expensive, or time-consuming. But they do need to be *fun*. Some examples:

- Save a few dollars by taking advantage of early-bird specials at local restaurants with menus and prices that cater to seniors. Eating dinner before 6:00 in the evening has an added advantage: It allows sufficient time for food to digest before your loved one goes to bed.

✗ Visit a local zoo, botanical garden, museum, or art gallery during off-peak hours. Call ahead to find out about any special events as well as discounts on admission rates (especially for seniors). Also confirm that the facility is accessible to people with disabilities. When you get there, find the restrooms first, so you know where they are if you need them.

✗ Spend a late morning or early afternoon at a local park. Your loved one will enjoy watching the people and absorbing the sights and sounds of nature. If he's able, the two of you can go for a short walk—though just being outdoors is relaxing and therapeutic. You might even want to pack a lunch, if the weather is cooperative.

✗ Attend a local production of a play or musical, especially if your loved one knows someone in the cast. Many communities have their own theater groups. Schools and churches put on performances, too.

✗ Make a trip to the community library. Few activities are more mentally stimulating than reading. And it's easy on aging eyes, with large-print books and books on tape widely available.

✗ Enroll your loved one in an art or crafts class at a local school, studio, or parks and recreation program. Be sure to arrange for transportation, if necessary.

FOR MORE INFORMATION

If you're thinking of taking a vacation with your loved one, start your planning with a visit to the following Web sites. They offer lots of helpful advice for elderly and disabled travelers.

• Access-Able Travel Source at **www.access-able.com**

• TravelSource: Disabled Travel at **www.travelsource.com**

Take Action... KEEP THE HAPPY IN HOLIDAYS

Family get-togethers and fun seem like they ought to go hand-in-hand. Often they do. But at times, like during the holidays, the atmosphere might feel more *Sopranos* than *Leave It to Beaver*. All the planning and preparation is stressful enough, especially for the host. Mix in any preexisting family tensions, and the celebration can quickly turn sour.

But caregiving can cast a holiday gathering in an entirely different light. Family traditions take on new significance. Family rifts might be set aside for the sake of the care recipient. Everyone may seem to genuinely appreciate the time together.

How can you keep your clan's gatherings festive, without a

Point of View

"My father, Luther, is 93 years old. Occasionally, I take him to the local shopping mall or a restaurant. Before we leave the house, I make sure he's wearing a badge around his neck that contains his contact and medical information in case we should get separated. I want him to feel comfortable, so I made a badge for myself, too. I jokingly tell him that we look like a couple of conventioneers."

—KARL SMITH,
Newark, Delaware

lot of stress? Glasgow recommends following these holiday ground rules.

- First and foremost, maintain realistic expectations. You have a lot on your plate already, and you can do only so much. Give yourself permission to not have a "perfect" holiday.

- Begin preparations as far in advance as you can. This heads off stress in the long run. If any of the guests haven't seen your loved one for a while, you'll want to contact them beforehand to explain the sorts of physical and behavioral changes they should expect.

- Request help if you need it. Often people don't pitch in simply because they aren't asked to.

- Plan the gathering with respect for the care recipient's needs. For example, if the person is accustomed to eating at certain times of the day, schedule the holiday meal accordingly. During the festivities, try to keep a lid on noise levels, and be sparing with decorations and blinking lights.

- Consider a small gathering, especially if your loved one has dementia. He may feel overwhelmed in the presence of a large group.

- Reevaluate your family traditions and continue the most meaningful ones as much as possible. Against the upheaval and uncertainty of a caregiving situation, traditions are a stabilizing force. Everyone in the family—and especially the care recipient—identifies with them and draws comfort from them.

- Gently encourage the care recipient to participate in the festivities. Be sure to include him in conversations. Engage him in a comforting activity, such as looking at old photo albums and reminiscing.

- Refrain from bringing up family disagreements, even though all the key players may be present. You're together for only a few hours, and you don't want to spoil the holiday with a confrontation. Instead, suggest setting up a time for a family meeting or a one-on-one conversation.

✗ Avoid serving alcohol to your loved one if he's taking any kind of medication, and especially if he has Alzheimer's or another degenerative disease. The combination of rich food and alcoholic beverages can cause confusion and hyperactivity in those with dementia.

Take Action... CELEBRATE SPECIAL OCCASIONS

In the context of a caregiving situation, birthdays and other special occasions—like Mother's Day and Father's Day—seem more important than ever. Certainly they present a wonderful opportunity to honor your loved one. Time and togetherness may be the greatest gifts you can give. Here's how to package them.

✗ Prepare the person's favorite meal, using his "special recipe." Invite everyone else in the family to come to dinner dressed in their Sunday best.

✗ Take a drive to a place that holds special meaning for your loved one. Try to stay on country roads and avoid fast-moving highways. Instead of listening to the radio, engage in a "trip down memory lane" conversation.

✗ Dig out old family photo albums and spend the day leafing through them with your loved one. Ask questions about the photos to get him talking, then let him reminisce.

✗ Give your loved one a massage, gently rubbing his neck, shoulders, and back. For comfort, he can sit at a table and lay his head on a cushy pillow. Play soft music to help him relax.

✗ Make arrangements for family members and friends to call with their best wishes. You might want to set up a phone schedule, so everyone has a chance to talk with the person of the hour.

Take Action... INVOLVE FAMILY THAT'S FAR AWAY

In our highly mobile society, with family members living miles—even continents—apart, holidays and special occasions may be the only times everyone can gather together. But physical

EXPERT OPINION

"As a physician who travels a lot and an only son, I knew that I could not adequately care for my 96-year-old mother, Irene, in my home. She lives in an assisted living center just 3 miles away. We spend quality time together. Just this morning, I went to the center and had breakfast with her in the big dining room. We chatted with some of her friends. Even if I'm traveling, I call her every other day. I advise my patients who are caring for sick spouses, parents, or grandparents of the importance of spending time with them. It's one of the best gifts you can give a loved one."

—DALE L. ANDERSON, M.D., an urgent care physician in St. Paul, Minnesota

Point of View

"My husband, Jerry, can't get around much now—he needs a walker and has trouble maintaining his balance—so taking long trips by airplane or car is no longer feasible. Fortunately, we have a time-share condo that's only about 2 hours from our home. Every August, we invite our children and friends to visit us there. We cook meals, share stories, and laugh a lot. Both my husband and I look forward to these annual getaways."

—MARY SHANDY,
Costa Mesa, California

distance needn't prevent families from spending quality time with their loved ones, particularly those who are receiving care. Thanks to technology, interacting across the miles can't get much easier. For example:

✗ Encourage relatives who live far away to call the care recipient on a regular basis, ideally once a week. They can use these conversations to share good news and fond memories.

✗ Have family members make audio or video recordings for the care recipient. Youngsters, in particular, will get a kick out of taping their messages. For the care recipient, hearing or seeing their loved ones on tape can provide wonderful mental stimulation, not to mention a healthy laugh or two.

✗ Request photos from faraway family birthday parties, anniversary celebrations, and other special events. Family members can explain what's happening in the pictures when they talk with the care recipient over the phone.

✗ If your loved one is mentally and physically able, teach him to use e-mail as a way of staying in touch with family members. Some Internet services such as Web TV are easy to operate and don't require a lot of computer knowledge. "Learning something new can be very exciting and satisfying for a care recipient, especially someone who is homebound," Glasgow says.

PART FIVE

Reaching Out for Help

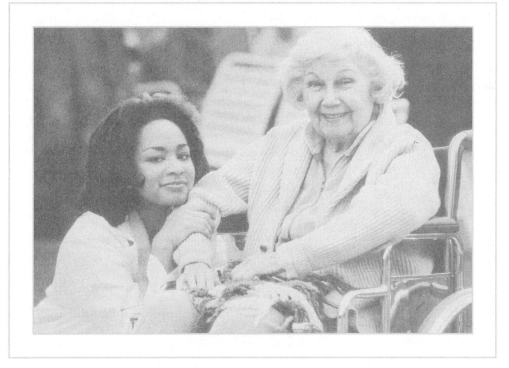

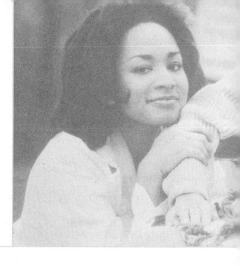

CHAPTER 19

COMMUNITY-BASED CAREGIVING

What You Need to Know

- Before you make your first phone call, give some thought to the kinds of assistance your loved one requires. Are you looking for transportation? Telephone check-ins? Adult day care? Write it down.

- Begin your search for support services with the Area Agency on Aging. The staff there can help guide you through the maze of community resources, directing you to the ones you need.

- Contact local churches as well as any veterans groups and/or fraternal orders to which your loved one belongs. Many such organizations offer support services.

- If you get tangled in bureaucratic red tape, consider hiring a professional care manager. You will pay a fee, but it's worth saving on stress.

I n caregiving, community services can be lifesavers. They give care recipients a choice between staying at home and moving into assisted living facilities. They protect caregivers against burnout by providing support for a range of tasks. And they provide guidance for anyone dealing with caregiving's complex legal and financial issues.

True, finding the right services for your loved one's situation and coordinating them on the person's behalf takes time and effort. You may need to make a lot of phone calls or go through a maze of referrals before you reach the appropriate person or organization.

This is where a geriatric care manager or social worker can help immensely. Either professional can assess your loved one's

FOR MORE INFORMATION

The National Association of Professional Geriatric Care Managers operates a nationwide referral network. To request a list of current members by geographic region, you can call **(520) 881-8008** or visit **www.caremanagers.org**.

To find a qualified social worker in your area, call the National Association of Social Workers at **(800) 638-8799**, or visit the organization's Web site at **www.socialworkers. org**.

needs, match available resources to your situation, and—perhaps most important—put you in touch with the right people in the right places. Your loved one's physician may be able to refer you to a qualified geriatric care manager or social worker in your area. If your loved one is being released from the hospital, ask her discharge planner for a recommendation.

Keep in mind, too, that some family service organizations—such as Catholic Charities, Lutheran Services, Jewish Family and Children's Services, and the Veterans Administration—will provide case management for a fee (often on a sliding scale, based on income) or for free. Your loved one must meet certain age and income requirements to be eligible.

Take Action... MAKE THE MOST OF AVAILABLE RESOURCES

The kinds of support services available to caregivers and care recipients tend to vary from one community to the next. (The names of these services can vary, too, though recognizable categories of assistance exist.) In general, people in urban and suburban areas may have better access to a more expansive network of caregiving resources than people in small towns and rural areas. But even there, you should be able to find basic support services, such as meal delivery, telephone reassurance, and the U.S. Postal Service's Carrier Alert program.

The following strategies can help you make the most of the services offered in your area.

✗ Determine which services your loved one needs and which you can provide. As mentioned above, a geriatric care manager or social worker can assist with this task. But you and your loved one may decide to handle it yourselves if the person's needs are rather simple and straightforward—for example, she needs help with housework or lawn maintenance.

✗ Do research to find out what kinds of services are available where you (or your loved one) live. Again, you can do this with guidance from a geriatric care manager or a social worker, or you can tackle it on your own. Some community resources, like the Area Agency on Aging (AAA), provide information and referrals for a range of services. (We'll talk more about the AAAs in just a bit.) With a little phone work, you may be able to find a grocery store that offers free delivery, or a hairstylist or manicurist who makes house calls.

✗ Assess the quality of the available services. Even if you are getting a referral from a physician or the AAA, you need to check out the service provider for yourself. Conduct your own interviews. Visit facilities like senior centers and adult day care centers unannounced to see how clean they are and what sorts of activities are going on. If at any point in this process a provider seems hesitant or refuses to answer certain questions, take that as your cue to move on.

✗ Inquire about the fee for every service, and expect a clear answer. If you don't get one, it's best to continue your search. Also, be sure to get the fee in writing before you sign a contract with any service provider.

✗ Ask whether your loved one qualifies for free or subsidized services. If the person is a veteran, for example, he may get many services at no charge. Sometimes free or subsidized assistance is available only short term.

✗ Find out whether your loved one's insurance will pay all or part of the fee for a particular service. In general, Medicare and Medicaid coverage for community services is rather limited. Private insurance may be more generous, but you'll need to contact your loved one's insurer with questions about his policy.

Through this entire process, involve your loved one as much as possible. The person may be more likely to accept assistance—and to realize you can't do everything by yourself—if he's included in the decision making to the extent possible. If you think it would help, you could ask someone whom your loved one respects and trusts—like a close friend or a member of the clergy—to participate in discussions of caregiving issues.

With all this in mind, let's take a closer look at some of the support services commonly available for caregivers and care recipients.

EXPERT OPINION

"For a long time, we've had a program in Albert Lea [Minnesota] where seniors are given a chance to call in to the fire department on a daily basis. If they don't call the fire department, the fire department calls them. So every day seniors have contact with someone, and if they have a problem or an emergency, we have a chance to deal with it very quickly. This is just one way that we can keep tabs on the seniors of Albert Lea, and it's relatively inexpensive."

—THE HONORABLE GIL GUTKNECHT, Congressman, First District, Minnesota

What's Available in Your Community?

Make a photocopy of this chart. Then as you talk with various providers about the caregiving resources in your community, fill in each column with the information you gather. It can help you (in consultation with your loved one) compare services and decide which ones best suit your situation.

Resource	Contact Person	Available Services
Area Agency on Aging	_____	_____
Church organizations	_____	_____
	_____	_____
Veterans agencies and organizations	_____	_____
	_____	_____
Fraternal organizations	_____	_____
	_____	_____
Senior center	_____	_____
YM/YWCA	_____	_____
Meal delivery programs	_____	_____
	_____	_____
Transportation services	_____	_____
	_____	_____
Telephone reassurance	_____	_____
Carrier Alert program	_____	_____
Health insurance counseling	_____	_____
	_____	_____
Support groups	_____	_____
	_____	_____

Fee	Covered by Insurance?	Notes
_____	☐ yes ☐ no	_____
_____	☐ yes ☐ no	_____
_____	☐ yes ☐ no	_____
_____	☐ yes ☐ no	_____
_____	☐ yes ☐ no	_____
_____	☐ yes ☐ no	_____
_____	☐ yes ☐ no	_____
_____	☐ yes ☐ no	_____
_____	☐ yes ☐ no	_____
_____	☐ yes ☐ no	_____
_____	☐ yes ☐ no	_____
_____	☐ yes ☐ no	_____
_____	☐ yes ☐ no	_____
_____	☐ yes ☐ no	_____
_____	☐ yes ☐ no	_____
_____	☐ yes ☐ no	_____
_____	☐ yes ☐ no	_____
_____	☐ yes ☐ no	_____
_____	☐ yes ☐ no	_____

To find the Area Agency on Aging in your loved one's community, you can look in the blue pages of the phone directory, in the "Guide to Human Services." You can also call the national referral number, the Eldercare Locator, at **(800) 677-1116** or visit **www.eldercare.gov**.

People who use this service, which is operated by the National Association of Area Agencies on Aging, have access to more than 4,800 state and local information and referral service providers, identified for every ZIP code in the country. The database also offers telephone numbers for Alzheimer's hotlines, adult day care and respite services, nursing home ombudsman assistance, consumer fraud, in-home care complaints, legal aid, elder abuse/protective services, Medicare/Medicaid/Medigap information, tax assistance, and transportation.

AREA AGENCIES ON AGING

As mandated by the federal government's Older Americans Act, every state must have an agency devoted exclusively to protecting the welfare of older citizens. This agency—which might be called the Commission on Aging, Department of Aging, or Office of Aging—is charged with establishing and overseeing regional and county offices to serve an area's senior population. These local offices are known as Area Agencies on Aging.

Consider your loved one's AAA a point of entry in the search for caregiving resources. AAAs plan, implement, and coordinate services that enable older adults in need of care to live independently. Some services are provided by the AAAs directly, while others are subcontracted to local providers. The best way to find out what's available where your loved one lives is to call the agency directly.

The services offered by Area Agencies on Aging, depending on location, include the following. (Some of these will be covered in more detail a bit later in the chapter.)

Information and referral assistance. Every AAA has trained staff answering its phones. These professionals can direct you to the services that may help most, based on your loved one's situation.

Client assessment. Someone from the AAA staff can evaluate your loved one's needs and eligibility for services. This can be done either over the phone or in person at your loved one's home.

Care management. Based on a physical, psychological, and social assessment of your loved one, the AAA staff can recommend a plan of care that includes community services. The plan might also call for medical treatment, if necessary.

Senior centers. AAAs often sponsor these centers, where older adults can enjoy social and recreational activities. Some senior centers serve meals; others provide adult day care for older people who are functionally impaired. (For more information on adult day care, see chapter 20.)

Meals on Wheels. Through this low-cost service, volunteers deliver well-balanced prepared meals to people who can't shop or cook for themselves. For someone who's homebound, the deliveries are a welcome opportunity for social contact. And the daily visits by volunteers may provide some peace of mind for caregivers.

Transportation. The AAA staff can help you arrange rides for your loved one to destinations such as the doctor's office or the supermarket.

Health insurance counseling. AAAs can help beneficiaries understand their options and rights under Medicare, Medicare+Choice, and Medicaid. They can also provide information on Medigap and other insurance alternatives. This service is available by phone.

Caregiver support. The recently established National Family Caregiver Support Program helps those who help others. Through the AAAs, it provides caregiver training, individual counseling, group support, and respite care (either free or for a fee), among other services.

Beyond all these resources, AAAs may offer home health care, housekeeping assistance, telephone reassurance, and emergency response systems. Some also have elder abuse prevention programs, which intervene in situations of abuse, neglect, or self-neglect.

CHURCH ORGANIZATIONS

Some organizations with religious affiliations have caregiving resources similar to those offered by the AAAs. You might choose a religious group over the AAA and other providers because you feel its services will better align with your (and your loved one's) values and principles. Then again, maybe the organization has a more convenient location or hours. Or it's the only provider where your loved one lives.

You might even perceive the services of a religious group as entitlements. "People have a sense of being part of us, and expect more from us, possibly because they've contributed to our financial drives in the past," notes Harry Citron, a licensed clinical social worker for Jewish Family Services of Baltimore.

You don't need to belong to a particular church to take advantage of a religious group's caregiving resources, since most of these organizations will assist anyone of any faith. Some are under contract with government agencies, which means their services are fairly secular.

Here's a sampling of organizations with religious affiliations and the caregiving resources they offer.

FOR MORE INFORMATION

To locate Catholic-based caregiving support services in your loved one's community, look in the white pages of the phone directory for Catholic Family Services, Catholic Community Services, Catholic Charities, or Catholic Social Agency. Or visit www.catholiccharitiesusa.org/states. It identifies service providers by state.

If you're interested in Lutheran-based caregiving support, contact Lutheran Services in America at (800) 664-3848 or www.lutheranservices.org.

The Association of Jewish Family and Children's Agencies has an online Elder Support Service Directory that lists service providers and contact information by state. You can view the directory at www.ajfca.org. For other Jewish-based caregiving resources in your loved one's area, look in the white pages of the phone directory for Jewish Family Services.

- Catholic-based programs for the elderly are available through organizations such as Catholic Family Services, Catholic Community Services, Catholic Charities, and the Catholic Social Agency. The programs vary by location, but typically include senior centers, adult day care, transportation, and counseling.

- Lutheran Services in America sponsors a variety of community-based caregiving resources, including senior centers, adult day care, telephone reassurance, and transportation. The organization also operates nursing homes.

- The Association of Jewish Family and Children's Agencies does client evaluations and assessments, as well as case management. Its other programs include home and telephone check-ins, meal delivery, shopping assistance, respite care, counseling, and crisis assistance. These services vary by location.

When contacting these organizations, keep in mind that their services aren't necessarily free. Often they assess fees on a sliding scale, based on income.

VETERANS AGENCIES AND ORGANIZATIONS

If your loved one is a veteran or a veteran's dependent, you'll definitely want to look into the support services and benefits available through veterans agencies and organizations. (Before you do, make sure you have all the necessary military discharge papers handy.)

At the federal level, health and medical programs for veterans are the responsibility of the Veterans Health Administration and the Veterans Benefits Administration, both agencies of the U.S. Department of Veterans Affairs (VA). The VA may be best known for operating hospitals, outpatient clinics, and nursing homes. But it offers many other services as well, including geriatric evaluation and management, home care, adult day care, respite care, and hospice care.

Depending on your loved one's veteran status, income, and other criteria, some VA-sponsored programs may be free, while others will require co-payments. Veterans who are at least 50 percent disabled because of a service-related illness or injury may be eligible for VA-financed home health care coverage. To qualify,

---

FOR MORE INFORMATION

If your loved one hasn't looked into veterans benefits or services before, here's what to do.

- For inquiries about health benefits, call the U.S. Department of Veterans Affairs (VA) at **(800) 827-1000**, or go to the Web site **www.va.gov**. On the home page, click on "Compensation and Benefits." At the bottom of that page, click on "Facilities Locator." This will direct you to the VA office in your loved one's area.

- For information about medical services, call **(877) 222-VETS** or go to the VA Web site. On the home page, click on "Health"; then scroll down and click on "VHA Facilities Locator." This will identify VA hospitals, clinics, and nursing homes in your loved one's area.

In addition, your state Department of Veterans Affairs can provide locations and contact information for state-run veterans homes, along with eligibility requirements. For a telephone number, look in the blue pages of the telephone directory.

the services must be authorized by a physician and must be provided through the VA's network of hospital-based home care units. The coverage does not apply to nonmedical services, such as housekeeping assistance.

The VA also gives financial support to state-run veterans homes. These facilities primarily provide nursing home care, though some may offer domiciliary (residential) care—available to veterans who cannot live independently because of medical or psychiatric disabilities—and adult day care.

Veterans organizations such as the Veterans of Foreign Wars (VFW) and the American Legion operate independently of the VA. Both advocate on behalf of their members (who pay membership fees) and support many community services. Both also help veterans to understand their government benefits.

With 2.8 million members, the American Legion is the larger of the two organizations. Members belong to local "posts," which will readily pitch in to help a veteran who's having trouble with his benefits claims. Some posts may provide services like telephone reassurance and transportation. If your loved one is a member, call his post to find out what services are available.

Like the American Legion, the VFW will go to bat for members tied up in the bureaucratic red tape of benefits claims. Membership has other perks, too, like life insurance and senior discounts. While local posts sometimes are viewed as social clubs, they're much more than that. "The VFW offers many opportunities not just for socializing but also for meaningful volunteer work," says Jerry Newberry, the VFW's national director for communications and public affairs. "The members of each post are encouraged to come up with new and creative ways to use their facilities, including activities that benefit not just them but the entire community."

FRATERNAL ORGANIZATIONS

Perhaps your dad is a longtime dues-paying Elk, Eagle, or Raccoon. If so, his local lodge might offer some assistance now that he's in need of care. Most likely, the assistance will take the form of phone check-ins, home visits, and transportation. But some fraternal organizations offer much more.

FOR MORE INFORMATION

The Veterans of Foreign Wars (VFW) has trained service officers who know the complexities of the law and will intervene on behalf of a member who has been denied veterans benefits. To learn more about this service, you can call the National Veterans Service hotline at **(800) VFW-1899** or **(202) 543-2239**. You can also visit the VFW Web site at **www.vfw.org**.

FOR MORE INFORMATION

Fraternal organizations are listed in the Yellow Pages under "Fraternal Orders." Check there for the telephone numbers you need.

The Masons (or for women, Eastern Star) is the largest fraternal order in the United States. In about 30 states, the grand lodge—a statewide administrative body—sponsors services for elderly members that include assisted living and nursing home care. Contact the grand lodge in your loved one's state to find out whether such services are available there.

For other fraternal organizations, your best bet is to contact the local lodge directly. You can also try calling the lodge officers, if your loved one can provide their names and phone numbers.

SENIOR CENTERS

If you're concerned about an older loved one who's home alone during the day with not much to occupy her time, you might try to interest her in visiting her local senior center. These centers can fulfill your loved one's need for company and activity. In fact, the services they provide are sometimes referred to as social day care.

Some senior centers are small social clubs that operate out of church basements. Others are large, publicly funded programs that offer a range of stimulating physical, social, and recreational activities, including exercise classes, movies, games, lectures by guest speakers, current events discussions, computer training, arts and crafts classes, and field trips. Health services—like blood pressure screening and blood sugar monitoring—may be made available to clients. Meals and snacks may be provided, too.

FOR MORE INFORMATION

Your loved one's Area Agency on Aging can tell you about the services provided at local senior centers. You can also check with the centers directly. They're listed in the blue pages, under "Guide to Human Services."

In general, senior centers are free and open to all elderly residents of any age, income, and health status, though some cannot accommodate people with dementia, mobility problems, or incontinence (unless your loved one can manage that herself). For some special activities or services, a fee may be charged. Hours of operation vary from center to center.

YM/YWCAS

YM/YWCAs count older adults among their most loyal members. More than 60 percent of Ys have health and fitness programs—especially aquatics classes—that are geared toward the senior population. Many have their own senior centers and social clubs. And they present numerous volunteer opportunities for those older people who are willing and able to share their time and talents.

A growing number of YM/YWCAs are offering adult day care programs that include an array of health-oriented activities, as well as arts and crafts. Some Ys have child day care, which means kids and adults get to mingle for some activities—a winning situation for both generations.

The YM/YWCAs vary in their accommodations for people with physical limitations and disabilities, though many now have chair lifts or ramps for their pools. You'll need to call the local Y to find out what's available there.

MEAL DELIVERY PROGRAMS

Meals on wheels has become a generic term for any program that delivers prepared meals directly to a person's door. These

FOR MORE INFORMATION

To learn more about the programs and activities that your local YM/YWCA offers, you can contact the organization directly. It should be listed in the white pages of the phone directory.

Caregiving around the World

Norwegians believe that seniors should remain in their own homes for as long as possible. To that end, communities provide innovative health and social services around the clock. One example is a Meals on Wheels program that delivers seven frozen meals each week, saving money on delivering one hot meal every day. Another example is a nursing home that sets aside two beds for seniors displaced by household emergencies, such as a power outage. Also, when a person reaches age 67, she receives a letter from the local senior center inviting her to become a member. Transportation is provided by volunteers.

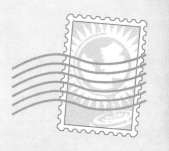

POST CARD

FROM NORWAY

programs—one uses Meals on Wheels as its official name—are available in most parts of the country, usually through senior centers, religious organizations, or hospitals. The majority are funded by the federal government through the Older Americans Act. For this reason, the meals must meet certain nutritional standards, providing one-third of the Recommended Dietary Allowances for adults age 65 and older. (Incidentally, meals served at senior centers must comply with this guideline, too.)

Typically, each delivery includes a hot lunch and a cold, bagged dinner. Often the meals are distributed by volunteers who have been trained to watch clients for signs of a medical problem or other trouble—a bonus benefit for care recipients and caregivers alike. The cost for delivery is nominal, usually no more than $5 a meal. Some programs provide meals for free or simply request a donation.

Some meal delivery programs limit their eligibility to homebound or low-income residents. If your loved one doesn't qualify, you may have other options. For example, some cooks and caterers will deliver a week's worth of meals at a time, or even prepare the food right in your loved one's kitchen. And some organizations offer meal services for people who have special dietary needs because of medical problems like diabetes and renal failure. Ask your loved one's physician or dietitian about the availability of these services.

Another option is to have frozen meals delivered by mail. One program recommended by the National Meals on Wheels Foundation is Home Cooking for You, which prepares healthful homestyle meals and ships them nationwide. Of course, your loved one would need to heat the meals himself.

TRANSPORTATION SERVICES

In a caregiving situation, transportation can be a major issue—especially if the care recipient isn't able to leave the house by herself, much less drive anywhere. Chances are you're too busy to be a full-time chauffeur. But just as likely, your loved one has appointments that she just can't miss. Besides, you probably don't want her spending hours at home alone simply because she has

---

FOR MORE INFORMATION

The Meals on Wheels Association of America can refer you to meal delivery programs that serve your loved one's community. Call **(703) 548-5558** or visit the Web site at **www.mowaa.org.**

FOR MORE INFORMATION

Information on Home Cooking for You is available by phone at **(800) 235-7070** or online at **www.homecookingforyou.com.**

no way to get where she'd like to go. So where can she find some reliable "wheels"?

The AAA that serves your loved one's community may provide transportation to and from adult day care, senior centers, shopping malls, and specific appointments. In some cases, a van or bus will pick up a group of people on a set day and take everyone to a predetermined destination, such as the supermarket. In other cases, a driver takes a person door to door for individual appointments and errands.

Some community transportation services are free, while others may have a nominal fee or ask for a donation. Many of the buses and vans are wheelchair accessible.

If the services offered through AAA don't meet your loved one's needs or schedule, you might be able to find a private driver, perhaps a retiree who's looking to make some extra cash. Check with your loved one's church or fraternal organization, if he belongs to one. Just make sure the person you hire is licensed, insured, safe, and dependable.

TELEPHONE REASSURANCE

As its name suggests, telephone reassurance involves prescheduled calls to homebound older adults to reduce their isolation and monitor their well-being. Often the caller is a volunteer senior citizen, who may ask routine questions such as "Did you take your medications today?" or "What did you eat for lunch?" If something doesn't seem right, or if the person doesn't answer the phone, the volunteer will alert you or another person designated as a contact.

Telephone reassurance services are available through AAAs, religious groups, senior centers, and other public or nonprofit organizations. Home health care agencies may offer phone check-ins as well, for a fee.

CARRIER ALERT PROGRAM

Through the Carrier Alert program, you can authorize your loved one's letter carrier to watch for any unusual or unplanned accumulation of mail. Should the carrier notice anything suspi-

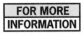

FOR MORE INFORMATION

Look in the Yellow Pages under "Limousine Service" to see the sorts of private transportation options available in your loved one's community. You needn't hire an actual limo; you may be able to find a reasonably priced sedan service.

FOR MORE INFORMATION

If you'd prefer to arrange phone check-in services through a private home health care agency, look in the Yellow Pages under "Home Health Services" to see what's available in your loved one's area.

cious, a postal supervisor would contact the AAA where your loved one is registered. The AAA would try to contact your loved one by phone. If he cannot be reached, the agency would alert the designated emergency contact. If that person can't be reached, the AAA would send someone to your loved one's home to check on him.

Carrier Alert is a free program offered by the U.S. Postal Service. To sign up for it, contact your loved one's AAA, or ask his letter carrier for information.

HEALTH INSURANCE COUNSELING

Every state has a Senior Health Insurance Assistance Program (SHIAP) or Health Insurance Counseling and Advocacy Program (HICAP) staffed by information specialists or trained volunteers. These people are available to help Medicare beneficiaries and their families understand their options and rights under Medicare, Medicare+Choice, and Medicaid, and to provide information about Medigap and other insurance options. Usually consultations are handled over the phone, though they may be done in person.

Additional services offered by SHIAP or HICAP vary from state to state. They may include comparisons of health insurance and managed care plans, assistance with medical bills and insurance claims, and information on long-term care insurance.

Many AAAs participate in SHIAP or HICAP either by offering health insurance counseling directly or by subcontracting it through another provider. We'll discuss health insurance and benefits more thoroughly in chapter 24.

SUPPORT GROUPS

Support groups are wonderful resources for caregivers and care recipients who want to talk with other people in the same situation as theirs. Perhaps more than anyone else, group members understand and sympathize with what you're going through. Their own experiences produce real-world advice on how you can cope.

The best support groups emphasize what you can do for

FOR MORE INFORMATION

New York State runs a good Web site that features contact information for health insurance counseling programs in many other states. You can check out the Web site at **www.hiicap. state.ny.us/home/ hiassist.htm.**

FOR MORE INFORMATION

To find out which support groups are available for your loved one, try the National Self-Help Clearinghouse at **www. selfhelpweb.org** or the American Self-Help Clearinghouse Self-Help Sourcebook at **www.mentalhelp.net/self help.** You can also look in the blue pages of the phone directory, under "Support Groups."

yourself, and what you can gain by doing for others. Some groups offer their members respite care. Others allow members to borrow medical equipment such as canes, wheelchairs, and hospital beds.

If your loved one has a particular medical problem, you may be able to find a support group just for people with that illness and/or their families. Groups exist for Alzheimer's disease, cancer, stroke, Parkinson's disease, and just about any serious condition you can name.

Some support groups have been established specifically for caregivers. For example, Children of Aging Parents sponsors 63 groups nationwide. And the Well Spouse Foundation, which targets spousal caregivers, has 40 groups nationwide. If neither organization has a group in your area, you can always start one of your own.

If you have access to a computer, don't overlook the many support groups online. For a list of what's available, visit Elder-Care Online at www.ec-online.net or Empowering Caregivers at www.care-givers.com.

FOR MORE INFORMATION

For caregiver support, contact either of the following organizations.

• Children of Aging Parents, 1609 Woodbourne Road, Suite 302A, Levittown, PA 19057. Phone: **(800) 227-7294** or **(215) 945-6900**; Internet address: **www.caps4 caregivers.org**.

• Well Spouse Foundation, 610 Lexington Avenue, #814, New York, NY 10022-6005. Phone: **(800) 838-0879**; Internet address: **www.wellspouse.org**.

CHAPTER 20

HELPING HANDS FOR THE CAREGIVER

What You Need to Know

- A growing number of caregiving families are taking advantage of home care services. For the most part, these services are less expensive than residential care, and they allow a loved one to remain at home longer.

- A home care agency can help coordinate services on your loved one's behalf. You can also hire home care providers who work independently of agencies.

- Most health insurance programs cover a very limited number of home care services. But with a little digging, you may be able to find services that are provided free or for a reduced fee.

- For caregivers, adult day care and respite care offer a welcome break from day-to-day responsibilities and can help protect against burnout.

You do your best to care for your loved one. You're up with the sun to put in a load of his laundry. You call at lunch to make sure he has taken his medication. You rush home from work to make him a healthy dinner. By bedtime, you're exhausted—and after too little sleep, you start all over again.

Like many caregivers, you may be realizing that you can't squeeze 48 hours' worth of responsibilities into a 24-hour day—plus have time for your family, your job, and yourself. It only leaves you tense and exhausted. You know you need help.

Fortunately, help is available. In fact, home care is among the fastest-growing trends in health care. The reason? Quite simply, most people who become care recipients would rather stay in their own homes than move into residential care. While comfort and familiarity may be their primary motivators, the economics make sense, too: Most home care—with the exception of round-the-clock skilled nursing—costs less than the care provided in nursing homes, most assisted living facilities, and hospitals.

In general, home care services are available 24 hours a day, 7 days a week. The care providers may work by themselves or as a team on a shift, part-time, hourly, or as-needed basis.

Each year, more than 22,000 agencies nationwide provide home care services to more than two million people with physical disabilities, chronic health problems, dementia, or terminal illnesses. And as the American population ages, the number of home care agencies is expected to grow.

But assessing all the services provided by these agencies and choosing the ones that best match a loved one's situation can seem overwhelming. As many caregivers discover, they need help finding help.

"Often family caregivers don't know where to turn," says Robert Bua, chief executive officer of CareScout, a Miami-based eldercare Web site. "So what do they do? They go on the Internet and do vast searches. On our Web site, we've had almost one million hits. That's people 'walking through our doors' in search of solid, trusted information on caring for their loved ones."

But the Internet isn't the only place to learn about home care. You can get information and referrals for home care agencies, as well as independent home care providers, from a number of organizations in your community. The Area Agency on Aging can facilitate your search (for more information, see chapter 19), as can your family service agencies and your local chapter of the Visiting Nurse Associations of America. Geriatric care managers, social workers, and hospital discharge planners are other good resources. (When evaluating prospective home care agencies, don't forget to use the Caregiver's Checklist on page 88.)

In this chapter, we'll explore six general categories of home care available to care recipients and their families.

- Home health care
- Homemaker services
- Live-in help
- Adult day care
- Respite care
- Hospice care

FOR MORE INFORMATION

To help narrow your search for a home care agency, look for one that is affiliated with one of these accrediting associations.

- Accreditation Commission for Health Care: **(919) 785-1214**

- Community Health Accreditation Program: **(800) 669-1656, ext. 242**

- Joint Commission on Accreditation of Healthcare Organizations: **(630) 792-5000**

- Homecare University: **(202) 547-3576**

Caregiver's Checklist

What Kind of Home Care Can Help Most?

In general, home care services are considered either "supportive" or "skilled." Using the following checklist, you can determine which services will be most helpful to your loved one (and to you). Simply mark each item "yes" or "no."

Supportive Services	Yes	No		Yes	No
Bathing, shampooing hair	☐	☐	Providing companionship	☐	☐
Using toilet	☐	☐	Providing transportation	☐	☐
Brushing teeth	☐	☐	Repairing or maintaining home	☐	☐
Dressing	☐	☐	**Skilled Services**	**Yes**	**No**
Doing laundry	☐	☐	Medical care	☐	☐
Making meals	☐	☐	Nutrition management	☐	☐
Washing dishes	☐	☐	Physical therapy	☐	☐
Vacuuming	☐	☐	Professional counseling	☐	☐
Monitoring medications	☐	☐	Emergency response systems	☐	☐
Assisting mobility	☐	☐			

You'll learn what they are, what they cost (and how to pay for them), and what you should look for when comparing providers. From there, you and your loved one can decide which services will be most helpful in your particular situation. Remember, they exist for the sole purpose of supporting caregiving families like yours. So don't hesitate to make the most of them.

HOME HEALTH CARE

Mary Hart is a visiting nurse for a home health care program in St. Paul, Minnesota. After 20 years of working in a hospital, she chose to switch over to home health care because of the growing demand for it, especially among older people. When she visits clients, she may take their blood pressure, or set up their medications, or administer their injections.

"So many of my clients are single, without families. They're in desperate need of neighborhood-type nursing care," Hart says. "They get to know me very well, and they depend on me to get them to their doctor appointments, or to call their doctors on their behalf."

The skilled nursing Hart provides is just one example of the services that might come under the umbrella of home health care. These days, clients can obtain all kinds of medical treatment and support on an in-home basis—whether they're looking for physical or occupational therapy, nutrition counseling, dental or podiatric care, or something else.

The makeup of your loved one's home health care team de-

The Home Care Patient Bill of Rights

The federal government requires that all people receiving home care services are informed of their rights. To that end, the National Association for Home Care has created a patient bill of rights, which is enforced by federal law. A home care patient is entitled to:

- Receive appropriate and professional care in accordance with physician's orders
- Choose care providers
- Be fully informed of all his or her rights and responsibilities by the home care agency
- Receive timely responses for service requests made to the home care agency
- Be given service only if the agency can provide safe, professional care at the level required
- Receive reasonable continuity of care
- Receive the information necessary to give informed consent prior to the start of any treatment or procedure
- Be advised of any change in the plan of care, before the change is made
- Refuse treatment within the confines of the law

and be informed of the consequences of his or her action

- Be informed of his or her rights to formulate advance directives as provided by state law
- Have health care providers comply with advance directives in accordance with state law requirements
- Be informed within reasonable time of anticipated termination of service or plans for transfer to another agency
- Be fully informed of agency policies and charges for services, including eligibility for third-party reimbursements
- Be referred elsewhere, if denied service solely because of his or her inability to pay
- Voice grievances and suggest changes in service or staff without fear of restraint or discrimination
- Receive a fair hearing when any service has been denied, reduced, or terminated
- Be informed of what to do in the event of an emergency
- Be advised of the telephone number and hours of operation of the state's home health hotline

EXPERT OPINION

"In general, home health aides and other personal care workers are considered low-skill labor, earning maybe $8 to $10 an hour. What we're finding is that because of demographic shifts across the United States, we're going to experience a shortage of these workers over time.

"Today, roughly 700,000 elders have no children or siblings to provide care for them. In another 20 to 30 years, that number is going to double. These people will need to rely completely on formal or paid caregiving systems."

—**MARC A. COHEN,** vice president of LifePlans, Inc., and president of the Center for Health and Long-Term Care Research, both in Waltham, Massachusetts

pends on her specific situation. In general, the key players may include the following:

Physicians. Some doctors still make house calls, especially for their homebound patients. More commonly, they'll work with home health care providers to identify a patient's needs and develop a plan for her care. According to Medicare regulations, the plan must be reviewed by the physician and home care agency officials at least every 62 days in order to remain eligible for coverage.

Registered nurses (R.N.s) and licensed practical nurses (L.P.N.s). If your loved one has a particular medical problem, a nurse can play a vital role in managing treatment. She's trained to check vital signs (such as temperature and high blood pressure), administer intravenous therapy, change wound dressings, and provide other skilled medical care.

Social workers. In caregiving, perhaps one of the most important functions of a social worker is to serve as a liaison between the family and available community resources. Sometimes these professionals act as case managers to coordinate a person's medical and supportive care. Social workers also can assess the emotional and social factors that may be affecting a care recipient's well-being and provide counseling, if necessary.

Physical therapists. As their title suggests, physical therapists use exercise, massage, and other techniques to restore the strength and mobility of patients whose physical abilities have been hampered by illness or injury. Physical therapy also does wonders for pain management and relief.

Occupational therapists. If your loved one has difficulty with routine tasks like eating, bathing, and dressing, she may work with an occupational therapist to relearn them, or adapt them to her abilities. The goal of occupational therapy is to improve function in everyday living.

Speech language pathologists. Sometimes people develop a speech disorder as a result of surgery, stroke, or another trauma. A speech language pathologist can provide training in speech skills, as well as in proper breathing technique, swallowing, and muscle control.

Dietitians. For some conditions, like heart disease and diabetes, a special diet may be part of the treatment plan. But good nutrition (along with adequate hydration) makes sense for anyone who wants to maintain the best health possible. That's where a dietitian can help, offering nutrition counseling and developing meal plans to help your loved one improve her eating habits.

Home health aides. These professionals can assist with routine personal tasks like getting in and out of bed, bathing, and dressing, as well as some household services. They are not trained to administer medications or provide other skilled medical care.

Companions. While they're not health care providers in the conventional sense, companions contribute a valuable service to home care. Basically, they act as adult sitters, spending time with care recipients who can't or don't want to be left alone. The two may play games, make crafts, watch television, or just enjoy each other's company.

With the exception of physicians, all of these health care providers can be hired through a home care agency. Some but not all states require these agencies to be licensed and to meet minimum standards of care. You're not obligated to go through an agency, however. Many professionals in the home health care field—including nurses, therapists, home health aides, and companions—choose to work independently. Just keep in mind that if you go this route, you're responsible for recruiting and hiring your home health care team, and for supervising their services. You'll want to check credentials to be sure each person has received appropriate training and is bonded.

Who Pays?

Because Medicare, Medicaid, and private health insurance pay for only certain home health care services, many caregiving families decide to pay out of their own pockets. But that may not be necessary. For example, some community organizations—local chapters of the American Cancer Society, the Alzheimer's Association, and the Easter Seal Society, among others—may have funds to subsidize home health care. And the U.S. Department of Veterans Affairs (VA) offers home health care coverage to eligible

FOR MORE INFORMATION

To find out whether any organizations in your loved one's community offer financial support for home health care, your best bet is to call the Area Agency on Aging. Look in the blue pages of the phone directory in the "Guide to Human Services," or check the Eldercare Locator at **(800) 677-1116** or **www.eldercare.gov**.

For information about veterans benefits, call the U.S. Department of Veterans Affairs at **(800) 827-1000,** or visit the VA Web site at **www.va.gov**.

EXPERT OPINION

"I would like to see church congregations develop a goal-centered, high-quality senior adult ministry program so that seniors don't get the leftover time in the pastor's schedule or the congregation's schedule. Most churches have programs for children, youth, stewardship, social ministry, evangelism, and worship, but not all have goal-centered programs for senior adults.

"Right now, at least 25 percent of most church members are senior adults. When we baby boomers become the seniors in our congregations, we are going to want high-quality programs."

—**THE REVEREND LOIS KNUTSON,**
visitation pastor for Our Savior's Lutheran Church in Montevideo, Minnesota

military veterans, with the conditions that the necessary services be authorized by a physician and provided through the VA's network of hospital-based home care units.

In Pittsburgh, the city's Veterans Administration Healthcare System has mobile geriatric units that travel to the homes of veterans in need of medical care. "The geriatricians on our staff attend to the specific needs of a very large segment of our veteran population," explains VA representative David Cowgill. "The vans allow us to reach those people who may not be physically able to get to our hospital, and who may not receive care if we did not go to them."

HOMEMAKER SERVICES

In addition to health care, many home care agencies offer homemaker services. They'll send someone to your or your loved one's home to do light cleaning, laundry, grocery shopping, meal preparation—pretty much anything that will help keep the household running. Perhaps the only thing they can't do is provide any sort of medical care.

Generally, homemakers work on an hourly or live-in basis. (We'll talk about live-in helpers next.) Their rates can range from minimum wage to $18 an hour, depending on the skill level and experience necessary for your particular situation. While the fees likely won't be reimbursed by Medicare, Medicaid, or private health insurance, they may be waived or adjusted on a sliding scale for people who are low income.

Like some home health care providers, some homemakers offer their services independently rather than through an agency. You'll need to screen the candidates yourself to find someone whom you and your loved one trust and feel comfortable with. Make sure the person is bonded, too.

LIVE-IN HELP

If you or your loved one has the living space and the financial resources (since the costs will most likely be out-of-pocket), you may consider hiring a live-in helper. This type of home care is best suited to long-distance caregiving situations, in which the primary caregiver can't be there in person and the care recipient needs round-the-clock support. In this arrangement, the family must provide the hired helper with room and board. In exchange, the helper can prepare meals, do light housekeeping, and perform other nonmedical services.

If you opt for live-in caregiving, you want to take the time to make sure you're choosing the right person for the job. Helpers work through agencies or as independent contractors. Officials of the National Association for Home Care offer these guidelines for effectively screening candidates.

- Conduct an in-depth interview with each candidate—in person, if that's possible. Be sure to cover all of the questions in the Caregiver's Checklist on page 254.

- Thoroughly explain all of the tasks the prospective caregiver will be expected to take on. Now is the time to find out whether the person is unable or unwilling to do certain kinds of work.

- If the candidate works independently, discuss salary, but avoid agreeing to pay wages in advance. Instead, offer to issue paychecks on a regular schedule, perhaps weekly or biweekly.

- Request references and check them carefully. Ask about the person's reliability, punctuality, and trustworthiness, as well as her ability to handle stress. Try to get some insight into her personality and her attitude toward those who are ill or elderly. If the person works independently, ask whether she is bonded.

Perhaps most important, be sure to include your loved one in the screening process, if he's able to participate. After all, he's going to be living with the person you hire. His opinion should carry as much weight as anyone else's.

"Ask your loved one how he feels about each candidate," advises Rich O'Boyle, founder of ElderCare Online and a member of the National Association of Geriatric Care Managers. "Always put the care recipient first, and never lose sight of what he likes and wants."

ADULT DAY CARE

Around the United States, adult day care centers are growing in popularity among caregivers who need to provide full-time as-

---

FOR MORE INFORMATION

The National Association for Home Care has a wealth of resources for those interested in live-in help and other kinds of in-home caregiving services. You can write to the association at 228 Seventh Street SE, Washington, DC 20003, or call **(202) 547-7424.** On the Internet, visit **www.nahc.org.**

How Qualified Is a Live-In Helper?

When you're interviewing candidates to provide live-in care for your loved one, be sure to get answers to the following questions, adapted from *Hiring Home Caregivers: The Family Guide to In-Home Eldercare* by D. Helen Susik, M.A.

1. Why are you interested in the home care field?

_____

2. What is your previous home care experience?

_____

3. What type of training have you received?

_____

4. Why did you leave your last position?

_____

5. Do you currently provide care for others? If so, how many clients do you have?

_____

6. How many hours per week will you be available to provide care for my loved one?

_____

7. How flexible is your schedule?

_____

8. Are you willing to perform light household chores such as cooking and vacuuming?

_____

9. What type of vehicle do you drive? Is it insured?

_____

10. Will you be able to run errands or take my loved one to appointments?

_____

11. How have you handled emergency situations in the past?

_____

12. How do you deal with someone who may resist care?

_____

sistance and supervision for their loved ones but who want to find an alternative to 24-hour live-in care. Currently, more than 4,000 of these centers are operating nationwide. They fall into three general categories: those that encourage social interaction; those that offer medical care (also known as adult day health care); and those that focus on Alzheimer's care.

The social day care centers offer a full slate of activities, from games and gardening to art classes and museum field trips. Some of these centers may assist with bathing and other personal care tasks. The medical day care centers expand on the personal care aspect, providing services such as blood pressure monitoring, physical and/or occupational therapy, and medication management (some of which may be covered by Medicare). Centers that specialize in Alzheimer's care tend to have more staff trained to assist people with dementia and more medical personnel than social day care.

Adult day care has advantages for both the caregiver and the care recipient. Caregivers can enjoy peace of mind knowing that their loved ones are in a safe and stimulating environment. As a bonus, they get a reprieve from their caregiving responsibilities to focus on other tasks or to treat themselves to a much-deserved day

Point of View

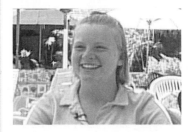

"I work at the Friendship Center because I love spending time with the elderly. I learn something new every day. Growing up, I wasn't around my grandparents very much. Now everyone at the center is like a grandparent to me."

—JAMIE ELTGROTH,
Santa Barbara, California

Calming Day Care Jitters

Anyone who has placed a child in day care can recall the overwhelming emotions of going there for the first time and leaving the little one behind. Those same powerful feelings—the guilt, the worry, the sadness—can resurface when an adult loved one enters a day care program.

Diane Feather sees it all the time. She's the director of caregiver family services for the Sheridan Senior Center in Sheridan, Wyoming. Recently, the center expanded its programs to include in-home assistance with personal care and housekeeping, transportation services for doctor appointments, and a program to deliver meals. But for 10 years, the cornerstone of the center has been an adult day care program called Daybreak.

Feather has noticed that when families bring their loved ones to day care for the first time, many are reluctant to leave. And some care recipients need to attend the program for several days before they settle in and feel comfortable there.

To help both care recipient and caregiver adjust to day care, Feather recommends easing into attending. Try 1 day a week to start, and increase gradually. "The caregivers, especially, need to remember that giving themselves a break can actually make them better at caregiving," Feather adds. "They shouldn't feel guilty about it."

The National Adult Day Services Association can help you find an adult day care program in your area. To contact the association or get a copy of its publication *Standards and Guidelines for Adult Day Care*, call **(866) 890-7357** or visit **www.ncoa.org/nadsa**. Closer to home, you may want to check with your Area Agency on Aging. The staff there can direct you to adult day care providers as well.

off. As for the care recipients, they respond well to the structured routines and opportunities for social interaction that are cornerstones of adult day care. In some cases, enrolling in an adult day care center can delay or even prevent placement in residential care.

But the benefits aren't limited to caregivers and care recipients. Many adult day care centers invite high school students to serve as volunteers. For those teens whose grandparents live far away or have passed away, the centers can bridge the generation gap, allowing them to meet and mingle with their elders.

If you're interested in adult day care for your loved one, experts recommend visiting a center several times, at different hours. Find out the history of the center, including the number of years it's been in operation and the qualifications of the director and staff. Make sure the ratio of staff to clients is adequate, and the environment is safe and secure. While the regulations governing adult day care centers vary from state to state, some "best practice" recommendations are outlined by the National Adult Day Services Association in its publication *Standards and Guidelines for Adult Day Care*.

A good adult day care center will assess your loved one prior to admission and develop a customized care plan that accommodates his medical and social needs. To follow through with the plan, the center should offer a full range of in-house services, as well as referrals to outside resources as necessary.

The cost of adult day care averages $50 a day. The actual fees can range from a few dollars a day for a limited or subsidized local program to more than $185 a day for a complex medical program that includes transportation, according to Mark S. Lachs, M.D., M.P.H., chief of geriatrics and gerontology at New York Hospital in Manhattan. In some states, Medicaid will pick up the tab for medical adult day care on behalf of beneficiaries who meet certain clinical and financial eligibility requirements. Most social adult day care is paid for out of pocket.

RESPITE CARE

Caregivers need time off from their caregiving responsibilities to relieve stress and prevent burnout. Whether you get the urge for a weekend getaway or a weeklong vacation, or your job takes you away from home, you can arrange for respite care during your absence.

In respite care, a trained professional will move in with your loved one and take over your caregiving role, whether for several hours or several days. As an alternative, you can place your loved one in a nursing home or residential care facility for a short-term stay.

These brief reprieves from a caregiving situation are healthy not just for caregivers but also for care recipients. Both of you can use an occasional break. Your loved one, especially, gets a chance to spend time with other people and to enjoy a change in his daily routine.

Despite these benefits, too many caregivers feel guilty, selfish, or ashamed for seeking out respite care, says Pauline Salvucci, founder and president of Self Care Connections in Cape Elizabeth, Maine. "Yes, asking for help is difficult. You're probably not used to doing it," acknowledges Salvucci, who cares for her 89-year-old mother at home. "Unfortunately, most caregivers take on the responsibility of caregiving without recognizing the ongoing necessity for occasional relief."

"I tell family caregivers that they must schedule 'away time' for themselves," adds Patricia McGinnis, executive director of the California Advocates for Nursing Home Reform in San Francisco. "Go to a movie or leave town for the weekend, whatever it takes. Otherwise, you risk getting ill or feeling stressed, isolated, and resentful."

Respite care does have one hitch: Medicare and most private health insurance policies won't cover it. Medicaid will reimburse the cost of short-term stays in nursing homes, but only for those who meet certain financial and functional eligibility requirements. To foot the bill, Salvucci suggests asking adult family members to contribute, say, $10 a week to a respite care fund. This allows relatives who live far away to pitch in with a loved one's care. Deposit the money in a bank account, so it's available when it's needed.

To find affordable, reliable respite care in your area, start by contacting your Area Agency on Aging, as well as local chapters of the Visiting Nurse Associations of America and the Alzheimer's Association. Primary care physicians and community hospitals can

FOR MORE INFORMATION

The Shepherd Centers of America train senior citizen volunteers to provide part-time respite care. Currently, more than 100 centers operate in communities throughout the United States. To learn more about this program, you can contact the organization by phone at **(816) 960-2022**. Or visit the Web site at **www. shepherdcenters.org**.

offer referrals, too. And don't forget to check with the churches and synagogues in your community. Some have volunteer respite care programs.

If you opt for in-home respite care, Salvucci recommends inviting the caregiver to visit with you and your loved one several times before a longer-term stay. You want the two of them to get acquainted with each other and to be comfortable while they're together.

"The care recipient should not feel like a stranger is in the house while the caregiver is away," Salvucci says. "You want a respite care provider who is attentive and patient, but not overbearing toward your loved one. And you need to spell out the provider's responsibilities in your absence."

HOSPICE CARE

If your loved one is terminally ill—generally meaning she has been given less than 6 months to live by a medical professional—you may want to contact your local hospice agency for help. Hospice professionals and volunteers serve as an extra pair of helping hands, offering care and compassion to your loved one during his last months of life.

Hospice may be best known for providing psychological and spiritual support for the terminally ill and their families. But it encompasses a much wider range of services, including skilled nursing care, respite care, social work support, and bereavement counseling. In addition, hospice workers are trained to answer questions about insurance benefits, funeral planning, and other end-of-life issues.

Once your loved one's physician authorizes hospice care, you'll need to schedule a consultation with the hospice team. If your loved one is able, he must sign consent and insurance forms that limit medical care to controlling symptoms and providing pain relief, without curative measures. (If your loved one can't sign for himself, you can do so on his behalf.)

Most hospices are state licensed and Medicare certified. Still, a physician's authorization is required for a patient to qualify for Medicare's hospice benefit, and the authorization must be renewed every 6 months. Medicare will pay for physician services,

FOR MORE INFORMATION

For a referral to a hospice care agency in your community, contact the National Hospice and Palliative Care Organization at **(800) 658-8898** or Hospice Link at **(800) 331-1620**. On the Internet, you can visit either organization's Web site: **www.nho.org** or **www.hospiceworld.org**.

skilled nursing, physical therapy, counseling, home health aide and homemaker services, and short-term respite and in-patient care, as well as medical equipment and supplies and medications for managing symptoms and controlling pain. Even with Medicare, you may be responsible for a small co-payment, according to the National Hospice Organization.

For families coping with the trauma of terminal illness, hospice can be a lifeline. Su Bonnet, a home health aide herself, remembers how hospice helped her and her parents as her mother, Judy, was dying of cancer.

Judy was diagnosed with pancreatic cancer in November 2000. When the cancer reached its final stage and was ruled inoperable, Judy's physician recommended hospice care.

"My mom did not want to die in a hospital, and my father promised to take care of her at home," Su, of Lake San Marcos, California, recalls. "When we began hospice care, my mother could no longer walk by herself and needed a wheelchair. She was losing weight, and she had a blood clot in her left thigh. The hospice workers were very kind and compassionate to my mother, and to my father and me."

With medical professionals and home health aides tending to Judy's physical needs, Su and her mom could enjoy private time together. Su would bring Judy fresh-cut flowers from the garden, make her iced coffee (her favorite drink), and brush her silver, silky hair. "Mom died on August 4, 2001, at age 73," Su says. "Thanks to hospice, my dad and I could honor her final wish—to die at home."

EXPERT OPINION

"Think of the revolution that has occurred in the average office over the past 20 years. By and large, all the menial, repetitive jobs have been replaced by technology. But in the field of caregiving, very little has changed. I think technology could have a major impact, improving the efficiency of caregiving without removing the ability of caregivers to interact with patients. I think the Internet will give us enormous potential for delivering care at a distance, but technology can't solve everything. [We need] a caregiving environment that's high tech and high touch."

—**EDWARD SCHNEIDER, M.D.,**
   dean of the Leonard Davis School of
   Gerontology at the University of
   Southern California in Los Angeles

CHAPTER 21

HOUSING OPTIONS BEYOND HOME CARE

What You Need to Know

- These days, a variety of housing options exist for care recipients. Each one is designed for people with specific needs and lifestyles.

- The best time to discuss your loved one's long-term living arrangements is well before she may require alternative housing.

- At many assisted living facilities and nursing homes, staffing shortages continue to be a source of concern. If you're looking into this sort of facility on your loved one's behalf, be sure to make note of staff-to-resident ratios.

- A stepped care community offers independent living arrangements, an assisted living facility, and a nursing home on one campus. Residents can move from one facility to another as their health and medical needs dictate.

For many caregiving families, the time comes when a loved one requires more supervision and support than they can provide at home. Unless the person made plans for his long-term care, the rest of the family faces a difficult, often heart-wrenching question: "Where will our loved one live?"

Years ago, that question was pretty much a rhetorical one. If a person's physical or mental health declined to the point where he failed to thrive with home care, his family's main alternative would have been nursing home placement, even if he didn't require 24-hour skilled nursing. But since the early 1990s, the number of housing options has grown considerably, driven by the demands of families who want an intermediate level of care for their loved ones.

"It's demographics at work," says Bruce Rosenthal of the American Association of Homes and Services for the Aging, a coalition of nonprofit social service organizations in Washington, D.C. "People are living longer, so the United States has more elderly than ever. And more are on the way, as the baby boom generation gets older. Compared with their parents, today's elderly are wealthier, better educated, and more consumer-savvy. They want choices, and the housing industry is responding. The latest innovations in housing cost less than nursing homes, and they also help preserve independence."

Take Action... PUT A HOUSING PLAN IN PLACE

The best time to review housing options with your loved one is *before* more advanced care becomes necessary. In fact, in an AARP survey, a clear consensus of older Americans said they want to discuss with their families what will happen should they become unable to live independently.

Of course, that doesn't make raising the issue any easier. "You're asking your loved one about a situation that she hopes never comes up. She may refuse to talk about it," says Gail Hunt, executive director of the Bethesda, Maryland–based National Alliance for Caregiving. "Still, you'd like to get some sense of the person's preferences while she's independent, so you can gauge whether they're changing as she begins to need help. Most people insist that they don't want to end up in a nursing home. Then as their health declines, they may become less resistant to the idea of residential care."

If you and your loved one haven't discussed her future living arrangements, and she's able to do so, you should seriously consider broaching the subject sooner rather than later. Use the following strategies to facilitate the conversation.

✗ Assess your loved one's abilities and circumstances. If you completed the Caregiver's Checklist on page 30, you may want to take another look at it now. Do you see a lot of categories with C and D responses? They're good indicators that your loved one requires frequent or ongoing assistance, perhaps beyond what can be provided at home.

Point of View

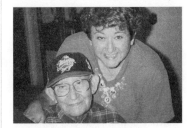

"I love my dad and felt I shouldn't abandon him. But I knew I had to place him in residential care—for my health, for my mother's health, and for him, too. He has very special needs, and I couldn't provide for him anymore. Placing him was heartbreaking. He took care of me all his life, and now I couldn't take care of him. But I just couldn't."

—ALICIA FRANCO,
Santa Barbara, California

FOR MORE INFORMATION

If you haven't contacted your Area Agency on Aging before, you can obtain a telephone number by looking in the blue pages of your phone directory, in the "Guide to Human Services." Another option is to use the Eldercare Locator by calling **(800) 677-1116** or visiting **www.eldercare.gov**.

For a referral to a qualified social worker or geriatric care manager in your area, check with one of the following organizations:

• National Association of Social Workers. Phone: **(800) 638-8799**; Internet address: **www.socialworkers.org**.

• National Association of Professional Geriatric Care Managers. Phone: **(520) 881-8008**; Internet address: **www.caremanager.org**.

✗ Talk with other family members about your loved one's situation. If they also completed the Caregiver's Checklist, as suggested in chapter 3, ask whether they marked any C and D responses, and if so, in which categories. Building consensus within the family can strengthen your case for recommending alternative housing to your loved one.

✗ Explore your housing options. Your Area Agency on Aging can fill you in on the facilities and services in your community and put you in touch with people who can provide additional information. If you prefer, you can hire a social worker or geriatric care manager to help evaluate and narrow your choices. Then you'll be prepared when you approach your loved one to discuss them.

✗ When you raise the housing issue with your loved one, make clear that you're doing so out of love and concern. Let her know that you're worried about her trying to handle too much by herself.

✗ Pose questions rather than making pronouncements. For instance, avoid saying "You can't live on your own anymore." Instead, ask "If something happened, and you couldn't live on your own anymore, where would you want to go?"

✗ Bring up the subject indirectly. Using the Caregiver's Checklist on page 30 as your guide, casually ask your loved one how she's managing those tasks you feel she's struggling with. "Are you doing okay with your grocery shopping?" "Do you have any problems cleaning the house?" "You take a lot of medications; how do you track all of them?" Then listen carefully to your loved one's replies; they may provide an opening for further discussion of her housing situation.

✗ Take your cues from your loved one's unsolicited comments. Older people, especially, tend to talk freely about their aches and pains, as well as other infirmities. You can use these kinds of complaints as springboards to a conversation about housing. "I'm sorry to hear your knee has been acting up. Do you think living in a home with so many stairs might be aggravating the problem?"

X If your loved one resists efforts to talk about her housing arrangements, don't force the issue. Sometimes a crisis must occur in order for a person to accept that she can't be by herself anymore. At that point, she'll be more open to your intervention—and you'll be ready to step in and help. In the meantime, be patient.

X If your loved one refuses to consider alternative housing, even though you and other family members feel she can't stay in her current situation, consider gathering the entire family for a group intervention. This sort of meeting must be handled with care; you don't want your loved one to feel she's being criticized or attacked, which will only make her more resistant to discussing her living arrangements. Encourage everyone to be gentle and respectful, but firm: "We're concerned about you, and we want to help you make decisions about your care."

X If your loved one won't listen to her family, enlist the aid of someone else whom she trusts. Perhaps a physician, a member of the clergy, or an old friend could convince the person that she can't wait much longer to talk about her housing preferences.

Keep in mind that as long as your loved one remains mentally competent, she can make her own decisions about her living arrangements, even if you don't agree with them. Your best bet is to educate yourself about the available services and facilities, so if the person asks for your help—and eventually, she will—you'll be ready. With that in mind, let's explore the more common housing options for those requiring care.

ACCESSORY HOUSING

If your loved one wants to continue living independently, even though you and your family feel she needs more supervision and support, accessory housing might be a suitable compromise. It could take the form of an apartment carved out of your basement—often called an in-law unit—or a small cottage behind your home. In either arrangement, your loved one would be close, but in a separate dwelling. She could share meals and participate

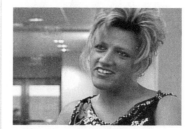

Point of View

"One night, my father woke up totally out of it and turned on the water in the bathtub. He flooded my house. My kitchen ceiling collapsed. The carpeting was destroyed. He had no idea what he'd done. That's when it got to be too much for me. When I finally placed him in a nursing home, it was a relief. I felt guilty, but it was a relief."

—PAM HADDAD,
Pittsburgh

FOR MORE INFORMATION

If you're thinking about remodeling your basement to include an apartment for your loved one, the book *Creating an Accessory Apartment* by Patrick Hare and Jolene Ostler can show you how. Look for it at your local library.

AARP also publishes information about accessory and ECHO housing. Call **(800) 424-3410,** or on the Internet, go to **www.aarp.org** and type "ECHO" in the search field.

in activities with your family as she chooses, while retaining her independence and privacy.

A freestanding accessory cottage can be built from scratch or purchased already assembled. The manufactured models—sometimes called ECHO units (for Elder Cottage Housing Opportunity)—are like conventional mobile homes, only smaller. They're moved onto your property and set up.

Installing an accessory unit can cost between $20,000 and $40,000, a significant investment for most caregiving families. The unit will increase your property value—an advantage if you're planning to sell your home, a drawback if you're already footing a hefty property tax bill. In addition to these issues, you need to consider the following:

• Is accessory housing allowed on your property? Zoning regulations or deed restrictions may prohibit it. Your municipality's zoning officer can help with this information.

• Is accessory housing acceptable to your neighbors? The last thing you want is to install an ECHO cottage in your backyard and get embroiled in a costly legal battle because of it. Explain your plans to your neighbors and find out whether you have their support.

• Do you need special permits, even if you're putting an accessory apartment in your basement? Be sure you have all the necessary documents before you begin work. Otherwise, you may face fines and removal of the new unit.

When Massachusetts resident Gail Finger decided to explore accessory housing for her parents, a local contractor offered to build a self-contained 526-square-foot, one-bedroom apartment for $65,000. "Then my father found out about the ECHO units," Finger says. "We got one completely installed—foundation, utilities, everything—for $35,000. The quality is exceptional. Meanwhile, my old house squeaks and creaks wherever we walk."

Even though her parents' living space is adjacent to her own, it's treated as completely separate. "We don't have a connecting doorway," Finger says. "If we want to visit each other, we must go outside and walk next door. It helps maintain everyone's privacy."

And if that privacy is threatened, Finger and her parents don't hesitate to let each other know about it. "A few times, my parents intruded a bit too far into my family life, and I had to tell them to back off," Finger recalls. "It was hard, but we grew closer because of it. Keeping silent would have bred resentments and driven us apart."

SHARED HOUSING

Think of college students renting a house together. Each person gets a private bedroom and has access to common areas like the kitchen and bathroom. All the residents are responsible for a portion of the household chores and bills.

That's shared housing. While an old concept for the young, it's a newer concept for the elderly—one whose time has definitely arrived.

In some cases, several older adults will form a group for the express purpose of buying or renting a home and sharing it. More commonly, someone who already owns or rents a home has extra rooms and invites others to move in.

According to the National Shared Housing Resource Center, shared housing is a good alternative for older people who function reasonably well on their own but want to reduce their living expenses. As a bonus, they'll get security, companionship, emotional support, and possibly a helping hand with routine tasks.

Like accessory housing, shared housing comes with its own set of issues. Zoning regulations may prevent groups of unrelated people from living together. Neighbors might object if the new residents make too much noise or take up too many parking spaces. Landlords may be reluctant to rent to a group. Remember, too, that if your loved one's living expenses decline in a shared housing arrangement, so may her government entitlements—notably any Supplemental Security Income payments she's receiving. (Supplemental Security Income, or SSI, is a government entitlement program for low-income elderly and disabled.)

Even so, shared housing is gaining in popularity among the older population. "I'd estimate that 40 percent of the people in shared housing arrangements are seniors," says Laura Fanucchi, West Coast coordinator for the National Shared Housing Resource Center. "This housing option can work very well for them,

FOR MORE INFORMATION

The National Shared Housing Resource Center publishes a directory of programs that help older people establish a shared housing arrangement. The organization has nine regional offices throughout the United States. To find the one that serves your area, visit **www.nationalshared housing.org.**

Information on shared housing is also available from AARP. Call **(800) 424-3410,** or on the Internet, go to **www.aarp.org** and type "homesharing" in the search field on the home page.

Outlook

"In the future, I think we'll see more women entering the workforce and more mobility of the workforce. As a result, I expect that caregiving by adult children, particularly women, will become increasingly difficult. My hope is that the societal response to these changes in geography and gender roles will be to create innovative ways of formal and informal caregiving. I think we may see more men providing caregiving, both as spouses and adult children, in the next 10 to 30 years. And I wouldn't be surprised if older people begin to take caregiving into their own hands. I imagine a world of 'families' of older persons living together to stay independent. I have fond memories of communal living from college days. I wouldn't be averse to going back to that."

—HOWARD FILLIT, M.D., executive director of the Institute for the Study of Aging in New York City

especially if they own or rent their homes. They can save on living expenses and get help with tasks like cooking, housekeeping, and lawn maintenance. Shared housing is a great way for seniors to live independently while giving each other the assistance they need."

ASSISTED LIVING

Somewhere between the independent lifestyles of accessory and shared housing and the round-the-clock care of nursing homes, you'll find the as-needed support of assisted living (AL) facilities. Usually, residents of these facilities must be able to walk, eat, bathe, dress, and perform other personal care on their own. Housekeeping is provided, as are meals (though some housing units may have kitchens, so residents can cook for themselves if they choose). An on-site medical staff monitors each resident's health and medications and can intervene in the event of a medical emergency. Educational, recreational, and social programs are offered as well, to engage the residents physically and mentally.

AL facilities evolved from the so-called board and care homes, a sort of pre-nursing home from the 1970s. The concept of AL developed in the 1980s, and since then, facilities have sprung up all over the country. According to *American Demographics* magazine, some 45,000 AL facilities were constructed in the 1990s. Some are decidedly no-frills, while others seem more like country clubs. Depending on the facility, units can be purchased outright or rented on a monthly or yearly basis.

Today, AL facilities serve as residences for some 1 million Americans. The cost for this kind of housing varies, but according to recent surveys by *Time* magazine and the National Association of Elder Law Attorneys, it averages $75 to $100 a day (or $2,250 to $3,000 per month). That's compared with $120 to $150 a day (or $3,600 to $4,500 per month) for nursing homes.

As common as AL facilities have become, they continue to be viewed with skepticism by much of the older population. "People seem to think that once they move in, they lose their independence," says Francine Moore of the Assisted Living Federation of America, a nonprofit organization that represents 6,000 AL facilities nationwide. "In fact, residents are encouraged to be as independent as they're able. Facilities vary in the services they provide, but most strive to be flexible because residents want choices, and because their need for help varies so much."

Shop Around before Signing

Like nursing homes, AL facilities have come under scrutiny in recent years, primarily because of quality-of-care issues arising from understaffing and poor staff training. In a 1999 General Accounting Office report involving 721 AL facilities in four states, 27 percent had been cited for quality-of-care violations more than 5 times, and 11 percent had been cited 10 or more times. The report also criticized the facilities for issuing contracts that are vague or misleading, or that lack important information about fees and services.

"Assisted living facilities are repeating the same mistakes so many nursing homes have made," says Janet Wells, director of public policy for the National Citizens' Coalition for Nursing Home Reform in Washington, D.C. "They grow too much too fast, paying too little attention to staffing and quality of care."

"Some AL communities do have problems," Moore acknowledges. "As with anything else, you need to explore assisted living with both eyes open. Visit several facilities to get a feel for them. And be sure to read their contracts carefully."

The staff of your Area Agency on Aging can provide information on AL facilities in your community. You can also seek referrals from family members, friends, physicians, members of the clergy, and local seniors organizations.

Once you find a few facilities that you're interested in, you can evaluate them using the Caregiver's Checklist on page 268. All the items in the checklist are important, but the fact is, no facility is perfect. "You need to focus on the criteria that you and your loved one consider top priorities," Moore explains. "Most prospective AL residents want a community that's affordable, that's organized to preserve their independence, and that has friendly residents and helpful staff, including medical personnel who can respond to emergencies. Beyond that, just remember to read the contract carefully." Even better, review the contract with an attorney, preferably one who specializes in elder law.

Keep in mind that every state has an agency responsible for inspecting, licensing, and issuing Medicare/Medicaid certification to residential care facilities. These agencies can tell you whether

(continued on page 273)

FOR MORE INFORMATION

Beyond your Area Agency on Aging, any of the following national organizations can facilitate your search for assisted living (AL) facilities.

• The Assisted Living Federation of America maintains a list of member facilities that can be searched by state, county, and city. To access the list, visit **www.alfa.org** and click on "Consumers." You can also call **(703) 691-8100**.

• The American Association of Homes and Services for the Aging publishes a member directory containing both AL facilities and nursing homes, as well as booklets on selecting a good facility. Call **(202) 783-2242**, or visit **www.aahsa.org**.

• CareScout/National Eldercare Referral Systems maintains a Web site, **www.NursingHomeReports.com**, that contains a wealth of information about AL facilities. To speak with someone directly, call **(800) 571-1918**.

• The Consumer Consortium on Assisted Living offers resources for prospective residents of AL facilities, including a checklist for evaluating facilities. Call **(703) 533-8121** or visit **www.ccal.org**.

Caregiver's Checklist

How Does an Assisted Living Facility Measure Up?

Many caregiving experts recommend visiting an assisted living facility several times before deciding to place a loved one there. When you go, be sure to take along the following checklist, adapted from the Consumer Consortium on Assisted Living in Arlington, Virginia. Answer as many questions as you can, then look back over the list, focusing on those responses you and your loved one feel matter most.

General

• How close is the facility to family and friends? (A good facility that's nearby might be a better choice than an excellent facility that's far away.) _____

• Is the facility accepting new residents? _____

    If not, what is the anticipated waiting period? _____

• What is the occupancy rate? (If it's unusually low, the quality of care may be poor.)_____

• Have any complaints been filed against the facility? _____

    _____

    If so, how were they resolved? (Contact your Area Agency on Aging or your local long-term care ombudsman for this information.) _____

• Is the facility licensed and certified by a state agency? _____

    If any problems were found, have they been corrected? (The facility should have the latest licensing inspection report.) _____

    _____

Costs

• What is the basic fee? _____

    What services does it cover?_____

• What additional services are available? _____

    At what extra charge? _____

• Is a deposit required? _____

    Is any of it refundable if you change your mind? _____

• If a resident is away for an extended period (perhaps in the hospital or visiting children), which fees still apply?_____

• When, how often, and why can fees be changed? _____

• When fees are changed, how much notice are residents given?_____

- If residents need financial assistance, is any available? _____

- Are residents required to carry renters insurance?_____

- If an accident destroys a resident's property, or if a resident damages property, who is responsible for cleanup, repair, and replacement? _____

Contracts

- Is the print large enough for an older person to read? (If not, ask for a large-print version.) _____

_____

- Does it specify basic fees? _____

    Extra charges? _____

- Does it explain refund policies in case of transfer, discharge, change in ownership, or closing? _____

_____

- Does it explain the responsibilities of the resident and the facility? _____

- Does it specify resident conduct that may result in a request to leave?_____

- Does it specify residents' rights? _____

- Does it outline a reasonable grievance procedure? _____

    An appeals process? _____

Staffing

- Is the staff friendly and interested in the residents?_____

- How many staff members work each shift? _____

    What are their responsibilities? _____

- How much training does the staff have? _____

    What kind of training do they have? _____

- How many residents are assigned to each direct-care staff member? _____

    What other duties does the direct-care staff have? _____

- Does the direct-care staff speak the residents' language? _____

- Do staff members have special training to deal with people in the early stages of dementia?_____

_____

- How does the staff deal with aggressive residents or wanderers?_____

- If residents don't like their direct-care staff, can changes be made? _____

- What is the staff turnover rate? _____

(continued)

Caregiver's Checklist
continued

Personal Care

• What assessment is done to determine a new resident's needs? _____

• Who assesses new residents? _____

    What are that person's qualifications? _____

• How often are residents reassessed? _____

• Does the facility customize daily schedules to accommodate residents' eating and sleeping habits and other preferences? _____

• How often are residents' quarters cleaned? _____

• Does the staff have a schedule for checking on residents' whereabouts and well-being? _____

• What happens when a resident's health status changes, making the person require more care? _____
_____

• How does the staff determine whether a resident who's in declining health must move to another facility that provides more advanced care? _____

• What if a person needs nursing home care but doesn't want to leave behind a spouse or partner? _____
_____

• Must residents have normal cognitive function? _____

    Are people with early-stage dementia accepted? _____

Health Care

• Does the facility provide a written plan of care for each resident? _____

• Who develops this plan? _____

• How often is it revised? _____

• Can residents and their families offer their input on the plan? _____

    If so, how? _____

• What if residents or their families disagree with some aspect of the plan? _____

• To what extent do staff members monitor residents' health? _____

• Is a nurse on staff? _____

    What are the person's hours and responsibilities? _____

• Is a doctor on staff? _____

    What are the person's hours and responsibilities? _____

• If doctors and nurses are not on staff, do they visit regularly? _____

    Are they on call? _____

• If a resident complains of illness, what happens? _____

• Under what circumstances do staff members call a resident's family or doctor? _____

• What safeguards ensure that residents get the right dose of the correct medication on the prescribed schedule? _____

• How are prescriptions filled? _____

• Must residents use the facility's pharmacy? _____

    If so, what do medications cost?_____

• Who reviews the residents' medications? _____

    How often does this occur?_____

Emergencies

• Who decides if 911 should be called? _____

• What kinds of medical emergencies have staff members been trained to handle? _____

• Does the staff know what to do in the event of fire, flood, and other nonmedical emergency? _____

Transportation

• Is transportation available for off-site shopping and other activities?_____

• Is transportation available for doctor and dentist appointments? _____

• What do transportation services cost? _____

• Is transportation accessible to people in wheelchairs? _____

Meals

• Does a nutritionist or dietitian review meals and plan special diets for residents who need them? _____

• When are meals served?_____

• What if a resident is late for a meal or misses it completely? _____

• If a resident wants to skip a meal regularly, is the person entitled to a refund?_____

• Can meals be delivered to residents' quarters? _____

    Does this cost extra?_____

• Can residents request special diets for ethnic or religious reasons? _____

• What snacks are available and when? _____

Activities and Socializing

• Does the facility have a weekly or monthly activity schedule? _____

• Who develops and supervises recreational activities? _____

    What is that person's training?_____

• Do the residents and their families have any input in planning activities?_____

(continued)

Caregiver's Checklist
continued

- How much freedom do residents have to walk the grounds? _____
- Does the facility have an enclosed outdoor area for residents with dementia? _____
- How are religious needs met? _____
    Does the facility have an on-site chapel? _____
    Is transportation available to religious institutions? _____

Accessibility

- Must residents be fully ambulatory? Or are canes, walkers, and wheelchairs allowed?_____
  _____
- Is the facility fully accessible to wheelchairs? _____

Safety

- Are floors covered with nonskid surfaces? _____
- Does the facility have regular fire drills? _____
- Does the facility have an emergency evacuation plan in place? _____
    Is the plan available to residents and their families? _____
- How does the emergency evacuation plan address people with disabilities?_____
- Does each room, including the bathroom, have a call button? _____
    How often are the call buttons checked to make sure they work?_____
- Do the windows have safety locks? _____
- Which doors are locked and when? _____
- Do the emergency exit doors have alarms? _____
- What measures prevent confused residents from wandering away?_____
- What measures protect residents' property from being damaged or stolen? _____
  _____
- Are background checks performed on all staff members? _____
    If so, what kind of checks? _____

Facility-Initiated Discharge

- Under what circumstances can a resident be asked to leave? _____
- How many days' notice is given? _____
    To whom? _____
- What are the steps in the appeal process? _____

certain AL facilities are licensed and certified, and what standards they must meet. All the records are open to the public.

NURSING HOMES

The main distinction between AL facilities and nursing homes is that the latter provide round-the-clock medical supervision and support, often in a more hospital-like setting. The typical accommodations are either a private room with bath or a two-person room with bath. Staff members help residents toilet, bathe, dress, eat, and socialize. Physicians and nurses are on staff and on call.

Currently, about 1.7 million Americans reside in nursing homes (also known as skilled nursing facilities). Anyone who lives to age 65 has a 50-50 chance of spending some time in one.

Most people think of nursing homes as permanent residences for those who need long-term care. But short-term stays have become quite common—especially among those who require some sort of posthospital rehabilitation, as after a stroke. Generally Medicare will pay for short-term stays, but not for most long-term care. Another federal program, Medicaid, will pick up the tab for that, provided that the patient meets a number of strict financial criteria. (Medicare, Medicaid, and other benefits programs are covered at length in chapter 24.)

Nursing Homes That Make the Grade

Wouldn't it be wonderful if someone rated every nursing home in the country? Thankfully, someone does: CareScout/National Eldercare Referral Systems, a Wellesley, Massachusetts, company that's funded by the insurance industry.

"For 4 years in a row, we've knocked on the doors of 17,000 nursing homes nationwide," says Robert Bua, chief executive officer of CareScout. "We've analyzed their inspection reports and given them letter grades from AAA to F.

"The bad news is, only 3 percent of homes earned a AAA rating, meaning that according to their inspection reports, they had no deficiencies in 4 years," Bua continues. "The good news is, 35 percent earned an A rating, meaning they had a few deficiencies that have been corrected. So you see, good nursing homes are out there. But you may have to search for them, and when you find them, they may cost a lot."

For a nominal fee, you can obtain copies of the nursing home evaluations prepared by Bua's company. For more information, call CareScout/National Eldercare Referral Systems at (800) 571-1918 or visit www.NursingHomeReports.com.

Federal law requires every state to have an Office of the Long-Term Care Ombudsman. It's responsible for sending inspectors to nursing homes to monitor their quality and investigate complaints. To track down your state's long-term care ombudsman, call the National Association of State Units on Aging at **(202) 898-2578.**

The National Citizens' Coalition for Nursing Home Reform is a consumer advocacy organization that supports the states' long-term care ombudsmen. To learn more about the organization's services, call **(202) 332-2275** or visit **www.nccnhr.org.**

The Nursing Home Compare Database, a service of Medicare, contains information about the performance of every Medicare- and Medicaid-certified nursing home in the United States. It also features a "Guide to Choosing a Nursing Home." The database is available at **www.medicare.gov.** If you don't have Internet access, call **(800) 633-4227.**

These days, nursing homes are a growth industry. According to a 2001 survey by the federal Agency for Healthcare Research and Quality, annual expenditures for nursing home care soared from $28 billion to $70 billion between 1987 and 1996.

Unfortunately, nursing homes have a rather spotty reputation. Many people remain wary of them because of well-publicized scandals about poor-quality care. In early 2002, the U.S. Department of Health and Human Services (DHHS) released a report stating that 90 percent of nursing homes have too few staff to provide adequate care. Currently, many homes have one aide for every eight to 14 residents, while the report recommends one aide for every five or six residents. The DHHS investigators estimate that reaching satisfactory staffing levels would cost an additional $7.8 billion a year.

Good nursing homes with adequate staffing do exist. But they're not the norm. Too many homes don't provide proper training for their staffs to develop the necessary caregiving skills. Nor do they offer satisfactory pay or other incentives for top-quality employees to devote their lives to such difficult work.

In the early 1990s, Janet Wells, director of public policy for the National Citizens' Coalition for Nursing Home Reform, placed her mother in a nursing home, where she remained for 10 years. "Staffing is key," Wells says. "Ideally, each resident should receive 4 hours of hands-on care every day from the nursing staff and nurse's assistants." She recommends looking carefully at the amount of time staff members spend directly caring for residents. Scrutinize recent state inspection reports, too.

Take Action... PLAY A PROACTIVE ROLE IN YOUR LOVED ONE'S CARE

Before you start shopping around for a nursing home, you need to ask yourself one question: "Does my loved one really require 24-hour, round-the-clock care?" If not, you should look into assisted living facilities instead.

On the other hand, if a nursing home seems like the best option, your first phone call should be to the Area Agency on Aging. The staff there can fill you in on nearby homes, and tell you whom to contact for further information. Be sure to ask others

(continued on page 279)

Protecting the Rights of Nursing Home Residents

Reports about nursing home neglect and abuse prompted Congress to pass the Nursing Home Reform Law, later supplemented by the Americans with Disabilities Act. The law is very explicit about the rights of nursing home residents. The following synopsis is adapted from the book *Nursing Homes: Getting Good Care There*, published by the National Citizens' Coalition for Nursing Home Reform.

Access to information. Residents have the right to:

- Information about all services and their costs
- Information about the facility's policies, procedures, rules, and regulations
- Assistance from the state's long-term care ombudsman in resolving problems
- Information about state inspections of the facility
- Assistance in cases of vision or hearing problems
- Information communicated in the language they speak

Participation in care. Residents have the right to:

- Review their medical records
- Receive appropriate care for and information about their conditions
- Refuse medications and other treatments and request alternatives, if available
- Participate in discharge planning

Making choices. Residents have the right to:

- Choose their physicians
- Participate in activities
- Participate in a residents' council

Privacy and confidentiality. Residents have the right to:

- Private, unrestricted communication (including phone calls, letters, and meetings) with family and friends

- Assistance from any individual or agency providing health, legal, social, or other services
- Confidentiality regarding personal, medical, and financial affairs

Dignity and respect. Residents have the right to:

- Freedom from mental and physical abuse
- Freedom from unnecessary physical and chemical constraints
- The same care as other residents, regardless of their payment source

Security and complaints. Residents have the right to:

- Present grievances to staff and administrators without fear of reprisal
- Have grievances resolved promptly and professionally
- Manage their personal and financial affairs, or delegate the task to someone else
- File complaints with the state for abuse, neglect, or mishandling of property

Transfers and discharges. Residents have the right to:

- Not be transferred or discharged except for medical reasons, if their actions threaten the health and safety of others, for nonpayment of fees, or if the facility closes
- Be notified of transfer at least 30 days in advance
- Know the reason for the transfer, the date it's effective, and the location to which they will be moved
- Appeal transfers and discharges
- A safe, orderly, well-prepared transfer or discharge

How Do Nursing Homes Compare?

You want to find the best nursing home for your loved one. The questions in this checklist—adapted from *Your Guide to Choosing a Nursing Home*, a publication of the Health Care Financing Administration (now the Centers for Medicare and Medicaid Services)—can help. Make several copies of the form, one for each home you plan to visit. Then compare your responses.

Certification

- Is the facility certified by Medicare and/or Medicaid? _____

- Is it licensed by the state? _____

- What do recent reports by the state's Office of the Long-Term Care Ombudsman say about the facility? (By law, all state inspection reports must be posted for residents and visitors.) _____

  _____

- If the most recent report found deficiencies, have they been corrected? _____

  If not, when will they be corrected? _____

The Facility

- Are rooms, bathrooms, and halls clean and well-maintained? _____

- Are bathrooms equipped with grab bars and other assistive devices? _____

- How does the facility smell? (Many residents are likely to be incontinent, so bathroom odors are inevitable. But they should not be overpowering.) _____

- Are spills and other mishaps quickly cleaned up? _____

- Are residents given choices for meals and snacks? _____

- Are meals served in a timely manner and at the proper temperature? _____

- Can the facility accommodate special dietary needs? _____

- Does the facility offer organized activities, such as exercise classes, bingo games, and sing-alongs? _____

  _____

- Can the facility accommodate your loved one's ethnic and religious preferences? _____

- Do residents have sufficient privacy? _____

- Can residents choose their roommates? _____

  If not, how are roommates assigned? _____

- How are roommate problems handled? _____

- Are exits clearly marked? _____
- Does the facility have an emergency evacuation plan? _____
- Does the facility have periodic fire drills? _____

Staffing

- What are staffing levels during the day? _____
- What are staffing levels at night and on weekends? _____
- Do the staffing levels the facility cites match the levels you see? _____
- How quickly does the staff respond to residents' needs? _____
- How often are doctors on site? _____
- Is a dentist available? _____

    If not, who handles the residents' dental care? _____

- Are mental health professionals available? (Ideally, a nursing home should have a geriatric social worker, psychologist, or psychiatrist on staff or on call.) _____
- Does a nutritionist or dietitian supervise residents' meals and snacks? _____

Personal Care

- Who is responsible for residents' assessments? (By law, nursing homes must assess a new resident within 2 weeks of her arrival and develop an individualized plan of care based on her needs.) _____

    What are that person's qualifications? _____
    _____

- How often is a plan of care revised? _____
- Are discussions of the plan open to residents and their families? _____

    Are these discussions scheduled so that families can participate? _____

- If your loved one has a specific medical problem, how will staff members address it? _____
    _____

- How does the staff handle behavior problems? _____

    Do written guidelines exist? _____

- How does the staff deal with incontinence? _____
- What are the facility's arrangements for hospitalization? _____
- How are medications dispensed, and on what schedule? _____

(continued)

Caregiver's Checklist

continued

• Are residents' weights regularly monitored? _____

    How much weight must a resident lose before the staff takes action? _____

• Is staffing sufficient to assist those who need help with eating? _____

• Is water easily accessible in residents' rooms, as well as in the dining hall and day room? _____

• Does the staff encourage residents to drink fluids and stay well-hydrated? _____

• Under what conditions can residents be chemically or physically restrained? _____

    _____

• Can restraint policies be negotiated or appealed? _____

• How do residents file advance directives pertaining to resuscitation and mechanical life support? _____

    _____

    How does the facility make sure that advance directives are honored? _____

• Under what circumstances can residents be asked to leave the facility? _____

    _____

    How much notice is given, and to whom? _____

Special Care Units

• Does the facility have a separate unit for residents who are confused or have dementia? _____

• What services make the special care unit "special"? _____

• How much extra does the special care unit cost? _____

• What is the staff-to-resident ratio? _____

• What special training does the staff of the special care unit receive? _____

• Do residents with dementia get to go outside regularly? _____

Visitation

• Do the visitation policies work for you and other family members? _____

• Can you meet privately with your loved one? _____

• Can family members take residents off site easily? _____

Notes

_____

_____

_____

for their opinions, too. You're bound to encounter someone who has had personal experiences with a particular facility.

Once your loved one is placed in a nursing home, you are no longer her primary hands-on caregiver. Still, your input can have a major impact on the quality of care she receives. To that end, experts offer this advice.

- Befriend the staff on every shift. You've been a caregiver, so you know how difficult it can be. It's even more so for nursing home employees, who must look after several people at once (and for not much pay). If you praise and support them, they are likely to take a more personal interest in your loved one.

- Talk with the staff about your loved one. The more they know about the person, the better able they will be to provide good care.

- Keep asking questions. Even after your loved one has settled in, continue to monitor her care and to express concerns as they arise.

- Get involved in the nursing home's family council, which monitors the facility's policies and practices and advocates for patients' rights. Not all facilities have these councils, though they're required under the Nursing Home Reform Law of 1987.

- If your loved one complains about the facility, take her comments seriously. Solicit specifics beyond "I hate this place." What exactly is the problem? Then discuss it with the staff.

STEPPED CARE COMMUNITIES

A stepped care community (sometimes called continuing care or life care) features several different kinds of housing—independent living arrangements, assisted living facilities, and nursing homes—all on one campus. Residents can move from one place to another as their health and medical needs change.

Some people start in independent living and work their way to more advanced care as their health declines. Others go back and forth between facilities. For example, if a person who's in independent living has a stroke, he may be transferred to the

Point of View

"You hear about people who make their spouses or children promise never to put them in nursing homes. That's an idea from the days when people stayed at home and family lived close by. Today, everyone works, and family is scattered. We have to face facts. I've told my children that if they need to place me, so be it. I've decided that if I end up in a nursing home, I'm going to make the best of it."

—**DIANE HARRIS,**
Billings, Montana

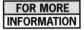

**FOR MORE
INFORMATION**

The AARP Web site has a helpful fact sheet on continuing care, with links to other useful sites. Visit **www.aarp.org/ confacts/housing/ccrc.html.**

nursing home, then to assisted living. Eventually, he may return to independent living.

Perhaps the greatest advantage of stepped care communities is their flexibility. They can accommodate anyone requiring any level of care. The cost of this sort of living arrangement can vary enormously, with entry fees ranging from $25,000 to $1 million and monthly fees in the thousands.

As for any other kind of residential care, the contract for a stepped care community should be reviewed carefully, in consultation with an attorney who specializes in elder law. Regulations for these facilities vary from state to state.

Hospice: Care for the End of Life

When modern medicine can't provide a cure, hospice provides the means to die with peace and dignity. Here the emphasis is not on treating an illness but on controlling pain and administering other palliative care toward the end of life. Emotional support, including grief counseling, also is available to patients and their families.

While the hospice concept has roots in ancient times, the first American facility opened relatively recently, in 1974. Since then, hospice has spread nationwide. Currently, more than 2,000 centers serve hundreds of thousands of people each year, either on site or through home care. Some hospices look like hospitals; others are more homey. Usually, their staffs include physicians, nurses, social workers, and counselors, among other health care professionals.

Hospice services are covered under Medicare, as long as a physician certifies that the patient is terminally ill, with a life expectancy of 6 months. (If the person survives longer, the physician must issue another certification in order to continue the Medicare benefit.) Some programs accept patients at diagnosis, which means they could receive care for a year or more. Hospice services may be covered under some long-term care insurance as well. Check your loved one's policy.

To learn more about hospice, or to find a facility in your area, contact one of the following organizations.

- The Hospice Association of America can answer basic questions about hospice care. Call (202) 546-4759, or visit www.nahc.org/HAA/home.html.

- The Hospice Foundation of America offers information and resources for hospice care. Call (202) 638-5419 or visit www.hospicefoundation.org.

- The National Hospice and Palliative Care Organization can help locate a hospice. Call (800) 658-8898 or visit www.nhpco.org.

PART SIX

Securing the Future

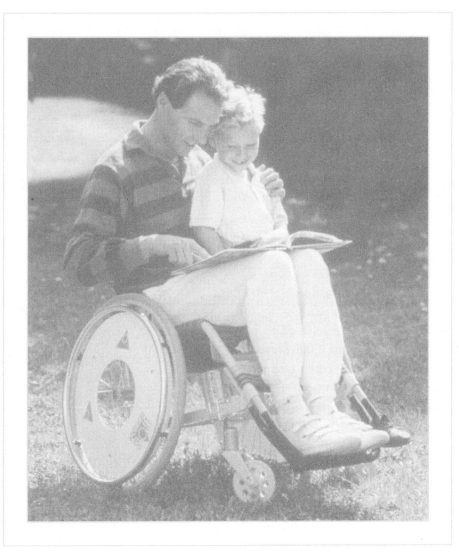

CHAPTER 22

WHEN TO CALL IN THE PROS

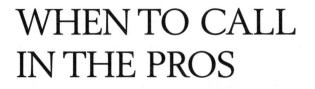

What You Need to Know

- Taking stock of your loved one's financial and legal affairs now can help guide decisions about his care down the road, especially in the event of a medical crisis.

- Experts recommend working with a financial planner and an attorney who specializes in elder law. They can assess your loved one's situation and make recommendations to ensure his long-term security.

- Look for financial planners and attorneys who are certified in their respective fields. Certification indicates that they've met certain educational and training requirements.

- Generally, financial planners and attorneys are paid for their services. But some organizations offer financial and legal advice for free or a reduced fee.

One look, and Tamara Barrett knew her grandmother was in trouble. Mary Ingold's family had noticed her increasingly odd behavior and forgetfulness but dismissed them as eccentricities typical of advancing age. At 71, Mary still had her sense of humor. She regularly followed tabloid accounts of celebrity mischief. "Always good for a laugh," she'd say.

But this day was different. When Tamara arrived at her grandmother's home, Mary opened the front door, wild eyed and shaking. Behind her, piles of envelopes and invoices covered the dining room table of her Seminole, Florida, home.

"I've got to pay the bills," Mary said as she paced around the table. Tamara watched her grandmother pick up stacks of papers and hold them to her chest before putting them down.

EXPERT OPINION

"If you are the caregiver, you really need to understand your loved one's financial situation and wherewithal, as well as the services he qualifies for versus those he must pay for. Sometimes you may feel uncomfortable digging into personal information, but you need to do it."

—**ELAINE BEDEL,** chair of the board of governors of the Denver-based Certified Financial Planner Board of Standards

Tamara flipped through the electric bills. Her grandmother didn't owe anything; in fact, she had credit. Curious, Tamara picked up the bills from the water, telephone, and insurance companies. Many of them also showed credits, with no payments due.

Under the influence of an early, undiagnosed stage of Alzheimer's disease, Mary had been double-, triple-, and quadruple-paying bills. What's more, she had continued paying for car insurance and an automobile club membership even though she had long ago given up her car. Even worse, she was missing a credit card.

The disorganized state of Mary's finances caught the attention of her three children, who soon placed their mother in an assisted living facility. Eventually, they would discover that Mary had paid more than $2,400 toward a life insurance policy worth only $1,500, and cashed in certificates of deposit totaling thousands of dollars to help a smooth-talking relative. And because Mary had no long-term care insurance, her children were forced to sell her house to pay for her care, leaving her impoverished when the money ran out.

The moral of this cautionary tale: If you haven't been keeping a watchful eye on your loved one's financial and legal affairs, you'd better start now. And get professional assistance, if you need to.

NO TIME LIKE THE PRESENT FOR PLANNING

As many a caregiver knows too well, caregiving presents all sorts of challenges beyond their control: a loved one who's in declining health, relatives who don't pitch in, bureaucracies that stonewall. Financial and legal planning is within your control. By getting some sense of your loved one's business situation now, you can ensure her security for the long run. At the very least, you'll avoid surprises and hasty decision-making in the event of a crisis.

Ideally, your loved one has taken steps on his own to get his business affairs in order. This sort of planning can never begin too soon. In fact, it should kick off in a person's early twenties, with a living will, advises Nancy Coleman, director of the American Bar Association's Commission on Legal Problems of the Elderly in Washington, D.C. "Any of us could be in an accident or experience a serious illness," Coleman observes. "Age has nothing to do with it."

To reinforce Coleman's point, consider that the number of people requiring long-term care is just about evenly split between those under age 65 and those over age 65—5.6 million versus 6.6 million. Clearly, anyone who puts off their financial and legal planning until they're older is risking their and their families' future.

Of course, people's lives change with the passage of time. Any major life event—marrying, having children, buying property, losing a spouse—should serve as a cue to update financial and legal documents as necessary.

Even though planning far in advance of need is best, "anytime is better than never," says Charles Sabatino, president of the National Academy of Elder Law Attorneys, based in Tucson. "Families with many assets may have more choices, but even those who are low income must know what benefits they're entitled to and what measures they can take to ensure their dignity and autonomy."

FOR THE BEST ADVICE, ASK THE EXPERTS

As important as planning is, getting involved in a loved one's financial and legal matters can be logistically daunting, especially if you have a family and a full-time job in addition to all your caregiving responsibilities. It can be emotionally draining, too, clouded by your own anxiety and the care recipient's resistance to your "snooping" in his personal affairs.

"My heart goes out to people," says Elaine Bedel, chair of the board of governors of the Denver-based Certified Financial Planner Board of Standards, of caregivers' struggle to make the right financial and legal decisions on a loved one's behalf. "Seeking professional advice can really simplify a caregiver's life."

The best professionals for the job are financial planners and attorneys who specialize in elder law. These days, they're relatively easy to find; with the general population living longer and needing more care, the fields of elder finances and elder law are growing in popularity. Generally, people in these professions are paid for their services. But with a little sleuthing, you may be able to get assistance for a reduced fee, or even for free. (More on this later.)

Tapping into the expertise of financial planners and attorneys not only spares you a lot of stress, it also safeguards your loved

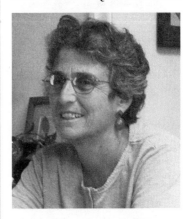

Point of View

"I was looking into some facilities in the Pittsburgh area. Well, my mother would have to spend all her money and then get Medicaid. That's how everybody does it. It's very complicated and hard to figure out."

—JONI RABINOWITZ,
Pittsburgh

EXPERT OPINION

"In the United States, for every three disabled people living in the community, only one is actually getting paid services. The vast majority of individuals, 80 percent of the population, are receiving help from family members."

—**MARC A. COHEN,** vice president of LifePlans, Inc., and president of the Center for Health and Long-Term Care Research, both in Waltham, Massachusetts

FOR MORE INFORMATION

The National Academy of Elder Law Attorneys maintains a list of member attorneys on its Web site, **www.naela.org**. Membership is open to any lawyer in good standing, though they must meet certain minimum criteria in order to be mentioned in the organization's "Experience Registry." This listing identifies lawyers with experience in various elder law specialties, from living wills to Medicare appeals.

Your Area Agency on Aging and local chapters of disease support groups can offer referrals to attorneys who specialize in elder law. Look up these organizations in the blue pages of your telephone directory, under "Guide to Human Services."

one against unintentional oversights and mistakes. So whom should you call—a financial planner or an attorney? Actually, experts recommend hiring both, if you can.

"Some attorneys who specialize in elder law also offer financial planning and/or money management services, though the ethics codes in most states require that the business components be kept separate from the law practice," Sabatino says. "Most attorneys are accustomed to working with financial planners in a team approach to eldercare."

Ultimately, which financial planner and attorney you hire will be influenced by many factors, ranging from the person's fees to her personal style. As with all the other professionals on your caregiving team, finding someone whom you and your loved one like and trust is paramount.

Take Action... LOCATE A QUALIFIED LAWYER

An attorney who specializes in elder law can offer guidance on a variety of legal issues that commonly arise in caregiving situations, particularly in the areas of taxation, benefits and pensions, health care, housing, and estate planning. In addressing these issues, attorneys typically work with other eldercare professionals, which means they can link their clients with a wide range of resources, Sabatino says.

When shopping around for an attorney, your greatest challenge may lie not in locating one but in narrowing your choices. The following tips can help.

✗ Start your search by soliciting referrals and recommendations. Your Area Agency on Aging can direct you to experienced, reliable attorneys who specialize in elder law. So can local chapters of disease support groups, as well as state and local bar associations. And don't forget to ask family members, friends, and colleagues; someone may be a client of an attorney you're considering. "Just don't use the Yellow Pages," Sabatino says.

✗ Steer clear of attorneys who handle any and all kinds of cases. Laws have become too complicated for any one person to be an all-around expert, Sabatino says. "A large

Caregiver's Checklist

How Does a Lawyer Rate?

During your initial phone conversation with a prospective attorney, be sure to ask the following questions, recommended by the National Academy of Elder Law Attorneys. (You may want to make several copies of this questionnaire, one for each candidate.)

1. How long have you been in practice?

_____

_____

2. Are you a member of the state and/or local bar association?

_____

_____

3. Does your practice have a particular specialty?

_____

_____

_____

4. Are you certified in elder law?

_____

_____

5. What percentage of your time do you devote to elder law?

_____

_____

6. Do you charge for the initial consultation? If so, how much?

_____

_____

7. What information do you want to see at the initial consultation?

_____

_____

_____

_____

firm may be able to handle many kinds of cases because it has a variety of experts on its staff," he explains. "But smaller firms and sole practitioners need to have a specialty. Elder law has become a special focus."

✗ Check whether an attorney has been certified by the National Elder Law Association, the approved certifying organization of the American Bar Association. According to Sabatino, the only objective measure of an elder law specialty is certification. Attorneys who are certified in elder law must meet certain experience criteria, provide references, and pass a daylong exam. Then they must be recertified every 5 years. Certification in elder law has been available only since the mid-1990s; so far, about 220 attorneys nationwide have earned it.

✗ If your loved one will be the client, include him in any meetings with prospective attorneys. In fact, the only reason he should not attend is if he's physically or mentally incapacitated or he has already appointed someone else to act on his behalf under a durable power of attorney. (We'll discuss durable power of attorney in more detail in chapter 25.)

✗ At your first meeting with a prospective attorney, ask whether she charges a flat or hourly fee, whether she bills

Legal Aid That's Easy on the Wallet

Some organizations offer legal services to older Americans for free or a reduced fee. Among the resources worth checking out:

- The Eldercare Locator, sponsored by the U.S. Administration on Aging, serves as a portal to more than 4,800 information and referral services, including legal assistance. Call (800) 677-1116 (available Monday through Friday from 9 A.M. to 8 P.M.) or visit www.eldercare.gov.

- By law, your Area Agency on Aging must provide legal aid to people over age 60 with economic or social need. You can find your local agency through the Eldercare Locator or in the blue pages of your telephone directory, under "Guide to Human Services." When you reach the agency, ask for information on programs such as Legal Assistance for Seniors.

- The Administration on Aging maintains a list of legal hot lines for people over age 60 at www.aoa.gov/Legal/hotline.html. The hot lines are staffed by attorneys, who may provide referrals to legal service programs or to practicing bar members. Some hot lines may charge nominal fees for their services.

Caregiver's
Checklist

How Does a Financial Planner Fare?

Finding a qualified financial planner requires some research on your part. You can start by asking prospective planners the following questions, recommended by the Certified Financial Planner Board of Standards. (Be sure to make extra copies of this questionnaire, so you have one for each candidate.)

1. What experience do you have?

_____

_____

2. What are your qualifications?

_____

3. What services do you offer?

_____

4. What is your approach to financial planning?

_____

_____

5. Will you be the only person working with me?

_____

6. How will I pay for your services?

_____

7. How much do you typically charge?

_____

8. Could anyone besides me benefit from your recommendations? (This question could disclose possible conflicts of interest.)

_____

9. Have you ever been publicly disciplined for any unlawful or unethical actions in your professional career?

_____

10. Can I have the details of the services to be provided in writing?

_____

For a more detailed list of questions, along with a checklist for interviewing financial planners, visit the Certified Financial Planner Board of Standards Web site at www.cfp-board.org.

To verify a financial planner's certification, you can call the Certified Financial Planner Board of Standards at **(888) CFP-MARK** or visit **www.cfp-board.org**. On the Web site, you can enter your ZIP code to locate a certified planner in your area. You'll also find a list of questions to ask during your initial interview.

Other good resources include the following:

• American Institute of Certified Public Accountants, Personal Financial Planning Division, **www.cpapfs.org**

• American Society of Chartered Life Underwriters and Chartered Financial Consultants, **(800) 392-6900**

• National Association of Personal Financial Advisers, **(888) 333-6659**

for additional expenses, and how long she'll need to complete your legal work. If her terms are satisfactory, get them in writing. Also find out whether she'll update you on any changes in the law that could affect your situation.

✗ If you don't like an attorney's answers to your questions, or you just don't feel comfortable with her, resume your search. You need to find someone you feel good about in order for your relationship to be positive and productive.

FINDING A FINANCIAL PLANNER

Like attorneys, financial planners have specialties—everything from investments to insurance. You'll need to do some research to find the best candidate, but it's worth the effort. A qualified planner can evaluate your loved one's financial situation, set priorities, make and implement recommendations, and monitor them. "In addition, a financial planner should be able to determine how long your loved one's resources will last, how much he can spend on care, and whether he should purchase long-term care insurance," says Bedel, who's also the owner of Bedel Financial Consulting in Indianapolis.

When you meet with a financial planner for the first time, go armed with a list of questions about her credentials and services, Bedel says. A qualified candidate will be certified in financial planning, as indicated by the initials C.F.P. after her name. To earn certification, a person must take college courses in financial planning, acquire at least 3 years of professional experience, and pass a 2-day examination. She must also complete 30 hours of continuing education every 2 years.

Be sure to ask about compensation, too. Some financial planners charge flat or hourly fees, while others receive commissions on client investments. Still others collect fees and commissions.

CHAPTER 23

MANAGING FINANCES

What You Need to Know

- To help ensure your loved one's financial security, set clear financial goals. Then you can devise a saving and spending plan based on those goals.

- In order to make any financial transactions on your loved one's behalf, you need his authorization, ideally in the form of a durable power of attorney for finances. Another option is joint ownership of his bank accounts.

- Your loved one can reduce his living expenses simply by taking advantage of the many federal and state benefits earmarked for care recipients.

- A reverse mortgage can turn what may be your loved one's biggest financial asset, his home, into a source of income. But the pros and cons of this kind of loan must be weighed carefully.

When her mother was diagnosed with early-stage Alzheimer's disease, Phyllis Bernstein didn't want to believe it. But the signs were there. On one occasion, Esther Bernstein started a fire when she lit an oven stuffed with paper bags to warm a meal. Later, she told her daughter the oven had switched on by itself. On another occasion, when Esther was hospitalized after a fall, she didn't recognize her surroundings.

But the real heartbreaker was her checkbook. "It had crossed-out words, and amounts with no payees," Phyllis recalls. "It didn't even look like her handwriting."

This discovery was all the more painful because Esther, now in her eighties, had been a successful bookkeeper. "It was her life," Phyllis says. "She's a great lady."

Phyllis is quite accomplished in the world of finance herself.

EXPERT OPINION

"Talking with your parents about long-term care is every bit as important as discussing sex with your children. The risk of silence is just too great. You need to have a family conversation in which everyone acknowledges that long-term care may be in the future, that it is very expensive, and that getting access to quality care at the appropriate level in the private marketplace requires early planning."

—**STEPHEN MOSES,** president of the Center for Long-Term Care Financing in Seattle

FOR MORE INFORMATION

Fraud artists often target people who are elderly or ill with their telemarketing scams, home repair schemes, and other cons. If you suspect your loved one has been victimized, report it to the National Fraud Information Center by calling **(800) 876-7060** or visiting **www.fraud.org**. This organization, which is affiliated with the National Consumers League in Washington, D.C., will alert the appropriate law enforcement authorities.

She's a CPA and a personal financial specialist, a designation awarded to only 3,000 of the 330,000 CPAs nationwide. She runs her own firm, Phyllis Bernstein Consulting in New York City, and is a consultant to the American Institute of Certified Public Accountants.

Yet despite her impressive credentials, Phyllis felt overwhelmed when she first took over her mother's bill paying. "While in the hospital, my mom had one test after another, so all these bills were coming in," she says. "And they kept coming for months, 15 to 20 of them."

But for Phyllis, the situation presented a greater challenge than tracking bills and writing checks. "If it had been somebody else, . . ." she says, her voice trailing off. "But she's family. I'm emotionally connected. It's hard."

TAKING ON THE MANAGER ROLE

Stepping in to help with a loved one's financial affairs *is* hard. But sometimes it's necessary. In fact, experts recommend intervening even before you notice any of the following red flags.

- A checkbook that lacks entries for payees and/or amounts

- Checks that have bounced

- Bills that have been overpaid, perhaps months in advance

- A utility that's shut off because of nonpayment

- Credit card statements that list unexplained charges, suggesting misuse—and not necessarily by your loved one

- Any large or repeated expenses that point to possible fraud

Of course, just acknowledging the need for financial management and planning can touch a nerve in caregiver and care recipient alike. Caregivers may become angry or resentful if they're accused of prying, or fearful if they're called upon to make decisions that affect a loved one's standard of living. Those who are caring for their parents may feel a sense of loss about the change in familial roles that accompanies the transfer of financial responsibility.

As for the care recipients, they worry about losing control of their personal finances, which they've handled on their own from the time they entered adulthood. They likely perceive outside intervention as a threat to their independence. Or they simply may not feel comfortable disclosing their financial affairs, even to immediate family.

These are normal reactions, according to experts; with the right approaches, they can be overcome. For example, if your loved one seems resistant to even talk about finances, try expressing your concerns in terms of their impact on someone else the person cares about, suggests Suzanne Mintz, cofounder and president of the National Family Caregivers Association, based in Kensington, Maryland. You might say, "We need to make sure the money you've set aside for the grandkids is protected."

Another option is to enlist a non–family member your loved one trusts—perhaps a close friend or a member of the clergy—to initiate the conversation about finances on your behalf. Or you could go a more surreptitious route: Dig up a newspaper or magazine article telling the story of a family who neglected to do any financial planning and leave it lying where your loved one will see it.

For your part, if you're feeling stressed by the prospect of managing your loved one's finances, you might get some peace of mind by joining a support group. You'll be introduced to others who have been in your shoes and can help you cope. If you're not able to attend meetings in person, or you don't feel comfortable doing so, you may want to check out support groups and caregiver chat groups online.

Remember, too, that you can get professional assistance, whether you hire your own financial planner or you seek advice from a government agency or nonprofit organization. Any of these resources can provide much-needed financial expertise, as well as an objective viewpoint on the care recipient's situation. That alone might appease any apprehensions that you and your loved one are experiencing.

FINANCIAL PLANNING BEGINS WITH CLEAR GOALS

Before you get into the details of organizing your loved one's financial affairs, the two of you need to look at the big picture by

FOR MORE INFORMATION

To locate a support group in your area, start by checking with your Area Agency on Aging or with local chapters of disease-specific organizations. Both are listed in the blue pages of your telephone directory, in the "Guide to Human Services."

Another resource is the National Family Caregivers Association, which educates and supports those who care for loved ones who are elderly, disabled, or chronically ill. Call **(800) 896-3650**, or visit **www.nfcacares.org**.

If you're interested in online support, you can find a listing of caregiver chat groups at **www.ec-online.net**, the Web site for Eldercare Online.

EXPERT OPINION

"A significant number of caregivers die while caring for a family member. Caregivers must take time for themselves so they can be there in the long run. This is a race, but it's a marathon, and caregivers need to learn how to pace themselves."

—**DONNA BENTON, PH.D.**, director of the Los Angeles Caregiver Resource Center at the University of Southern California

clarifying the person's financial goals. They involve much more than paying the bills on time every month. "Think short term and long term," Mintz advises. "The longer your loved one requires care, the more she's going to have to spend. And the costs may rise as her health declines."

Just estimating those costs can be a real eye-opener. Consider that in 1999, the median income for senior households (singles or couples age 65 and older) was $22,812, while the average fee for nursing home care was $56,000. Generally, home care (except for round-the-clock skilled nursing) and assisted living facilities are less expensive, while continuing care communities run higher. But all the rates may rise from year to year because of inflation.

While pondering your loved one's financial future, you should be contemplating your own, too. "Parents of kids with special needs are very aware that they most likely will die before their children. But people caring for parents or spouses may not consider that possibility," Mintz says. "Contemplating the 'What if . . . ?' is important to ensure your loved one's financial security in the event of crisis."

Mintz recommends addressing two important questions as part of the goal-setting process, no matter how uncomfortable they may be. First, who will look after your loved one and her finances if you become incapacitated or die? And second, who will look after you and your finances if you become ill or disabled?

Keep in mind, too, that as primary caregiver, you may end up picking up the tab for some of your loved one's expenses. A survey by the National Alliance for Caregiving and AARP found that families caring for elderly relatives spend an average of $171 per month on caregiving expenses. Mintz adds that caregiving families pay out 11.2 percent of their income for medical expenses, compared with 4.1 percent for the general population.

"People expect Medicare to cover a lot more than it actually does," Mintz says. "For example, it doesn't pay for adult diapers, which can cost more than $1,000 a year. It will pay for a certain range of wheelchair, but if you want a lightweight chair or perhaps a fully electric bed, Medicare doesn't pick up the tab for those kinds of upgrades."

What Are Your Loved One's Financial Goals?

The whole purpose of financial planning is to ensure a loved one's long-term financial security. But the definition of financial security can change dramatically once caregiving enters the picture. To help shape (or reshape) your loved one's goals, take a few moments to answer the following questions.

1. How do you and your loved one plan to pay for his long-term care?

_____

_____

2. Does the person want to stay at home for as long as he's able?

_____

_____

3. If your loved one's health declines, is residential care a possibility?

_____

_____

4. Do you think your loved one needs to reduce his expenses to save for long-term care?

_____

_____

5. Would the person benefit from having a savings and spending plan?

_____

_____

6. If your loved one lives far away, do you want him to move closer, or would you move closer to him?

_____

_____

7. If you were to die or become incapacitated first, what would happen with your loved one's finances and care?

_____

_____

_____

_____

Take Action... LAY THE FOUNDATION FOR LONG-TERM SECURITY

Once you and your loved one have determined where she should be heading financially, you can begin figuring out how she'll get there. Along the way, you may end up taking on a number of money management tasks—not just paying bills but also making bank deposits, monitoring spending, tracking investments, preparing tax returns, and filing benefits claims. To prepare for the job ahead, and save time and hassle in the long run, implement the following strategies now.

✗ Make sure your loved one has given you the necessary legal authority to act on her behalf. With a document called a durable power of attorney for finances, the person can appoint you as her financial "caretaker," authorizing you to handle her money matters should she become incapacitated. She wouldn't be signing away her own decision-making powers; as long as she's competent, she remains in charge of her financial interests. (To learn more about power of attorney, see chapter 25.)

✗ If your loved one has reservations about executing a durable power of attorney for finances, ask her to name you as joint owner of her bank accounts. That way, you can make deposits and write checks on her behalf. Another way to obtain legal access to her accounts is by being designated her "deputy" or "agent." This option should be discussed with an attorney who specializes in elder law, because of potential liability issues and limits imposed by the Federal Deposit Insurance Corporation (FDIC) on insured accounts.

✗ Obtain a duplicate key to your loved one's safety deposit box and authorization to use it. And if she doesn't have a box, encourage her to get one. It may be the best place to store certificates of deposit, savings bonds, deeds, wills, and other important documents.

✗ Create a system for organizing and tracking medical bills, benefits statements, insurance claims, and other papers pertaining to your loved one's health care. Just one doctor's office visit can generate a flood of paperwork from when services are provided to when they're paid for. To stay on

FOR MORE INFORMATION

To find an attorney who specializes in elder law, check with your Area Agency on Aging or the referral service of your local bar association. Both should be listed in the blue pages of your telephone directory, under "Guide to Human Services." Another good resource is **www.naela.org**, the Web site for the National Academy of Elder Law Attorneys.

top of it all, you need a filing system that's logical and accessible, for you and whomever else may need to use it. For ideas, see chapter 10.

✗ If you have primary responsibility for your loved one's finances, keep other family members informed of decisions and transactions to avoid disputes down the road. Perhaps you could send them monthly reports detailing the cash flow. Or get them involved by delegating certain tasks. For example, if someone in your family has an accounting background, he might be willing to prepare your loved one's tax returns.

✗ Remember to solicit your loved one's opinion before pursuing any financial actions on her behalf. She's entitled to play an active role in the decision-making process, and she should be encouraged to do so. It reinforces her sense of self-worth and independence—and it might help build trust between the two of you, as she sees you working to protect her interests.

Take Action... ASSESS YOUR LOVED ONE'S FINANCIAL SITUATION

Once you've laid the groundwork for managing your loved one's finances, your next step is to take a thorough inventory of his assets, income, and expenses. After all, you can't ensure your loved one's future financial security without getting a clear picture of his current situation. It will drive many of the decisions the two of you need to make.

If the very prospect of finding and documenting all your loved one's financial information seems daunting, take heart: Most caregivers feel the same way, says Sharon Luker, owner of VSR Financial Services in Plano, Texas, and a certified financial planner who specializes in eldercare. Your best bet is to use some sort of worksheet, like the Caregiver's Checklists on pages 298 and 300, or a computer software program. Luker has one that can project a person's income and expenses up to age 100. "The reality is, people are living a lot longer," she notes—and she has her own family history to back her up. Her grandmother lived to 103, her great-aunt to 96.

Point of View

"My mother and father worked their whole lives. They bought a house after the war. That's what we're spending now, money from the sale of the house. It costs a fortune, $4,000 a month, for my mother to receive home care in her own apartment. That's the way she wants to live. When the money runs out, we'll have to see whether we can afford it."

—PHYLLIS BERNSTEIN, New York City

How Much Has Your Loved One Saved?

Your loved one's assets and income help determine her ability to pay for her long-term care. For each applicable item in the list below, simply write the total value or annual payment in the middle column.

Asset	Total Value	Notes
Checking accounts		
Savings accounts		
Certificates of deposit		
Retirement accounts		
Life insurance policies		
Stocks and bonds		
Other investments		
Home equity		
Automobile		
Personal property, such as jewelry and collections		
Cash on hand		

Income Source	Annual Payment	Notes
Social Security benefits		
Veterans benefits		
Pensions		
401(k) distributions		
IRA distributions		
Annuities		
Dividends		

Itemizing your loved one's assets and income sources should be fairly straightforward. By comparison, expenses are more variable and, therefore, easy to over- or underestimate. To make your figures as accurate as possible, be sure to do the following:

✗ Develop an expense history using your loved one's canceled checks and check register from the past year or two. On a piece of paper or a computer spreadsheet, organize the payments into general categories such as groceries, utilities, and credit cards. Note the date and amount of each payment, as well as the payee. You're looking for those expenses that occur on a regular basis—whether monthly, quarterly, or annually. Once you've identified them, mark them as either fixed or flexible. (Fixed expenses are those that must be paid, such as income taxes; flexible expenses can be reduced or eliminated entirely.) Then transfer this information to the Caregiver's Checklist on page 300.

✗ When tabulating expenses, leave out vehicle-related costs such as loan payments, insurance, fuel, and maintenance. Chances are your loved one will stop driving eventually, so these expenses will no longer apply. (In fact, if the person needs assistance with his finances, he probably shouldn't be getting behind the wheel.) The good news is, if the vehicle is fully paid for, it's an asset that can be sold for cash.

✗ If your loved one is on Medicare, be sure to account for any premiums, deductibles, and coinsurance he must pay out of pocket. Supplemental insurance policies may cover all or part of these costs, but they have premiums and deductibles as well. Be aware that some low-income people may qualify for state-sponsored programs that pick up the tab for Medicare deductibles and coinsurance. (We'll discuss Medicare, Medicaid, and other health care benefits and insurance options in chapter 24.)

✗ Consider whether you'll need to do any home remodeling to accommodate your loved one's changing physical abilities. By installing ramps, expanding doorways, and making other structural modifications, you foster mobility and independence—which could postpone or even prevent your loved one's placement in residential care. You may be able

(continued on page 302)

FOR MORE INFORMATION

To learn more about state programs that cover out-of-pocket Medicare expenses, call **(800) MEDICARE** and ask about the Medicare Savings Programs. You can also visit the Medicare Web site at **www.Medicare. gov/Basics/HelpToPay.asp.**

The Social Security Administration can provide current figures for Medicare premiums, deductibles, and coinsurance. Call **(800) 772-1213** or visit **www.ssa.gov.** You can also look up the local office in the blue pages of your telephone directory, under "Guide to Human Services."

Caregiver's Checklist

How Much Is Your Loved One Spending?

By completing this expense inventory, you can see at a glance how your loved one spends his money—and where he can cut back to save for his long-term care. Write the dollar figure for each applicable item in the "Monthly," "Quarterly," or "Annually" column.

Fixed Expenses	Monthly	Quarterly	Annually	Notes
Mortgage or rent				
Homeowners or renters insurance				
Property taxes				
Utilities				
Water/sewer				
Phone				
Cable				
Garbage removal				
Medicare (premiums, deductibles, coinsurance)				
Supplemental insurance (premiums and deductibles)				
Prescriptions				
Life insurance				
Long-term care insurance				
Income taxes				
Credit card payments				
Personal loan				
Business loan				

Flexible Expenses	Monthly	Quarterly	Annually	Notes
Home maintenance				
Lawn maintenance				
Snow removal				
Food				
Clothing				
Toiletries				
Haircuts				
Newspaper delivery				
Books/magazine subscriptions				
Pet food and care				
Organization memberships				
Charitable contributions				
Presents				
Miscellaneous (use space below)				

The National Council on Aging sponsors a free online service that can assess your loved one's eligibility for benefits within seconds. Just go to **www.benefitscheckup.org**, and type in the person's age, ZIP code, and other requested information. (Because the service is anonymous, you won't need to provide a name or Social Security number.) The person's profile will be compared against a database of 1,000 programs, including health care, financial assistance, and legal counseling. You receive a list of those programs that match your loved one's needs, interests, and location.

The Pharmaceutical Research and Manufacturers Association of America sponsors a prescription program for people considered low-income. To learn more, visit the organization's Web site at **www.phrma.org**.

to finance the necessary upgrades through grants or low-interest loans from community organizations. Your Area Agency on Aging should have this information.

Take Action... CUT COSTS WHILE ENHANCING CARE

If your loved one has more money going out than coming in, the two of you can work together to pare her expenses. Fortunately, Luker says, the older generation has skills and experience in tightening purse strings. For baby boomers, it can be a challenge. "They're accustomed to spending as they please," Luker observes. "But once they understand the financial strain of long-term care, they can change their habits rather quickly."

That said, paring expenses doesn't necessarily mean giving up nonessential purchases. Older people, especially, could ease their financial load just by taking advantage of the many federal and state benefits they're eligible for—like nutrition services, home energy discounts, and property tax relief. According to the National Council on Aging, some 3.7 million seniors who qualify for food stamps don't receive them. Another 3 million are missing out on Medicaid benefits, and 1.2 million haven't applied for their Supplemental Security Income payments.

Other cost-saving strategies that you and your loved one may want to consider include the following:

✗ Contact your Area Agency on Aging or your local health department to find out about discounted or free services for care recipients, and possibly for caregivers.

✗ Call your loved one's utility companies to ask whether she's entitled to reduced rates or weatherization assistance.

✗ Shop around for the best phone rates and encourage your loved one to make long-distance calls during off-peak hours.

✗ If your loved one isn't enrolled in a prescription program, look into whether she would qualify. Currently, 29 states sponsor programs that help pay for medications. In addition, some pharmaceutical companies offer reduced prices for people considered low income. Your loved one's pharmacist or physician should be able to provide names and telephone numbers for participating companies.

X Scan all bills, credit card statements, and insurance claims for overcharges.

X Consult a tax expert or the Internal Revenue Service about tax credits for care recipients and caregivers.

X To save on postage, arrange for the electronic payment of regular bills, like utilities.

X Arrange for direct deposit of your loved one's Social Security checks and other benefits payments. That way, all the money goes straight into a bank account.

X If your loved one has disability insurance, find out whether the policy covers the costs of physical therapy or other health care services.

X Check with local educational facilities about services available to the public. For example, the students at a vocational school may do low-cost haircuts or home repairs as part of their training. Likewise, students at a dental college may provide reduced-fee or free dental care.

X Buy staple household items in bulk. And clip coupons, perhaps enlisting the assistance of a teenage son or daughter or another family member.

USING INVESTMENTS TO YOUR ADVANTAGE

Streamlining your loved one's expenses is just one way to save toward his long-term care. Enhancing his assets and income is another. You wouldn't want to try anything risky with his nest egg, of course. But he could get extra cash from some of his current investments.

For example, you might check your loved one's life insurance policy to see whether it will pay a specified portion of the death benefit in advance. Some policies do. If your loved one is terminally ill, you could turn over the policy to what's called a viatical company. Investors pay a percentage of the policy's face value (which is taxable) and take over the premiums. Then when your loved one dies, they collect the benefits.

FOR MORE INFORMATION

If you or your loved one has questions about his taxes, you can get help through one of the following services, sponsored by the Internal Revenue Service (IRS) and staffed by trained volunteers.

• Tax Counseling for the Elderly (TCE) is for people age 60 and older, primarily those who are homebound or institutionalized. If your loved one is unable to get to the nearest TCE location, he can ask for someone to come to his home.

• The Volunteer Income Tax Assistance Program serves the elderly and disabled, as well as those with low or fixed incomes.

To learn more about these programs, including their availability in your area, call the IRS at **(800) 829-1040**. Be prepared to navigate a number of voice mail menu options before you reach a live person.

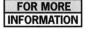

FOR MORE INFORMATION

For detailed information on reverse mortgages, including explanations of the different types, a loan calculator, and advice on choosing a lender, visit AARP's Web site at **www.aarp.org/revmort**.

FOR MORE INFORMATION

To locate lenders that offer reverse mortgages, call the National Reverse Mortgage Lenders Association at **(202) 939-1760** or visit **www. reversemortgage.org**. The Web site features a wealth of information about these loans.

Often a person's biggest asset is a home, especially one that's owned outright. (If it's mortgaged, remember that your loved one could lower his monthly payments by refinancing the loan or applying for a home equity loan.) But deciding to sell should not be done in haste. After all, leaving behind all those memories won't be easy.

Even if your loved one seems enthusiastic about moving elsewhere, actually doing it can be traumatizing. For older people, especially, just changing rooms is unsettling. "They're thinking, 'Left turn, left turn, and the first door is mine,'" Luker says—but suddenly, they're ending up in the wrong place.

As an alternative to selling, you and your loved one could pursue a reverse mortgage—even if his home isn't fully paid for. These loans can be costly and complicated, which is why experts recommend consulting a financial advisor before applying for one.

Basically, a reverse mortgage functions exactly as its name suggests: The lender makes payments to the borrower, who can use the money at his discretion. This kind of loan is available to people age 62 and older, provided they can apply and sign for it themselves. They can opt to receive lump-sum payments, monthly payments, a line of credit, or a combination of the three.

The amount of a reverse mortgage depends on the applicant's age, the home's equity and location, and interest rates. Among the conditions for approval:

- The home must be the applicant's principal residence.
- The home must be structurally sound.
- The borrower must continue to pay property taxes and insurance.
- The loan must be repaid with interest when the borrower sells the home or moves out. If the person dies, the loan would become the responsibility of the estate or the heirs, who would get to keep the home.

Your loved one can choose from among four kinds of reverse mortgages. The least expensive, the Home Equity Conversion Mortgage, is available through the Federal Housing Authority. The others are the Home Keeper, offered by Fannie Mae, and the Equity Guard and Cash Account Plan, both from the Financial Freedom Funding Corporation of Irvine, California.

If your loved one decides to apply for a reverse mortgage, he can expect to pay for a credit report; origination, appraisal, and monthly service fees; closing costs; and insurance. He can cover these costs with an advance on the loan—which, of course, increases the amount he owes.

Keep in mind that in some cases, reverse mortgage payments can affect Medicaid and Supplemental Security Income benefits. This is another reason to seek financial counsel before signing anything.

IF YOU NEED ASSISTANCE . . .

If you're feeling uncertain about any aspect of your loved one's finances, or you're worried about making potentially costly mistakes, you can get help. A number of resources are available, depending on your loved one's needs and ability to pay for services.

In some states, AARP offers free money management assistance to older and disabled people who are considered low-income. To qualify, their liquid assets can't exceed $30,000, and their annual income can't exceed $19,560 for a single person or $27,679 for couples. Your Area Agency on Aging can provide more details on this program.

If you or your loved one can afford to pay for money management assistance, you might consider hiring a geriatric care manager. Generally, these professionals have backgrounds in gerontology, nursing, social work, or counseling. They can assess your loved one's needs, develop a plan for her care, and identify resources to help pay for it.

Another option is to seek out the services of a daily money manager, who can help set up a budget, pay bills, file insurance claims, and handle assorted other financial tasks. These professionals charge by the hour, based on the complexity of the work—whether it's balancing a checkbook or tracking income and expenses.

As with geriatric care managers, a daily money manager should be screened thoroughly before he's hired. Look for someone who's a member of the American Association of Daily Money Managers, which requires references and adherence to a code of ethics. Also find out whether any consumer complaints have been filed against him or his employer. Your local Better Business Bureau or consumer protection agency will have this information.

FOR MORE INFORMATION

The National Association of Professional Geriatric Care Managers lists members on its Web site, **www.caremanager.org**. To contact the organization directly, call **(520) 881-8008**.

FOR MORE INFORMATION

To learn more about the services provided by daily money managers, call the American Association of Daily Money Managers at **(301) 593-5462** or visit the organization's Web site at **www.aadmm.com**.

CHAPTER 24

WADING THROUGH THE BENEFITS MAZE

What You Need to Know

- While public programs and private insurance plans provide benefits for medical and long-term care, rarely, if ever, is just one of these resources sufficient to fully fund the costs of care.

- To determine whether your loved one has adequate coverage, review all his benefits and policies—ideally, in consultation with a financial planner or attorney. You want to identify gaps in coverage as well as areas of over-insurance.

- Medicare covers only basic medical expenses. It does not pay for the vast majority of services and supplies necessary for long-term care.

- Long-term care insurance sometimes picks up the tab when Medicare doesn't. But these policies vary considerably in terms of benefits and costs.

In any plan to pay for a loved one's long-term care, benefits programs play an indispensable role. Without them, only the very wealthy could afford the enormous expense of looking after a person who is elderly or ill. But mobilizing the proper resources will take some research and strategizing.

While every case is unique, in general, a single source of funding wouldn't begin to cover the costs of providing decent care. Instead, caregiving families must rely on a combination of public programs and private reserves to make ends meet. Figuring out who will pay for what is among the most crucial of your caregiving tasks—and the sooner it's done, the better off your loved one will be.

Many people believe that when they retire, Social Security and Medicare will pay for everything they need. Only after they become care recipients do they realize these benefits alone aren't nearly enough. They—and their caregivers—end up spending more out of pocket, which not only eats up their savings but also limits their options for care.

For a large segment of the senior population, Social Security payments are the primary source of retirement income. But they're intended as supplements to other financial resources. Given today's cost of living, they barely cover the recipient's most basic expenses, let alone caregiving bills.

As for Medicare, it was conceived as a means of ensuring adequate medical care for seniors. But that was in the 1960s, when the average life expectancy was shorter and the range of available treatments much narrower. In the years since, the definition of "adequate" care has changed quite a bit, as has the cost.

Without Medicare, many people couldn't afford medical care at all. So the program does serve a vital purpose. Still, it requires large deductibles and co-payments for many services and supplies. And it doesn't cover certain key expenses, like most prescription drugs.

What's more, Medicare has no provisions for caregiving costs, or for personal care that isn't deemed a medical necessity—such as assistance with walking, eating, using the bathroom, and other tasks of daily living. If a person lacks other benefits to cover what Medicare won't, he's left with two options: paying the expenses out of pocket, or spending down virtually all his savings to qualify for Medicaid.

This dilemma becomes particularly evident when considering long-term care, either in a residential care facility or at home. Medicare will foot the entire bill for up to 20 days in a nursing home, but only if admission is related to prior hospitalization. After 20 days, patients must cover a large portion of the charges themselves. After 100 days, Medicare pays nothing.

In terms of home care, Medicare will pick up the tab for rehabilitation and other health care services that a doctor has prescribed. It won't pay for custodial care, personal assistance like preparing meals and running errands, or necessary home modifications like installing wheelchair ramps.

The best way to avoid shelling out huge sums of money, and to safeguard your loved one's financial future, is to make sure he

Outlook

"So many of the issues caregivers face—emotional, medical, and otherwise—are made worse by our country's failure to address the financing of long-term care. Until we come to grips with this, caregivers will continue to be caught between their wishes and obligations to be good caregivers and the consequences of doing so.

"I believe the financing of long-term care should be handled the same as the financing of acute care. It should be an insurance expense that everyone contributes to and that employees match, preferably under the Medicare program."

—**PETER J. STRAUSS, ESQ.**, elder law and trust and estates attorney, author, and adjunct professor of law at New York Law School in New York City

EXPERT OPINION

"A woman who retires at age 62 is looking at another 25 to 30 years of life. And she should plan for that. The mistake a lot of people make is that they believe they can rely on publicly financed medical care. It does exist, and it does pay. But it offers zero choices. As long as millions of people have zero choices, you're going to have a regimented, centralized, institutionalized pattern of long-term care."

—**WILLIAM H. THOMAS, M.D.,**
caregiving advocate and founder of the Eden Alternative in Sherbourne, New York (www.edenalternative.com)

has a comprehensive insurance strategy in place. It may not cover everything, but at least it can help ease the financial burden of long-term care.

For example, many Medigap policies—which, as their name implies, can plug some of the holes in Medicare coverage—will pick up deductibles, co-payments, and other out-of-pocket costs. Private health insurance through retirement plans, spousal benefit programs, and other sources can help defray expenses, as can private long-term care insurance and prescription drug plans. We'll explore all of these options here.

If you're feeling uncertain at the prospect of deciding which options make the most sense for your loved one, your best bet is to seek the advice of as many people as possible. Talk with family members and friends who've been down the same path, as well as financial advisors, benefits counselors, and other professionals who understand not only the general caregiving landscape but also your loved one's specific situation. With their input, you can assemble a network of resources that will cover most of your loved one's caregiving expenses and reduce his—and your—financial liability.

SOCIAL SECURITY

When an employer withholds Social Security taxes from an employee's paycheck, that money goes into a federal fund that supports four different benefits categories, not just retirement income. Disability, family benefits, and survivors benefits all fall under the Social Security program. Benefits payments are based on past earnings.

Supplemental Security Income (SSI), a separate program for the low-income elderly and disabled, is administered by the Social Security Administration but paid for through general tax revenues. It is intended to guarantee these populations at least a minimal income to cover basic living costs. SSI benefits do not depend on past earnings.

When Congress created Social Security in 1935, it didn't envision the program as a substitute for other sources of retirement income, such as pension plans and personal investments. But as mentioned earlier, many Americans reach retirement age expecting to live off their Social Security payments.

To qualify for Social Security, people accumulate "credits" through their years in the workforce. They can earn up to four credits per year and generally need 40 credits to begin collecting benefits. In the meantime, they're splitting the costs of Social Security taxes with their employers, who match their employees' withholdings. People who are self-employed must foot the full amount of the taxes themselves.

Over the years, Social Security has been updated and expanded to reflect our nation's changing demographics and economics. In general, retirement payments equal about 40 percent of a person's lifetime earnings. But to save money for anticipated future demands on the Social Security program, the age for full retirement has slowly been rising. People born before 1938 can begin collecting full benefits at age 65, while those born after 1959 won't be eligible until they reach age 67.

If a person chooses, he can begin collecting Social Security benefits at age 62, though not in the full amount. By the same token, he could slightly increase his payments for every month he puts off collecting benefits once he's eligible for full retirement, up until age 70.

The disability benefits available through the Social Security program can help anyone who has earned the full amount of Social Security credits and has been sidelined by a physical or mental illness. To qualify for these benefits, a person must be unable to perform most kinds of work for at least a year.

The Social Security program also makes payments to the families of its beneficiaries. Possible recipients include spouses who've reached age 62, younger spouses who are involved in caring for minor children, and the children themselves. If a beneficiary dies, the surviving family members—including the spouse (or even an ex-spouse), children, and parents—may be entitled to survivors benefits, depending upon the circumstances.

MEDICARE

The country's largest health insurance program, Medicare offers hospital and medical benefits primarily to people age 65 and older, as well as to some younger people with disabilities. Currently, 39 million Americans participate in the program, which

FOR MORE INFORMATION

To learn more about eligibility requirements and other issues pertaining to your Social Security benefits, call the Social Security Administration at **(800) 772-1213** or visit the Web site at **www.ssa.gov**. You can also call your local Social Security office; it's listed in the blue pages of your telephone directory.

EXPERT OPINION

"When it began in 1935, Social Security wasn't intended to cover what it covers today. But Congress has always made the necessary changes so that the program could grow and accommodate the greatest number of people. I would expect the same to happen with Medicare. But the changes will evolve; they won't be instantaneous."

—**MICHAEL REYNOLDS**, district manager for the Marshall, Minnesota, district office of the Social Security Administration

FOR MORE INFORMATION

For answers to any questions about Medicare benefits and costs, you can talk to a customer service representative on the agency's 24-hour hotline, (800) 633-4227. You might also want to visit the Web site www.medicare.gov. From there, you can download documents on all aspects of Medicare and access the "Medicare Personal Plan Finder" to help select the most suitable coverage.

has been in operation since 1966. It's administered by the Centers for Medicare and Medicaid Services, formerly known as the Health Care Financing Administration.

While Medicare covers a wide range of expenses and services, navigating through the system can seem daunting because it offers so many options. In addition to what is called Original Medicare, people in many states can choose Medicare+Choice plans. These fall into two basic categories: Medicare Managed Care and Medicare Private Fee-for-Service. Both kinds of coverage are available through private insurance companies who receive reimbursement from the government and oversee the delivery of benefits.

Original Medicare

Original Medicare has two parts: A, for hospital benefits; and B, for medical benefits. In general, seniors qualify for these benefits if they or their spouses were legally employed for at least 10 years. Part A is free; Part B requires a monthly premium.

Those already receiving Social Security benefits when they reach age 65 are enrolled in Medicare automatically. Everyone else must apply for coverage. A person who doesn't qualify for Part A through employment may be able to get the coverage by paying premiums.

To ensure timely enrollment, experts recommend contacting your local Social Security Administration office at least several months before a person's 65th birthday. Delayed enrollment in either Part A or Part B can result in higher premiums.

Trying to make sense of Medicare benefits can test the patience of even the most insurance-savvy caregiver. Although policies and payment schedules change from year to year, the following general guidelines can help.

Medicare Part A. Part A pays for in-patient care at Medicare-certified hospitals. The program imposes limits on length of stay and dollar value, and it doesn't cover the costs of private rooms or private-duty nurses unless they are deemed medical necessities. Part A also pays for temporary rehabilitation services at skilled nursing facilities following a hospital stay for illness or injury, but not for full-time residential care.

Depending on the circumstances, Part A might cover some

skilled nursing and rehabilitative services at home rather than in a residential care facility. It might also pick up the tab for wheelchairs and other assistive devices. For patients with terminal illnesses, Part A will pay for care in a hospice program. (For more information on hospice, see chapters 20 and 21.)

Medicare Part B. Anyone who qualifies for Part A is eligible for Part B, which requires a monthly premium payment. Some people may opt not to purchase the coverage, particularly those with health insurance through a retirement plan, a spouse's employment, or some other resource. Part B pays for a variety of medical services, including doctor and emergency room visits, some rehabilitative care, laboratory tests, some medications, and preventive measures such as mammograms and vaccines.

In 2002, the monthly premium for Part B was $54, a figure that likely will rise every year. That said, people who put off purchasing Part B may end up paying even more in the long run, because the premium rises by 10 percent for each year someone is eligible for coverage but doesn't enroll.

Where the Program Falls Short

While Original Medicare has expanded over the years, large gaps in coverage remain. What's more, many physicians don't like dealing with the Medicare bureaucracy or being underpaid for their services.

In a nutshell, what Medicare reimburses doesn't come close to what most doctors charge. While many "accept assignment"—that is, they consider Medicare's fee payment in full (they're called participating physicians)—others do not. Those who collect from Medicare and then bill for their services besides usually are limited to a 15 percent surcharge, for which the patient is responsible.

Sometimes Medicare beneficiaries prefer to see doctors who don't accept Medicare payments at all. In such cases, the patients sign private contracts with their physicians of choice, and they must foot the entire bill themselves, either out of pocket or through private health insurance.

If a Medicare-approved provider refuses to file a claim for a medical or hospital service, or if Medicare rejects a claim, you have the right to challenge that decision. And challenging it is the first step toward getting part or all of it reversed.

(continued on page 314)

Outlook

"I believe this country needs a social insurance model of comprehensive long-term care that really shares the burden with families and friends. Too many families burn out, and too many older spouses die of 'broken hearts' because of their caregiving responsibilities. We need to be careful about asking families to do even more than they are right now."

—**LYNN FRISS FEINBERG,** deputy director of the National Center on Caregiving at the Family Caregiver Alliance in San Francisco

Original Medicare: An Overview

To give you a better idea of what Original Medicare covers (and what it doesn't), the following charts break down the Part A and Part B benefits for 2002. Keep in mind that these benefits change from year to year. If you have any specific questions about coverage and costs, your best bet is to contact your local Medicare office directly.

Medicare Part A

Part A helps pay for hospital stays, skilled nursing care, home health care, and hospice care as well as blood for transfusions.

Benefit	Beneficiary Pays
Hospital expenses, including semi-private rooms, meals, general nursing, and other hospital services and supplies. *Note:* Medicare does not cover the cost of a private room (unless medically necessary),a television or telephone, or private-duty nursing.	• $812 per day for up to 60 days of hospitalization • $203 per day for days 61 to 90 of hospitalization • $406 per day for days 91 to 150 of hospitalization • All costs beyond 150 days
Skilled nursing care after a related hospital stay of at least 3 days, including semi-private rooms, meals, and rehabilitative services	• Nothing for the first 20 days • Up to $101.50 per day for days 21 to 100 • All costs beyond 100 days
Home health care for prescribed treatment and for rehabilitation, including part-time skilled nursing care, physical therapy, occupational therapy, speech therapy, and some medical equipment and supplies	• Nothing for Medicare-approved services • 20 percent of Medicare-approved costs for medically necessary equipment
In-home hospice care, including medical and support services and medications for pain relief and symptom control	• Nothing for Medicare-approved services • $5 for outpatient prescription drugs • 5 percent of Medicare-approved costs for inpatient respite care
Pints of blood transfused during a covered stay in a hospital or skilled nursing facility	• All costs for the first 3 pints of blood • 20 percent of costs for subsequent pints

Medicare Part B

Part B helps pay for medical services, laboratory tests, and other health care services.

Benefit	Beneficiary Pays
Medical services, including doctor appointments (but excluding routine physical exams), diagnostic tests, second opinions for surgical procedures, medical equipment, outpatient mental health care, and outpatient physical, occupational, and speech therapy	• $100 deductible per calendar year • 20 percent of Medicare-approved amount after the deductible • 20 percent of all outpatient physical, occupational, and speech therapy services • 50 percent of outpatient mental health care
Clinical laboratory services, including blood tests and urinalysis	• Nothing for Medicare-approved services
Preventive services, including bone density measurements, colorectal cancer screening, diabetes services and supplies, glaucoma screening, mammograms, Pap smears and pelvic exams, prostate cancer screening, and some vaccinations	• In most cases, 20 percent of the Medicare-approved amount

What Isn't Covered

As of 2002, the Original Medicare program does not include benefits for the following:

- Custodial care at home or in a nursing home
- Health care obtained while outside the United States
- Routine or yearly physical exams
- Many screenings and vaccinations
- Outpatient prescription drugs
- Dental care and dentures
- Routine eye care
- Hearing exams and aids
- Routine foot care and orthopedic shoes
- Cosmetic surgery
- Acupuncture

Here's how it works: If a provider says Medicare doesn't cover a particular service or procedure, you or your loved one should request that the claim be filed anyway. If it is rejected, the notice you receive will include instructions on how to fight the decision.

Your local Social Security Administration office can assist with filing an appeal. While it may seem like a hassle, research indicates that a significant percentage of challenges result in at least a partial reversal of the initial decision.

Medicare+Choice

In addition to its original coverage, Medicare contracts with private insurers to underwrite Medicare+Choice plans. Those who qualify for Medicare can purchase any of the Medicare+ Choice plans offered in their area; the availability of this insurance depends upon the state or city of residence. As mentioned earlier, the two basic types of Medicare+Choice coverage are Medicare Managed Care and Medicare Private Fee-for-Service.

While Medicare+Choice plans generally provide benefits beyond Original Medicare, like more coverage for prescription drugs and hospital stays, some—not all—may require a premium on top of the standard monthly fee for Original Medicare Part B. They may have other administrative rules that plan members must follow as well, such as pre-notification of a planned hospitalization. Members are guaranteed all the coverage allowed under Medicare, and they retain their right to appeal unfavorable decisions on claims.

Most Medicare Managed Care plans function like HMOs (which we'll discuss a bit later in the chapter). Usually, plan members have limited deductibles and co-payments, but in exchange, they must agree to use designated physicians and health care providers. Most members have primary care physicians and can see specialists only upon referral.

Some Medicare Managed Care plans include an option called point-of-service. It allows members to receive care from physicians, hospitals, and other providers not in the plan's network. This benefit generally requires an additional payment but ensures increased flexibility in making health care decisions.

Medicare Private Fee-for-Service plans function like traditional health insurance policies, as well as Original Medicare. Plan members select their own health care providers, and the insurer reimburses a portion of the costs. Private Fee-for-Service plans offer the maximum in choice and benefits. But the plans themselves determine the patient's fee structure, so their total costs may be higher than Original Medicare.

Weighing the Options

Determining whether Original Medicare or one of the quasi-private plans is best for your loved one's situation requires careful evaluation. But even after you make a decision, you can change your mind. Once a year, beneficiaries have the opportunity to switch plans or to rejoin Original Medicare. Likewise, if a private insurer withdraws from the Medicare+Choice business (it has an annual "window" to do so), its plan members can choose any other coverage, including a return to Original Medicare.

Medicare recipients who have low incomes and limited savings, but who don't meet Medicaid's financial eligibility requirements, may qualify for Medicare Savings Programs. These state-based plans vary in their provisions, but they're relied upon by millions of Medicare recipients to cover some or all of Medicare's premiums, deductibles, and co-payments. Currently, benefits are available to those who have Medicare Part A, $4,000 or less in assets ($6,000 for a couple), and about $1,300 or less in monthly income (about $1,700 for a couple). These figures may change slightly from year to year.

MEDIGAP

Even when people have Medicare coverage, they usually end up paying a fair number of expenses out of pocket, including co-payments on hospitalization and other basic benefits, deductibles, a portion of doctor's fees, and prescription drug costs. That's why many decide to purchase what are called Medigap policies—private health insurance that helps pay for what Medicare itself does not.

Medigap policies can go a long way toward defraying the costs of medical care. Still, they don't offer comprehensive medical benefits. Like Medicare itself, Medigap is no substitute for a decent long-term care policy. (You'll read more about long-term care insurance in just a bit.)

People interested in purchasing Medigap coverage can choose

EXPERT OPINION

"We must have a strong Medicare program as part of the fabric of our society. It has to be the basis for everything else we do. But it's going to face tremendous demands, with 77 million baby boomers going into retirement in the year 2010. That's why I have proposed private-sector programs, such as tax credits for long-term care insurance, a $3,000 tax credit for family caregiving, and additional services for which the impetus comes from grassroots organizations."

—THE HONORABLE CHUCK E. GRASSLEY, senior senator from Iowa

EXPERT OPINION

"Because long-term care and caregiving assistance programs are in the Medicaid system, anyone who's just slightly above the poverty level doesn't qualify. Even when people do qualify, they end up in a very costly and inflexible situation that doesn't provide respite for the caregivers themselves. Under Medicaid, the care recipient can receive paid care for a certain number of hours a day. But the unpaid caregiver—the person who's providing care 18 hours a day—isn't entitled to anything. We need to start viewing the caregiver as a primary need source, too."

—**MICHAEL S. RABIN,** first deputy commissioner of the New York City Department for the Aging

from up to 10 different plans, depending on where they live. Federal law requires the insurance companies that underwrite these plans—ranging from Plan A, the most basic, to Plan J, the most comprehensive—to include a standard selection of benefits in each one. Insurers can add benefits over and above the approved minimum, if they wish. For this reason, the prices for each plan can vary. Not all plans are available in all states.

Take Action... CHOOSE THE BEST MEDIGAP POLICY

Despite the standardization among Medigap plans, deciding on a policy requires the same careful research and thought that goes into any insurance purchase. Consider the following advice before you start shopping around.

✗ Make sure your loved one actually needs a Medigap policy before investing in one. It may be an unnecessary expense for someone who is likely to become eligible for Medicaid in the near future or who has private health insurance that covers more than regular Medicare.

✗ If possible, purchase a Medigap policy within 6 months of your loved one's enrollment in Medicare Part B. By law, insurers cannot deny coverage or exclude pre-existing conditions during that time period. After 6 months, however, companies have much greater latitude to assess higher premiums for an applicant, reject an applicant altogether, or include stringent restrictions and exclusions that severely undermine the point of getting the policy in the first place.

✗ Start exploring your options early. Once your loved one becomes eligible for Medigap coverage, he may feel pressured to choose a plan quickly, only to end up with one that doesn't suit his needs or budget. By getting a head start on your research, you and your loved one will have time to thoroughly evaluate the plans available in your area.

✗ When comparing Medigap plans, consider each insurer's corporate history and financial stability. Your state's insurance department should have extensive information on the various companies, including records of consumer complaints and any sanctions imposed by the state.

✗ Once your loved one settles on a Medigap policy, take time to read the documents thoroughly. By law, customers are entitled to a 30-day "grace period" in which to review new insurance coverage. If you or your loved one isn't satisfied with the policy's provisions, return it with a request for a full refund.

MEDICAID

For those struggling to figure out how to pay for medical and long-term care, Medicaid can be a lifesaver. The program—run jointly by the federal and state governments—covers many expenses that Medicare won't, most notably extended nursing home care and many prescription drugs.

Federal regulations stipulate that a person who qualifies for Medicaid can own a home and some personal property but have no more than a couple of thousand dollars in cash savings. (The guidelines vary if the person is married.) Beyond that, each state sets its own standards as far as who is eligible and what requirements they must meet.

At minimum, Medicaid must pay for hospital services, doctors' fees, diagnostic and laboratory tests, and skilled nursing care in a facility or at home. In many states, the benefits also cover social work, dental and eye care, medications, and prosthetic limbs, among other services and supplies.

As you might imagine, Medicaid's generous benefits come at significant cost. Because the program's fees for health care providers fall below standard third-party reimbursement rates, many physicians and residential care facilities are reluctant to accept Medicaid patients. As a result, many of the providers that do accept Medicaid patients are overwhelmed, which raises the risk of substandard care.

This doesn't mean, as some would believe, that a residential care facility housing Medicaid recipients won't provide a decent living environment. Nor does it mean that many well-regarded facilities automatically reject applicants with Medicaid benefits. Many do limit the proportion of Medicaid recipients to perhaps 5 to 10 percent of their resident populations—which is why, if you're thinking about residential care for your loved one, you should select a fa-

FOR MORE INFORMATION

You can find out more about Medicaid eligibility guidelines, enrollment procedures, and benefits by visiting **www.hcfa.gov/medicaid/ mcaicnsm.htm**. This is the official Web site of the Health Care Financing Administration, the federal agency that oversees Medicaid.

FOR MORE INFORMATION

To find a certified financial planner in your area, visit **www.cfp-board.org**, the Web site of the Certified Financial Planner Board of Standards. You can search the organization's member database by ZIP code.

cility and get on its waiting list well in advance of need. (For more information on residential care options, see chapter 21.)

You've probably heard of people having to "spend down" their savings in order to meet Medicaid's eligibility requirements. If your loved one is in this position, be aware that he may be able to shield more of his assets than you might think. A good financial planner—one who's familiar with state and federal regulations, as well as your loved one's situation—can offer invaluable advice on trusts, gifts to heirs, and other legal options for preserving resources while ensuring eligibility for benefits. (To learn more about hiring a financial planner, see chapter 22.)

PRIVATE HEALTH INSURANCE

For care recipients who don't qualify for Medicare or Medicaid, or for anyone who wants more coverage than is provided by those government programs, private health insurance can bridge the gap to quality, affordable health care. Policies vary considerably in terms of their premiums, benefits, restrictions, and exclusions. Often they're made available as components of larger benefits packages, like those offered by employers to current and retired employees.

In fact, many older care recipients have excellent health coverage through a corporate retirement plan, union membership, or veterans program. Younger care recipients may be named as dependents on a spouse's or parent's medical plan, making them eligible for benefits.

Regardless of its provisions, virtually every health insurance policy falls into one of two broad categories: managed care or fee-for-service. Of the two, fee-for-service has been around longest. But managed care has become quite common, particularly in the last decade or so.

A managed care plan provides comprehensive health coverage for its members, in exchange for a monthly premium. Perhaps the best-known of these plans are the HMOs.

With managed care, each member selects or is assigned a primary care physician, who becomes the gatekeeper for medical services. Generally, members can see specialists only if they get referrals from their primary care physicians. All medical services, except in emergencies or other special circumstances, are provided through physicians and hospitals that participate in the managed care network. Because of this arrangement, managed care plans are able to hold down their premiums and other costs, though members may be assigned copayments and other small charges.

Almost since its inception, managed care has drawn criticism for restricting patient access to physicians and other health care providers. Another concern is that because participating physicians receive a fixed monthly fee for every plan member in their practices, they're under considerable pressure to see as many patients as possible, which could undermine quality of care.

By comparison, fee-for-service plans—also called indemnity plans—allow members to consult any physician or health care provider they wish. But this freedom of choice comes at a price: Invariably, fee-for-service is more expensive than managed care. Besides having higher premiums, the plans seldom pay what doctors actually charge, which means patients must make up the difference.

A third category of medical plan, called a preferred provider organization (PPO), combines elements of managed care and fee-for-service—and, therefore, falls between the two in terms of premiums. Basically, PPOs cover the costs of services provided within their own networks of physicians and hospitals. But they'll also pay for some services obtained from non-network health care providers at the choosing of members.

Since all three categories of health coverage have their advantages and drawbacks, you and your loved one need to compare plans carefully. Perhaps your most important consideration is whether you're looking for a comprehensive policy or you just want to plug holes in the rest of your loved one's health coverage. Even if the person got his insurance through a retirement plan or another benefits package, you need to know what it covers and how it dovetails with other medical benefits. You want to be sure the person isn't over- or underinsured, especially if he's paying premiums.

LONG-TERM CARE INSURANCE

Good residential long-term care—and even marginal residential care, for that matter—can cost $40,000 a year or more, depending on a facility's location and the selection and quality of its

Point of View

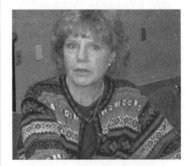

"I would love to have a dollar for every time an insurance company tells me, 'A wife can do that.' I'm willing to do the caregiving tasks, but I can't do all of them. I don't want the insurance companies to care for my husband—I just want them to care *about* my husband."

—MARY ANN NATION,
Franklin, Ohio

The Partnership for Long-Term Care

Several states, including California and New York, have established what is known as a Partnership for Long-Term Care. In this program, each state outlines what it considers important criteria for long-term care insurance policies, such as a minimum daily reimbursement rate, a grace period for late premium payments, and income protection. Insurance companies that offer policies meeting the approved criteria may market those policies as official partnership products.

The Partnership for Long-Term Care initiative was spearheaded by the Robert Wood Johnson Foundation (RWJF), a national philanthropic organization devoted to improving the health and health care of all Americans. To learn more about the initiative, and to find links to the various state programs, you can visit the RWJF Web site at www.rwjf.org.

services. Many people stay in these facilities not just for 1 or 2 years but for 10 or even 20.

Of course, a majority of care recipients would rather stay at home than go into residential care. Generally, home care isn't quite as costly, but expenses can easily add up to $10,000 to $20,000 a year. The less outside assistance caregiving families can afford, the more responsibilities the caregivers must take on themselves.

The fact is, few families can pay for long-term care without some sort of financial aid. Even the most well-to-do can run through their assets quickly if one of their own requires home or residential care. And the costs of such care tend to rise over time, though not just because of inflation. As a person's health declines, his need for services and support increases proportionately.

Long-term care insurance evolved as a means of helping to defray long-term care costs while protecting the care recipient's assets. While these policies have been around for decades, the market has been a relatively small one. Experts estimate that private insurance and Medicare combined pay less than $5 of every $100 spent on nursing homes nationwide. The balance is covered by the care recipients themselves or, once they spend down their savings, by Medicaid.

As the nation's population has gotten older, its long-term care insurance options have expanded considerably. Today's policies offer a much wider range of benefits, and they're not quite as expensive as they once were. Of course, the premiums are based to some degree on a person's age and health status. In fact, those already in need of extensive care probably wouldn't qualify for new policies. But if your loved one is in reasonably good health, long-term care insurance is at least worth considering.

Keep in mind that this type of insurance isn't for everyone. For example, if a person is likely to run through his savings and qualify for Medicaid within a year or so of entering residential care, a long-term care policy would be an unnecessary expense. The same is true for someone who doesn't have substantial assets to protect, especially since he probably won't be able to afford the premiums for first-rate coverage in the first place.

The most basic long-term care policy can cost well over $1,000 a year, with more comprehensive coverage running as much as $3,000 to $4,000 a year. A plan that features a higher daily coverage level, a longer benefit coverage period, a home health care option, and increases in benefit levels to offset inflation may have higher premiums but could provide significant savings on the back end.

Take Action... FIND THE RIGHT LONG-TERM CARE POLICY

If long-term care insurance seems like a good investment for your loved one, finding the right policy is key. The following strategies can help.

✗ Decide which policy features matter most to you and your loved one. Do you want inflation protection, premium waivers, home care benefits? What other provisions can protect your loved one's financial interests while ensuring quality long-term care? Having a clear idea of what you're looking for can simplify your search for the best policy.

✗ Avoid buying the first policy you hear about just because it sounds good. You're making an important financial decision; take time to shop around and compare policies. And don't hesitate to call insurance companies with your questions. You should understand every benefit, restriction, and exclusion before making a decision.

✗ Ask family members and friends whether they've purchased long-term care insurance. If they've already ventured into the marketplace, their experiences and insights can help guide your search.

✗ When sorting through the vast array of policies and benefits, work with an insurance agent whom you trust. A good agent is an invaluable resource, while a bad one can spell financial disaster. You want someone who puts a lot of effort into assessing your loved one's health status, financial status, needs, and preferences. Steer clear of an agent who seems to be exerting undue pressure to purchase a particular policy.

✗ Before making a decision, look into an insurer's financial rating. Your state's insurance department should maintain thorough records on all companies offering long-term care

(continued on page 324)

FOR MORE INFORMATION

The United Seniors Health Council, a program of the nonprofit National Council on the Aging, has published several helpful booklets on long-term care insurance. You can view the council's library online at **www.unitedseniorshealth. org/html/pubs_bookshelf. html**. Or you can write to 409 Third Street SW, Suite 200, Washington, DC 20024.

How Does a Long-Term Care Policy Compare?

When selecting a long-term care policy, you and your loved one need to decide which kinds of coverage best match his situation. Every extra benefit can raise the premiums, often significantly. By the same token, a stripped-down plan that provides only the most basic coverage could end up being a waste of money, which your loved one can ill afford.

The following questionnaire can help evaluate the various kinds of long-term care policies available in your state. You may want to make several copies, so you can complete one for each policy you're considering.

Question	Notes	Answer
What is the policy's daily maximum allowance for care?	Today's policies specify either a daily or a monthly maximum amount that they will pay for long-term care services. The policyholder chooses this amount at the time he purchases the policy. The higher the limit, the higher the premium. Choose a limit carefully, keeping in mind the actual cost of care in your loved one's area.	
Does the policy offer inflation protection?	This is extremely important, since the cost of long-term care will increase over time. Purchasing an automatic inflation protection rider will raise the maximum allowance for care by a stated amount every year, without affecting the premium. The purchase of such a rider does increase the level cost of the policy as well. Some policies may offer what's known as a CPI-type inflation rider, which allows policyholders to purchase extra coverage at specified intervals— usually every 3 years. With this type of rider, adding coverage will affect the premium.	
Does the policy include benefits for home care? If so, for which services?	Today's policies offer coverage for home care, ranging from homemaker services to skilled nursing. Most policies require that home care be provided through a licensed agency, though some allow for payments to unlicensed caregivers or even family members. Explore the options and costs before deciding which coverage best matches your loved one's needs.	

Question	Notes	Answer
What is the policy's elimination period?	An elimination period, also known as a waiting period or deductible, is the number of days the policyholder must pay for care before the policy kicks in. This period—which can range from 0 to 100 or even 365 days—is selected at the time the policy is purchased. The longer the elimination period, the lower the premium. When making a decision, be sure to consider the out-of-pocket costs as well as the premium. Often a shorter elimination period makes more sense, if the premium difference is minimal.	
What is the policy's lifetime cap on benefits?	Some policies may provide benefits for only a certain length of time, anywhere from 1 to 10 years. Others offer unlimited benefits. The policyholder chooses a limit at the time he applies for a policy. As the cap on benefits increases, so does the premium, with unlimited coverage being the costliest. Some policies may express their caps in terms of dollars rather than years or days. Simply divide a policy's daily maximum allowance into its lifetime cap to determine how long the coverage will last.	
What triggers the payment of benefits?	In general, today's policies will kick in (1) if the insured needs help with two or more activities of daily living (ADLs) or (2) if the insured needs supervision because of severe cognitive impairment. Tax-qualified policies—those that allow certain tax benefits for the insured—use both benefit triggers with the condition that any ADL impairment is expected to last at least 90 days. Policies that are not tax-qualified may use both benefit triggers, plus they may require a doctor's certification that care is medically necessary.	
Is the policy guaranteed renewable?	Almost all of today's polices are guaranteed renewable, which means an insurance company cannot cancel coverage because of an insured's declining health or advancing age. In fact, the only grounds for cancellation are nonpayment of premiums. The insurance company does have a limited right to raise premiums, but it must be done on a class basis with the permission of the Insurance Department in the state where the policy is filed.	

The National Academy of Elder Law Attorneys maintains a listing of members on its Web site. Go to **www.naela.org** and click on "Locate an Elder Law Attorney." You can search for an attorney who specializes in long-term care.

insurance. You can find out how many policies a company has issued, how quickly it processes claims, what kinds of consumer complaints (if any) it received, and how those complaints were resolved. Also review the credentials of the company's top executives and trustees: Do they inspire confidence or concern?

✗ Once you choose a policy, read it from start to finish *before* your loved one signs—ideally, with help from an elder law attorney who knows long-term care insurance. If anything remains unclear, call the insurance agent or the insurer's customer service department for an explanation. Remember, contract interpretations often hinge on the meaning of one or two words. You want to be sure the policy guarantees all the benefits your loved one has been promised. If it comes up short, don't buy it.

✗ If your loved one buys a long-term care policy only to discover that it's not what he expected, cancel it right away. Ask the insurer to refund the premium payment. Be aware that the grace period for cancellation varies from state to state.

✗ Through this entire process, document all of your research. Take notes during conversations, including the name and contact information of every person you speak with—professionals and laypeople alike. Date your notes so you can refer back to them easily. Keep copies of all paperwork pertaining to your loved one's long-term care coverage in an easy-to-find file.

PRESCRIPTION DRUG PLANS

The cost of prescription drugs has risen rapidly in recent years, and the trend probably will continue for the near future. The result is that medications account for an increasingly large percentage of our personal medical expenses. This can be a particular problem for the elderly, who often find themselves taking an ever larger number of drugs to improve or maintain their health.

Unfortunately, Original Medicare does not cover the cost of prescription medications, with the exception of some oral cancer drugs. Some Medicare+Choice policies offer a prescription benefit, as do some Medigap policies.

While the issue of prescription drug coverage has received national attention, it has yet to be addressed at the federal level. Meanwhile, more than half the states have either enacted or are in the process of enacting pharmaceutical assistance programs. Most of these plans target those in the elderly and disabled populations who have limited financial resources but do not meet the low-income requirements of Medicaid. Each state maintains its own specific, and often complicated, formula for determining eligibility.

Because these are state-run programs, they vary widely in their provisions. Most will pay for a broad range of prescription medications, and possibly a selection of over-the-counter drugs. Some seek to limit their costs by focusing on medicines for certain conditions, such as heart disease, diabetes, or Alzheimer's disease.

In general, pharmaceutical assistance programs require co-payments. Often they're a flat rate of a few dollars per prescription, but they can be substantially higher, especially if they're calculated according to the cost of a drug. Most plans do not carry deductibles.

Because states regularly modify or update the guidelines for their pharmaceutical assistance programs, your best bet is to check regularly on the eligibility requirements and benefits of the plans in your area. The federal government may well develop its own program, though for now, observers can only speculate about when that would happen and what the plan would include.

Depending on your loved one's situation, he may qualify for low-cost or free medications through other resources. For example, many states subsidize programs that target populations with certain conditions, such as heart disease, kidney disease, and AIDS. Sometimes these programs specifically provide for the distribution of prescription drugs to those who can't afford them. Local governments and non-profit agencies may sponsor drug distribution plans of their own, although financial considerations almost always limit their ability to reach large numbers of people.

Even some pharmaceutical companies offer low-cost or free medications to those who meet certain eligibility requirements. While these programs can be helpful, they often require a lot of paperwork for patient and physician alike. It may not be worth the time and energy, since the programs often are limited to a short-term supply of a particular drug.

FOR MORE INFORMATION

To learn more about the pharmaceutical assistance programs available to your loved one, as well as Medicare+Choice and Medigap plans offering a prescription drug benefit, visit **www.medicare.gov/ Prescription/Home.asp.** You can search for information by zip code or state.

FOR MORE INFORMATION

People who are considered low-income may qualify for prescription assistance through the Pharmaceutical Research and Manufacturers Association of America. To find out more about this program, visit **www.phrma.org.**

CHAPTER 25

LEGAL ASPECTS OF CAREGIVING

What You Need to Know

- Though it's not essential, consulting an attorney can help ensure the validity and comprehensiveness of your loved one's legal preparations.

- The laws governing wills, advance directives, and other legal documents for end-of-life care can vary from state to state. Researching the rules and regulations in your loved one's home state is critical.

- Even if your loved one has a will and other important legal documents in place, they should be reviewed periodically—and updated if necessary—to account for changes in life circumstances, family relations, and personal matters.

M y mother has a living will. Must she designate someone to make medical decisions in case she'd become incapacitated?"

"My father's finances are a mess, but he won't accept help from anyone. How do I get legal authority to intervene?"

"My husband wrote his will by hand. Is that acceptable?"

As a caregiver, you already may be wrestling with these kinds of questions about your loved one's legal affairs. If you aren't yet, you will. Actually, helping your loved one make legal preparations for a time when she may not be able to speak for herself is among your most important caregiving tasks. The sooner the two of you get the necessary paperwork in order, the better off you'll be.

Of course, no one enjoys talking about issues like estate planning and end-of-life care. But addressing these issues forthrightly—ideally, while your loved one is mentally alert and able—allows the person to determine her own future. She can choose the kind and level of care she wants to receive, which could help prevent disputes between family members, or between family and physicians. She can also make plans for the assets she holds, to ensure her long-term financial security and to minimize squabbles over who inherits what after her death.

GETTING HELP FROM THE EXPERTS

Unless you're an attorney yourself, you may feel uncomfortable about diving into legal waters, especially when someone else's health and welfare are at stake. The good news is that you can get help. Some matters, like executing a living will, you probably can handle on your own with research into your state's laws and guidance from government agencies and nonprofit organizations that provide caregiving support, like AARP or your local Area Agency on Aging. Others, like structuring your loved one's assets to minimize taxes and the inconveniences of probate, may require a lawyer's expertise.

These days, hundreds of attorneys around the country specialize in what is known as elder law. The National Academy of Elder Law Attorneys, a professional association, has a roster of about 4,000 members. A good elder law attorney should be able to advise you not just on estate planning or health care decision-making but on the entire range of legal issues that an older care recipient—or, indeed, anyone concerned about their later years—might face.

For example, elder law attorneys can help develop plans for efficiently utilizing the available health insurance options, including Medicare and Medicaid. They can handle cases of suspected age discrimination or financial abuse of an older person. They can explain the legal obligations of residential care facilities and take action to protect a patient's rights. They can offer guidance on establishing trusts to bypass inheritance taxes and on seeking conservatorships to protect a loved one's interests. And the list goes on.

While the elderly have had unique legal needs for a long time, elder law has evolved only in the past 10 to 15 years, with the

FOR MORE INFORMATION

The National Academy of Elder Law Attorneys can answer all sorts of legal questions that may arise in caregiving situations. It also can provide referrals to member lawyers. Call **(520) 881-4005** or visit **www.naela.org**. The Web site features an extensive list of links to agencies, associations, and other helpful resources.

If your loved one is receiving care because of a particular health problem, you may be able to get legal assistance through a nonprofit organization specializing in that problem. To find out what's available in your community, look in the blue pages of your telephone directory, in the "Guide to Human Services."

AARP runs a program that provides legal advice, including information on wills, advance directives, and other documents. Call **(800) 424-3410**, or visit the AARP Web site at **www.aarp.org**.

Your Area Agency on Aging also offers legal aid to people age 60 and over who meet certain eligibility requirements. Look in the blue pages of your telephone directory, in the "Guide to Human Services," or check the Eldercare Locator at **(800) 677-1116** or **www.eldercare.gov**.

general aging of the population. Even today, many people—especially those who could benefit from the services of an elder law attorney—are not aware of this specialty within the legal profession.

As a caregiving situation unfolds, you and your loved one may brush up against issues framed by a thicket of local, state, and federal laws—hundreds if not thousands of them. Inadvertently running afoul of them is not uncommon. Unfortunately, even small mistakes can lead to major inconveniences and expenses. Working with a good elder law attorney could prevent all that—and spare you unnecessary stress and uncertainty. (For advice on hiring an elder law attorney, see chapter 22.)

Of course, the elderly aren't the only ones receiving care. Many younger people require assistance and support because of disabilities or serious illnesses such as cancer, AIDS, or hepatitis C. While these care recipients face many of the same legal questions as their older counterparts—such as how to draw up durable powers of attorney and other documents—they may encounter other issues unique to their conditions. For this reason, they and their caregivers should consider consulting local chapters of condition-specific organizations, like the American Cancer Society. Often these groups can provide legal advice, or at least a referral to an attorney.

What if you and your loved one can't afford to hire an attorney? Many public agencies and nonprofit organizations for seniors—as well as those for other demographic groups, or for people with certain conditions—provide legal services at little or no cost. In addition, you and your loved one can take advantage of the voluminous self-help information and sample documents available in books and on the Internet.

But before the two of you make any final decisions, you must be convinced that you know the law well enough to safeguard your legal interests. If you have any doubt, checking with a lawyer could be a lot less costly than cleaning up a legal mess after your loved one can no longer speak for herself.

With that in mind, let's take a closer look at some of the key legal issues that may surface as part of your caregiving experience. We'll start with estate planning, which in many ways creates the framework for the rest of your loved one's legal affairs.

Legal Documents at a Glance

According to legal experts, each of the following documents plays a crucial role in your loved one's estate planning. If she hasn't drafted these papers already, she should—and the sooner, the better. (Trusts are not listed here because they're legal entities, not documents per se. But they're important nonetheless.)

Document	Purpose	Notes
Will	To distribute assets after death according to the deceased's wishes	A will must go through probate to determine distribution of property and payment of debts.
Letter of instruction	To convey a person's preferences regarding aspects of her estate not addressed in the will or other documents	Letters of instruction often include information about personal property with little economic value, like letters, family photo albums, and mementos, as well as guidelines for funeral or memorial arrangements, suggestions about asset management or other practical matters, and any final messages to loved ones.
Durable power of attorney for finances	To designate someone to handle financial matters in the event of any incapacity, including but not limited to terminal illness	The person executing the document can appoint someone to perform a specific task, such as signing checks, or to take on all responsibilities relating to assets and property.
Durable power of attorney for health care	To designate someone to oversee medical care in the event of incapacity, including but not limited to terminal illness	The designated person has access to the care recipient's medical records; in addition, this person may have to decide which course of treatment should be pursued or whether life-prolonging measures should be used.
Living will	To indicate whether doctors should use aggressive treatments to prolong life in the event of a terminal illness	A living will can spell out general principles or cite specific life-saving measures that the patient finds acceptable or unacceptable, such as being put on a respirator or being artificially fed and hydrated.

EXPERT OPINION

"As elder law attorneys, we have to look at all the ethical considerations of a situation and explain them to our clients. . . . We need to make sure that they're competent when they sign their documents, and that they think very clearly about whom they're choosing to represent their interests in the future."

—**JANET MORRIS,** elder law attorney for Bet Tzedek Legal Services in Los Angeles

THE BASICS OF ESTATE PLANNING

When you hear the words *estate planning*, you might conjure images of mansions, yachts, and other symbols of wealth. While money and property figure prominently in the process, it involves much more than that. And it's something everyone, not just the millionaires among us, should consider doing.

Unfortunately, many people put off estate planning much longer than they should, because they're daunted by the task and they don't like thinking about their own mortality. Some worry that their decisions will be final and irrevocable, and they're not ready to declare their intentions so absolutely. While these concerns are understandable, they can have serious consequences, especially if a person becomes incapacitated or dies without the proper legal documents in place. Family members may not be able to deposit pension checks or pay bills. Or they may disagree on decisions about their loved one's end-of-life care.

These sorts of problems only feed the stress of what can be a very trying situation. Yet with estate planning, they could easily be avoided. Perhaps your loved one will feel more comfortable with the process if she knows that, with a limited number of exceptions, she's free to make changes in her plan as long as she's mentally competent.

What's in an Estate?

As a caregiver, you probably will play a major role in your loved one's estate-planning decisions. To be an effective advisor, you must take into account the person's age, income, health status, relationships, and lifestyle, among other factors.

Broadly speaking, the elements of an estate plan address three categories of legal issues: distribution of property, preparations in the event of incapacity, and disposition of the deceased's remains.

The first of these, distribution of property, encompasses wills, trusts, and other means of transferring assets from the care recipient to someone else—possibly a spouse, a child, another relative, or a foundation or charity. It also includes naming beneficiaries for life insurance policies as well as retirement and pension accounts.

In the simplest sense, then, an estate consists of all a person's assets. It could be a $10 million stock portfolio and a substantial life insurance policy, or retirement benefits and a savings account with a few thousand dollars. Or it could be a treasured family memento—a beautiful piece of costume jewelry, a photo album, a hand-knit scarf—passed down from generation to generation. Though it may be worth nothing to anyone else, it holds enormous sentimental value for the family. In any event, it's an asset whose fate should be spelled out legally.

When the total value of an estate is substantial, inheritance taxes will be assessed. One of the objectives of estate planning is to minimize the amount heirs must pay. This means finding ways to reduce the official value of the estate to below the tax threshold—by establishing trusts and giving gifts, for example. A knowledgeable elder law attorney can explain your options.

The second category of estate planning, preparations in the event of incapacity, includes durable powers of attorney, living wills, and other documents that explain a person's wishes should she become unable to make her own decisions. These documents—collectively known as advance directives—either authorize someone else to make decisions on the person's behalf or instruct medical personnel about the use of lifesaving measures.

Incidentally, laws on durable powers of attorney, living wills, and other legal documents can vary from state to state. So if a person executes a power of attorney in Idaho, then moves to Georgia or New Mexico to live with a family member, she should find out whether the directive complies with the laws of her new state of residence. If it doesn't, she'll need to draw up a new one. A local social service agency or attorney can help assess a document's validity.

In terms of disposition of the remains, the third category of estate planning, some people prefer to leave those decisions to their families, while others provide very specific instructions for their funeral services and burial or cremation. Ideally, your loved one will plan for—and pay for—as much as possible in advance. This may seem unpleasant, but it allows the person to participate in the decision-making process and saves the family from having to agree on arrangements at a difficult and often emotional time. These days, most funeral homes offer preplanning services. Consider taking advantage of them.

Point of View

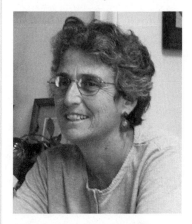

"[My mother's situation] has us looking at our own future, too. What are we going to need? What must we do to prepare? We haven't written our wills yet. We talk about it, and we understand we have to do it. Everything that happens with my mom makes us think about it even more."

—JONI RABINOWITZ,
Pittsburgh

WILLS

Of all the components of an estate plan, wills may be the best known since they have been around the longest. A clearly written will is an effective tool for ensuring the distribution of property according to a person's wishes and minimizing disputes among her heirs.

Many people put off drafting wills until they're sick, which means they may need help making decisions about who gets what. If the person you're caring for hasn't written a will, both of you can avoid a lot of hassle and expense by putting one together as soon as possible.

Even if your loved one already has a will, she should review it every couple of years to make sure it's up-to-date. Much can change in someone's personal life that will affect her decisions about the distribution of her property. Perhaps she has become a grand-

---

Understanding the Probate Process

The goal of probate is to ensure that a person's assets are distributed according to the instructions of her will—or, if she left no will, according to the laws of the state. Although executors can handle the probate process on their own, hiring an attorney can be helpful, especially if an estate is large and has many creditors. The estate will pay the attorney's fees, which can be 5 percent or more of the value of all the assets.

Of course, the simpler an estate, the simpler the probate process—not just for the executor but for the heirs as well. This means finding ways to remove some of the assets from the scrutiny of the probate court. (Often small estates can qualify for a streamlined probate process called summary administration. What constitutes "small" varies from state to state.)

For example, your loved one has the option of setting aside property in a living trust, which would not go through probate. Likewise, she could make tax-free gifts of up to $10,000 a year to as many people as she'd wish. The only drawback is that once she gives away the money, she has no legal claim on it. She'd have to rely on the recipient's goodwill in the event of an unexpected financial reversal.

Joint tenancy, or tenancy by the entirety, is another means of avoiding the probate process. When two people hold title to an asset and one of them dies, the survivor becomes the sole owner. In fact, in community property states, the communal assets often pass directly to the surviving partner.

Life insurance policies, retirement plans, and certain other financial instruments pay out directly to beneficiaries without going through probate. The same is true for payable-upon-death bank accounts, which your loved one can easily set up with a little paperwork.

mother, and she wants to leave mementos for her grandchildren. Maybe she has divorced or remarried. Perhaps she has acquired a valuable piece of artwork, and she wants it to stay in the family.

Not only can someone's personal life change, so can the laws pertaining to inheritance. The federal government periodically adjusts its threshold for paying inheritance taxes, which means your loved one may want to revise her will accordingly.

When a person dies, her will has to go through probate. This court process is intended to ensure that all the property is accounted for, that the provisions of the will have been fulfilled, and that any outstanding debts and taxes are paid. If the will names an executor, that person is responsible for taking the estate through probate. Otherwise, the probate court will appoint an executor—and not necessarily someone who knew the deceased.

The probate process is known for being time-consuming and expensive. It's also very public: A notice of the proceedings may be published in the local newspaper, and the will remains on file at the courthouse. For these reasons, many people look for ways to bypass probate. (To learn more, see "Understanding the Probate Process.")

If a person dies intestate—that is, without a will—sorting through the distribution of property becomes much more complicated, and potentially very expensive. In this situation, too, the probate court will name an executor to oversee the process.

Various states have specific laws governing the distribution of property in the absence of a valid will. So you may have no recourse, even if you believe the executor's decisions violate your loved one's wishes. If the person left behind minor children with no instructions as to who should step in to care for them, then the court will appoint a guardian—and it may not be anyone from the family.

Getting the Complete Picture

Before drafting a will, you and your loved one should compile a list of all the assets she has—real estate, bank accounts, stocks and bonds, prized family heirlooms, and so on. Keep digging until you're convinced your list is truly comprehensive. Often people forget about bank accounts that haven't been used, jewelry that has been stashed in the closet for years, and other items that would

What Assets Does Your Loved One Have?

The purpose of a will is to provide for the distribution of your loved one's property. To do this, of course, you need to know what that property is. The list below can help you take stock. Note that for some of the items, your loved one may already have designated beneficiaries. She may want to review and, if necessary, update those names as part of the will-writing process.

Real estate   _____

_____

Vehicles   _____

_____

Savings and checking accounts   _____

_____

Stocks and bonds   _____

_____

Annuities   _____

_____

401(k)/IRA accounts   _____

_____

Pension benefits   _____

_____

Social Security benefits   _____

_____

Veterans benefits   _____

_____

Life insurance policies   _____

_____

Personal property (for example,   _____
jewelry, furniture, artwork)   _____

count toward a person's estate. (If you wish, you can use the Caregiver's Checklist on page 334 to complete your inventory.)

If your loved one seems to struggle when deciding how to divvy up her property, you might reassure her by explaining that she can change her will at any time, as long as she's mentally alert and able. You could also point out that the more thorough and precise her instructions, the less likely conflicts and lawsuits will arise among her heirs.

The challenge in writing a will, of course, is trying to please everyone. Some beneficiaries may feel insulted or hurt if they don't receive what they wanted or what they believe they deserved. To inject a sense of fairness into the process, your loved one might provide instructions for passing on not just items of material value but also items of sentimental value to family and friends.

Another option is to involve all the potential heirs in the discussion of the will. This may not work for every family, especially those already in conflict about a loved one's care. But in the right circumstances, it can provide invaluable guidance in determining who gets what. Your loved one may not even realize that a particular lamp or blanket holds special significance for a certain family member. By letting everyone express their wishes, you give them a stake in the distribution of property that could help defuse disagreements later on.

Making It Official

A will can take various forms. Sometimes an oral will is considered legally binding, though defending it in court—should someone decide to challenge it—can be difficult. Many states accept handwritten wills that are dated and signed, but they, too, may be vulnerable to lawsuits, particularly if the handwriting is not completely legible.

The most reliable will is a printed one. Many self-help books and Web sites on legal matters offer a range of forms from which to choose. Some of these documents are relatively simple and straightforward, while others can be tailored to a person's circumstances as necessary.

Once your loved one writes, signs, and dates her will, make a copy for yourself and a copy for her attorney, if she has one. Then have the person file the original in a safe deposit box or another

FOR MORE INFORMATION

Nolo Press publishes a wide range of self-help books on legal issues of interest to caregivers and care recipients. The books include sample forms for wills, powers of attorney, and other documents. Call **(800) 728-3555** or visit **www.nolo.com**.

You can obtain state-specific forms from an organization called Choice in Dying. Call **(800) 989-9455** or visit **www.choices.org**.

Key Points about Wills

The laws governing wills vary from state to state. But no matter where your loved one lives, the following general guidelines can help ensure that her property is distributed according to her wishes.

- To avoid conflicts of interest and other potential legal problems, people who are named as beneficiaries of a will should not also sign it as witnesses.

- In some states, inheritance laws can override a will. For example, a spouse may be entitled to a certain percentage of the assets, even if the will specifies otherwise.

- Those named as beneficiaries on life insurance policies, 401(k) accounts, and other assets are entitled to those funds, even if a will states otherwise.

- Although many people write their wills without consulting attorneys, those with large and varied estates may want to seek legal advice on ways to reduce inheritance taxes and other costs for their heirs.

safe place, where both of you can find it. If she moves it without telling you, at least you'll have the photocopy as a backup.

Many people believe a will must be notarized to be legal. That isn't the case. On the other hand, a separate notarized statement signed by witnesses can simplify the probate process—especially in the event of any challenges—by helping to prove that the person was of sound mind when the will was drawn up.

TRUSTS

Unlike a will, a trust eliminates the probate process and possibly inheritance taxes, too. When property is transferred to a trust, the trust in effect becomes the legal owner. The grantor, or settlor—that is, the person who creates the trust—appoints a trustee, usually a person or a financial institution, to manage the property. The grantor also provides written guidelines for administration of the trust and designates beneficiaries, who eventually will receive the trust's assets.

The most popular category of trust is called a living trust because it's established while the grantor is alive. Often money and securities are the primary assets, though any kind of property is acceptable. In most cases, the trust is revocable; in other words, it can be changed or dissolved by the grantor unless or until the person is incapacitated. Upon the grantor's death, the trust's assets pass directly to the beneficiaries. While they must pay inheritance taxes, the transaction is not subject to review by the probate court, which can save a lot of time and legal fees.

In contrast, an irrevocable living trust cannot be changed once it is created. The biggest advantage of this kind of trust is that its assets aren't considered part of the estate, so the beneficiary doesn't have to pay inheritance taxes. Generally, an irrevocable living trust is used only by the wealthy, and then only in special circumstances.

Whether a living trust should be established, and whether it should be revocable or irrevocable, depend greatly on the size of the estate, the age and marital status of the grantor, relations among the heirs, and a host of other factors. You and your loved one may want to sit down with an attorney to discuss the pros and cons.

Along with the living trust, another broad category is the testamentary trust. Generally, the instructions for this kind of trust are outlined in a will, so it's established only after a person's death. The terms of a testamentary trust can vary, but in most cases, a third party manages the assets for the heirs and distributes funds as needed or mandated. This type of trust is useful for passing large sums of money to minor children without giving

---

Covering All the Bases

A letter of instruction is a non-binding statement that outlines a person's wishes beyond what is covered in her will and in other legal documents. The "official" papers cannot anticipate all eventualities, like what to do with the deceased's personal diaries. In these circumstances, a letter of instruction can prove helpful. Its provisions might include the following:

- Directions on preferred funeral, burial/cremation, and memorial arrangements
- Advice on what to do with private and possibly intimate effects such as diaries, letters, and other personal documents
- Suggestions on how to distribute prized family possessions that may have great sentimental but little market value, such as awards, costume jewelry, books, and dishware and cutlery
- Preferences for the future care of any pets, such as cats, dogs, or fish
- Information on where to find important documents such as the will and durable powers of attorney
- Guidelines for handling bank accounts, stock transactions, and other financial matters
- The names and contact information of the person's physicians, lawyers, and accountants, plus any other providers of professional services
- Recommendations to beneficiaries for maximizing the value of their inheritances
- Personal messages to loved ones or any other final thoughts

them control over the actual assets until they reach a certain age or fulfill obligations outlined in the will.

Although a trust is extremely effective at minimizing the hassles of probate, it isn't a substitute for a will. Even if someone establishes a number of trusts, she may have non-trust property that she must distribute. For this reason, many wills have a "pour-over" clause that covers all assets not set aside in trusts.

POWERS OF ATTORNEY

Beyond providing instructions for the distribution of her property, your loved one needs to appoint people to make decisions on her behalf should she become incapacitated. She can do this with a document known as a power of attorney.

Executing a power of attorney is the simplest way for a person to ensure her financial security and continuity of care. What's more, it's the best way to avoid the long and complicated court proceedings necessary to establish a guardianship or conservatorship, which requires proof that a person can no longer handle her personal affairs. (We'll talk more about guardianships and conservatorships later in the chapter.)

Simply put, a power of attorney designates one person to act in another's name. The signer of the document is called the principal; the designee is known as the agent, or the attorney-in-fact. A durable power of attorney continues even after the principal can't make rational decisions for herself.

Not all powers of attorney are created equal. Some go into effect as soon as they're signed. Others are "springing," which means they become valid only when the principal is no longer competent. Some are broad in scope, allowing the agent to make all financial and legal decisions. Others might limit the agent to signing checks or selling property.

In general, care recipients should have both a durable power of attorney for finances and a durable power of attorney for health care. Sometimes one person will take on both roles. But more commonly, a principal prefers to divvy up the responsibilities and choose the best person for each subject area.

Under a durable power of attorney for finances, for example, the agent might be a family member knowledgeable about money matters, or perhaps an accountant or a financial planner.

This person would have the authority to pay bills, sell assets, file taxes, submit insurance claims, and perform other necessary tasks to manage your loved one's financial situation.

Similarly, a durable power of attorney for health care—also called a health care proxy—empowers a person to make important medical decisions, such as what course of treatment should be pursued or whether life-prolonging measures should be used. Usually, this person has full access to the principal's medical records. For this role, your loved one would want someone who understands and respects her wishes regarding her health care.

Becoming Your Loved One's Voice

If your loved one grants you power of attorney for health care or finances (or both), sitting down and discussing her needs and preferences is absolutely essential. You don't want to sell her home if she'd rather unload her stock portfolio. Nor do you want to insist on surgery if she prefers palliative care at the end of life.

No matter how thorough your loved one is, she can't possibly provide written instructions for every conceivable—and inconceivable—caregiving scenario. You may find yourself in a situation in which you must make a decision based solely on what you think the person would want. The better you understand her wishes, the more confident you can feel about your choices.

What's more, by talking with your loved one, you reassure her of your heartfelt intentions to act in her best interests. Sometimes people hesitate to execute durable powers of attorney because they worry about relinquishing their decision-making abilities. Indeed, because power-of-attorney arrangements are not monitored, they can be vulnerable to abuse (and proving misconduct can be difficult and costly). Your loved one needs to know that as long as she's alert and able, she has a voice in her care—and if she becomes incapacitated, you'll speak on her behalf.

The guidelines for executing powers of attorney vary from state to state. Some require the signed document to be notarized; others want a copy filed with a government agency. Many allow the principal to limit the authority of the agent to specific situations and decisions.

You can find sample power-of-attorney agreements on the Internet and in self-help books. Before your loved one signs anything, though, the two of you should consult a lawyer who's

Outlook

"Three facts point to a pending crisis in caregiving. First, every 7 seconds a person turns 50. Second, one in every four households is involved in caring for a person over 50. And third, 30 percent of caregivers experience either physical or emotional effects. These facts are more alarming because they are accompanied by a shift in values. Younger generations are not volunteering and may turn to society to care for their parents. People age 60 and older are not *obligated* to honor, but they *care* enough to honor. The question is, will the boomers and those that follow feel the same?"

—**WILLIAM E. ARNOLD, PH.D.**, director of the gerontology program at Arizona State University in Tempe

Are Your Loved One's Legal Affairs in Order?

Organizing your loved one's legal papers does take time and effort. But you can streamline the process considerably by following this checklist.

☐ Prepare an inventory of all assets, including real estate, bank accounts, stocks and bonds, pension and retirement benefits, and family heirlooms.

☐ Help decide who should receive each and every asset.

☐ If your loved one has a will, review it together to make sure it reflects the person's wishes. If it doesn't, suggest she draft a new one.

☐ Determine whether your loved one could reduce the time and expense of probate by creating living trusts and other financial instruments.

☐ Confirm that the designated beneficiaries of life insurance policies, 401(k) plans, IRAs, and other accounts are consistent with your loved one's wishes. If not, have her update the names.

☐ Help select someone trustworthy and reliable as executor of the estate.

☐ Find out whether your loved one has prepared a durable power of attorney for finances and a durable power of attorney for health care. If she hasn't, encourage her to do so.

☐ Inform the prospective executor of the estate, as well as the agents for the durable powers of attorney, that they've been chosen for these roles. Ask whether they're able to accept the responsibilities.

☐ Discuss your loved one's wishes for end-of-life care, then help create a living will.

☐ Make sure that all legal documents conform to the laws of your loved one's state, and that they're signed and dated.

☐ Advise your loved one to store all her legal documents in one place that the two of you can access.

☐ Keep a signed copy of every legal document for yourself and for your loved one's attorney.

☐ Provide a copy of the will to the executor and copies of the durable powers of attorney to the designated agents.

☐ Send copies of the durable power of attorney for health care and the living will to your loved one's primary care physician and other medical personnel involved in her care, whether at home, in a hospital, or in a residential care facility.

☐ Ask your loved one to write down her preferences for funeral, burial/cremation, and memorial arrangements in as much detail as possible.

☐ Check to be sure your loved one has drawn up a letter of instruction to address any issues not covered by other legal documents.

familiar with the power-of-attorney laws in your state. If you and your loved one live in different states, the lawyer can help navigate the legal complexities of establishing and implementing power of attorney across the miles.

Along the same lines, your loved one should consider appointing a backup agent in case the primary agent is unavailable for some reason. Both of these people should keep copies of the power-of-attorney agreement on file in case they're called upon to make decisions on short notice. In addition, copies of a durable power of attorney for finances should go to banks and other financial institutions your loved one deals with; copies of a durable power of attorney for health care should be given to her primary care physician and other health care providers she sees regularly.

LIVING WILLS

Even if your loved one has executed a durable power of attorney for health care, she needs to prepare a living will as well. Both documents are known as advance directives because they provide instructions for the handling of a person's medical decisions in the event she can no longer speak for herself. But the documents differ in their primary functions: Where a durable power of attorney appoints someone else to make decisions on a person's behalf, a living will spells out the person's wishes, particularly with regard to end-of-life care.

Generally, a living will takes effect only when a patient is close to death because of illness or injury. In most cases, the document stipulates that if the chance of recovery is negligible, the person may be given pain relief but otherwise no aggressive treatment. On occasion, though, someone will craft a living will to specifically request the use of all life-sustaining measures.

While living wills tend to be broadly framed, some people prefer to spell out which measures they consider acceptable and which they don't want under any circumstances. For example, they may approve being fed intravenously but reject being hooked up to an artificial respirator.

These sorts of details can make preparing a living will an unsettling experience. Virtually no one likes to contemplate death, much less draw the line on end-of-life care. If your loved one

In Case of an Emergency . . .

If your loved one chooses, she can file what is known as a "do not resuscitate" order. This document directs paramedics and other medical personnel not to use lifesaving techniques in the event a person's heartbeat or breathing stops. It's different from a living will; in fact, many families are shocked to learn that their loved ones' living wills do not apply in certain medical crises.

Some states, such as Florida, have a standard form called a pre-hospital "do not resuscitate" order. It gives those with terminal illness the right to die without emergency medical intervention. The document must be signed by the patient or her representative as well as two physicians.

seems reluctant to make these sorts of decisions, you might remind her that in the absence of an advance directive, others will need to choose a course of action on her behalf. Often family members won't agree. Or the physician or hospital may refuse to suspend aggressive treatments because of ethical or legal concerns.

As with so many legal documents, the laws on living wills vary from one state to another. For example, consider the definition of the word *terminal*. In many states, a person who is in a deep coma that could go on indefinitely would not qualify as terminal, at least not as interpreted in a living will.

Likewise, some states may not view intravenous feeding and hydration as an extraordinary or aggressive treatment. In those jurisdictions, a person would need to use a living will to specifically instruct medical personnel to forgo such measures.

Because of the legal discrepancies between states, your best bet for creating a valid living will that accurately reflects your loved one's wishes is to consult an attorney who's familiar with the rules and regulations in the person's home state. If she already has a living will, double-check to be sure it complies with the prevailing legal requirements. And talk through the document with your loved one, so you know for certain what she wants and doesn't want.

Once the living will is final, make a copy for yourself so you have it in case you need it—as in a medical crisis, when your loved one may require emergency care. Also give copies to your loved one's primary care physician, to her hospital, and to any other health care providers for their files.

Remember, living wills and other advance directives do not automatically guarantee that your loved one's wishes will be honored. For these documents to fulfill their purpose, you and your loved one—and anyone else involved in her care—must prepare for their use.

GUARDIANSHIP AND CONSERVATORSHIPS

Watching someone you love slowly lose her ability to care for herself can be devastating. As long as she has executed durable powers of attorney, at least she can get help to manage her financial and medical matters.

But what if your loved one hasn't signed any power-of-attorney agreement? If you feel she poses a risk to herself or others, you may need to go to court to seek a guardianship. It's a last resort, but in the absence of a power of attorney, it may be the only way to safeguard your loved one's interests.

Two broad categories of guardianship exist. One, guardianship of the person, empowers someone to make decisions about an individual's medical care and similar personal matters. The other, guardianship of the property, authorizes someone to take charge of an individual's financial affairs.

Just like the laws themselves, the terminology pertaining to guardianships isn't consistent between states. The courts in some states describe the appointee as a *conservator* instead of *guardian*; others use the two terms interchangeably. Still others refer to the person handling personal matters as the guardian and the person managing the money as a conservator. In these states, while the jobs may be assigned separately, usually they're not. One person will serve as both guardian and conservator.

Of course, neither a guardian nor a conservator would be nec-

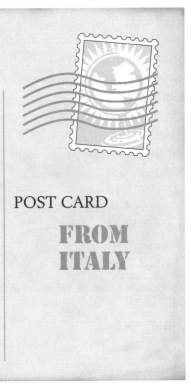

Caregiving around the World

Traditionally, the women in Italian families have taken on the caregiving responsibilities. If a parent or older relative is moved out of the home, the rest of the family may be subjected to criticism and gossip. But as more women enter the workforce, the family structure is changing. Today, the older people provide much of the care, with many "young old" Italians looking after their elders.

POST CARD

FROM ITALY

essary if a care recipient made her power-of-attorney appointments in a timely manner. Unfortunately, many people put off the task, or worse, they don't even realize they should do it. So if they're suddenly incapacitated—because of a stroke or an automobile accident, for example—their loved ones won't have legal permission to make decisions on their behalf.

Both guardianships and conservatorships have their disadvantages. To begin with, they require court proceedings, which can become very time-consuming and expensive. In addition, because the proceedings are a matter of public record, the intimate details of a care recipient's personal life and financial position may become widespread knowledge.

Beyond that, the care recipient has the right to defend herself against efforts to declare her incompetent. She's entitled to attend all the hearings, and to receive legal representation. If she can't afford an attorney, the court will appoint one on her behalf.

In determining whether a person needs a guardian or conservator, and who should fill those roles, the court has lots of discretion. It could choose the person who filed for guardianship or conservatorship in the first place. If several people are vying for the job, the court will choose the one who seems best able to handle the extra responsibilities and to act in the care recipient's best interests. If for some reason none of the candidates seems suitable, the court could bypass family and friends in favor of an attorney, a member of the clergy—perhaps someone who doesn't even know the care recipient.

But guardianship and conservatorship do offer one key protection that durable powers of attorney do not: They ensure that the guardian or conservator does not abuse his position. Even after making its appointment, the court continues to supervise the process, including reviewing—and sometimes approving—major decisions and transactions, such as the sale of property. It can even dismiss a guardian or conservator and appoint a replacement, if it determines such a move to be in the best interests of the care recipient.

Because pursuing a guardianship or conservatorship has so many legal implications, consulting an attorney is wise. He can explain the pros and cons of such an arrangement within the framework of your situation, as well as within the specific laws in your state.

PART SEVEN

Caring for the Caregiver

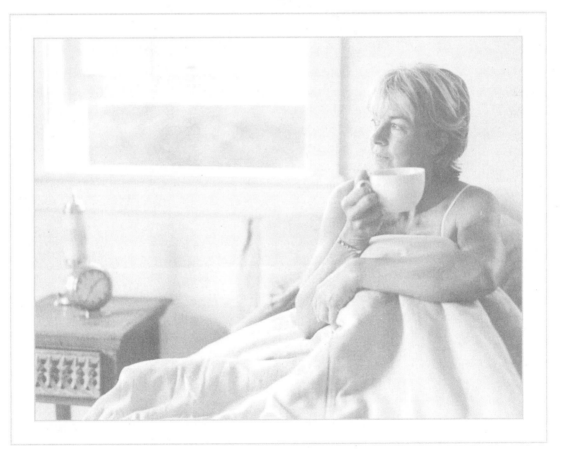

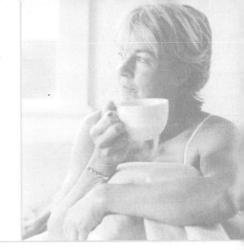

CHAPTER 26

FEELING BAD ABOUT FEELING BAD

What You Need to Know

- Before you can care for someone else, you must care for yourself. Otherwise, the emotional strain could contribute to physical illness.

- Powerful emotions like guilt, anger, and depression are common among caregivers. They're perfectly normal responses to the demands and uncertainty of the caregiving experience. They also can be managed.

- Getting support—whether from family and friends or a formal support group— is vital to maintaining emotional strength and balance. If you're not able to attend group meetings in person, you can always go online.

When running through their preflight safety instructions, flight attendants tell their passengers: "If you're traveling with someone who needs assistance, put on your oxygen mask first, then help the other person." Why your mask first? Because you can't help anyone else if you're struggling yourself.

It's a principle that applies in caregiving, too. Or at least it ought to. The reality is, most caregivers focus on their loved ones' needs to the exclusion of their own. While their devotion is admirable, they don't realize that they're setting themselves up for debilitating guilt, anger, depression—and, all too often, burnout.

Research has shown that the unrelenting emotional strain often associated with caregiving may take a physical toll as well, in the form of suppressed immunity. In one study, scientists at Ohio State University gave flu shots to 64 older people, half of whom were caring for a spouse with Alzheimer's disease. These shots work by stimulating the immune system to produce the antibodies that

Point of View

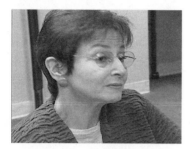

"The only thing really in your control is your attitude. If you live life angry and depressed, you miss the good parts. I've tried to make lemonade from my lemons. I can't do some things I'd like to do, but I have my pleasures. I read novels. I exercise regularly with a personal trainer, which has been extraordinarily beneficial. I take long walks every week with a friend. I'm a grandmother, and I love spending time with my granddaughter. I have a good friend who, like me, cares for a husband with MS. We talk several times a week."

—SUZANNE MINTZ,
Kensington, Maryland

prevent flu. In follow-up tests, the scientists found antibody levels to be adequate in just 37 percent of the caregivers, compared with 75 percent of the non-caregivers. The scientists concluded that the stress of caregiving had undermined immune function enough to impair antibody production.

This might help explain why caregivers seem to be at greater risk for illness than the general population. They do register more sick days because of upper respiratory infections, according to the scientific literature. And they tend to have lower scores on health self-assessments.

In fact, when Richard Schulz, Ph.D., a psychologist at the Veterans Administration Hospital in Pittsburgh, tracked more than 800 elderly people for 4 years, he found the death rate from all causes to be 63 percent higher among caregivers than non-caregivers. The wide margin may have resulted from a number of factors in the caregiving experience, but surely emotional distress was among them.

Time and again, studies have shown that the mind and emotions can influence physical health for better or for worse. This is why coming to terms with the often powerful emotions that surface in a caregiving relationship is so important. By acknowledging the normalcy of feeling bad, you actually help yourself feel better. In turn, you have more confidence in your ability to give care—which is good for you and your loved one.

With all this in mind, let's take a closer look at three of the most common emotions caregivers experience—guilt, anger, and depression—and the best ways you can cope with them. (We'll talk at length about stress management in chapter 29.)

CARING WITHOUT GUILT

Of all the emotions caregivers wrestle with, guilt is the most pervasive. "It's universal," says Joan Furman, author of *The Dying Time: Practical Wisdom for the Dying and Their Caregivers*. "Guilt is anger that people think they don't have a right to feel."

Indeed, when a person sacrifices so much to provide care for a loved one, guilt might seem like a misplaced emotion. Still, it's there. It may bubble up when you lose your temper with your loved one. Or when you take time for yourself. Or when you wish you had never gotten involved in your loved one's care.

"These feelings are very common," says Dolores Gallagher-Thompson, Ph.D., director of the Older Adult and Family Center at the Veterans Administration Medical Center in Palo Alto, California, and associate professor of psychiatry at Stanford University. "Having them doesn't mean that you're a bad person, or that you don't love the care recipient. Caregiving is enormously demanding. Negative emotions are inevitable—and so is feeling guilty because of them."

Sometimes guilt arises from a sense of inadequacy, adds Mimi Goodrich, L.C.S.W., of the Wellness Center in San Mateo, California. You want to be perfect, especially when caring for a loved one. Realistically, no one can achieve perfection. Still, in your own eyes, you're not good enough. And you feel guilty about it.

To deal with the guilt, Dr. Gallagher-Thompson suggests a do-it-yourself version of cognitive therapy that involves identifying and correcting erroneous thoughts before they bring you down. For example, if you start berating yourself for being inadequate, use the "good friend test": What would a friend say about your supposed shortcomings? Probably something like this: "You're in a tough situation. Caregiving is hard work. You've done remarkably well, better than most ever would. Sure, you've learned some things the hard way, and you have some regrets. But you've done your best. That's all you can do."

By being that friend to yourself, you can correct the distorted thinking that demands perfection. Your mind is free to acknowledge and embrace all you've accomplished. Suddenly, you realize you have little, if anything, to feel guilty about.

Of course, another powerful antidote for guilt is the support of friends and family, says Leslie Plooster, M.A., program associate for the Bethesda, Maryland–based National Alliance for Caregiving. They can reassure you that you're doing your best—and that your best is good enough.

Take Action... SEEK PERSONAL SUPPORT

When you're a caregiver, carving out time for positive, nurturing interactions with others might seem like a luxury you can ill afford. But you owe yourself that time. Without it, you may not

Point of View

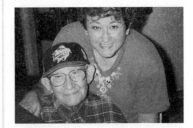

"**At first, I felt guilty going to a support group. I had to get past that; I had to accept that taking time for myself was okay. I go to the group thinking, 'I can't go on.' But I come away thinking, 'I can do this.'**"

—ALICIA FRANCO,
Santa Barbara, California

FOR MORE INFORMATION

To locate support groups in your area, start by looking in the blue pages of your telephone directory, in the "Guide to Human Services." You'll see listings for groups as well as for your Area Agency on Aging, which may have additional leads. Alternatively, you can find your Area Agency on Aging through the Eldercare Locator at **(800) 677-1116** or **www.eldercare.gov**.

Other organizations that offer referrals to support groups and general support for caregivers include the following:

• Children of Aging Parents: **(800) 227-7294; www.caps4caregivers.org**

• Family Caregiver Alliance: **(800) 445-8106; www.caregiver.org**

• National Alliance for Caregiving: **www.caregiving.org**

• National Family Caregivers Association: **(800) 896-3650; www.nfcacares.org**

have the mental resolve to deal with guilt and other negative emotions. Here's what to do.

✗ If you can't go out often because of your caregiving responsibilities, invite your friends over. They know you're stretched thin; they won't care if your house isn't immaculate or your refreshments aren't lavish. They'll be glad to see you, whether it's over wine and cheese or coffee and cookies.

✗ Even better, compare calendars with your friends to schedule regular afternoons or evenings out. By planning ahead, you have something to look forward to, and you can make arrangements for respite care.

✗ If you can't leave and your friends can't come over, get on the phone. Even a brief chat can help lift your spirits.

✗ Beyond your friends, draw strength from your faith. The congregation of a church or synagogue can provide the reassurance and encouragement you need to feel good about your caregiving role. Faith-based caregiving support services are sprouting up across the country.

✗ Join a support group. You don't even need to leave the house for meetings; just head into cyberspace. For homebound caregivers, Internet-based support groups are a godsend. Check with the Area Agency on Aging or with local chapters of condition-specific organizations. They should be able to recommend good support groups both in your community and online.

MANAGING ANGER

In caregiving situations, guilt and anger often go hand in hand. For instance, a caregiver may lash out at a family member who refuses to pitch in, then feel guilty about the outburst later. But in this case, getting angry serves a purpose. It allows for the release of pent-up emotions that otherwise might fester into physical illness.

That said, repeated angry episodes do more harm than good. Over time, they can set the stage for high blood pressure and heart disease, among other serious health concerns—just what a caregiver doesn't need. In fact, the constant presence of anger can make the caregiving relationship much more stressful for caregiver and care recipient alike.

To help caregivers manage chronic anger, Dr. Gallagher-Thompson and her colleagues developed a class called Coping with Frustration and Anger. It's based on cognitive-behavioral psychology—"cognitive" meaning cognitive therapy, "behavioral" referring to problem-solving techniques. Basically, the class teaches participants to tinker with their situations to minimize causes of anger—and to have more fun.

Instructors begin by affirming that anger is a perfectly normal emotion for caregivers. The key is to deal with it in a constructive way. Participants discuss the sources of their anger and their responses to it. They learn an exercise called the Instant Calming Sequence to defuse their anger on the spot. They practice cognitive therapy by self-correcting thoughts that are attached to unrealistic expectations. And they keep a log of situations that trigger their anger, so they can talk through possible solutions in class.

Just as important, participants receive instruction in using assertiveness rather than anger to express their needs and concerns. One lesson is a role-playing exercise, in which participants practice insisting—gently but firmly—that other family members follow through on their promises so the caregivers get a break from their responsibilities.

Those who've graduated from the class say they're much less hostile, and their families are much more supportive, than before.

Outlook

"Caregivers struggle with an inevitable conflict between their loved ones' needs and their own. Giving by the caretaker that is not matched by adequate receiving makes eventual burnout a certainty. Effective, sustainable caregiving now and in the future depends on meeting the caregiver's own needs for nurture, reassurance, support, and periodic respite. We need to find ways to refill the giver's emotional tank."

—ROY W. MENNINGER, M.D., chairman emeritus of the Menninger Foundation in Topeka, Kansas

The Instant Calming Sequence

Developed by Robert Cooper, Ph.D., a stress management psychologist from Ann Arbor, Michigan, the Instant Calming Sequence is the fast track to anger management. Dr. Cooper recommends using the technique as soon as you feel you're getting tense. With practice, you can relax within seconds.

1. Breathe smoothly, deeply, and evenly. You'll feel calmer right away.

2. Smile. Smiling sends nerve impulses from the facial muscles to the limbic system, the brain's emotional center. This shifts the entire nervous system toward calm.

3. Maintain good posture. When angry, people slouch, which amplifies negativity.

4. Visualize a wave of relaxation. Imagine you're in a hot shower, and your anger washes down the drain.

5. Take control. Forget feeling victimized, Dr. Cooper says. Instead, focus on coping.

EXPERT OPINION

"We teach the three Rs: relax, reconnect, rejoice. Caregivers can relax here. Most haven't felt carefree in ages. They rediscover who they are and reconnect with family they've neglected. As for 'rejoice,' we mean finding the positives in caregiving. Often the focus is on the negatives. But caregiving is a very important job. It's something to feel good about."

—**DONNA BENTON, PH.D.,** director of the Los Angeles Caregiver Resource Center at the University of Southern California

Though the class is offered in only a few locations around the country, you can incorporate its key elements into your self-care regimen. For example, you can learn the Instant Calming Sequence and practice it whenever you need to (see page 351). And you can keep your own "anger log," writing down situations that feed your anger and your reactions to them. Once you know your flash points, you can work on responding more constructively.

Beyond these self-care techniques, you can help head off angry outbursts just by taking regular breaks from your caregiving responsibilities. Arrange for respite care if you need to. "Time off is absolutely essential," says Percil Stanford, Ph.D., professor of gerontology and director of the Center on Aging at San Diego State University. "Do whatever you must to get away at least one night each week—or, even better, one entire day."

Your loved one's primary care physician may be able to recommend affordable, reliable respite care in your area. Many community hospitals offer referrals, too. Other possible resources include your Area Agency on Aging as well as local churches and synagogues, some of which sponsor volunteer respite care programs.

BEATING THE BLUES

Unlike guilt and anger, which can come on in an instant, depression tends to build up over time. What's more, it affects people in different ways. For about 5 percent of Americans, it takes the form of "the blues," a persistent down-in-the-dumps feeling. Another 5 percent suffer what physicians call clinical or major depression, the kind that can prompt thoughts of suicide.

Among caregivers, the rate of clinical depression runs much higher—18 percent, according to a Stanford University survey. It climbs to 46 percent among those who seek professional help for caregiving-related problems, many of whom have loved ones with dementia.

Depression has followed Suzanne Mintz through her caregiving experience. The Kensington, Maryland, resident was just 28 years old when her husband was diagnosed with multiple sclerosis in 1974. "The progression was slow, but steadily downhill," Mintz says. "Now he uses a wheelchair."

To help cope with her situation, Mintz joined forces with a

friend and fellow caregiver to found the National Family Caregivers Association. Still, she has had to weather four bouts of serious depression. "Life isn't fair," she says. "I got dealt a difficult hand."

For Mintz and other caregivers, the emotional strain of caregiving comes not from spending time on caregiving tasks or from coping with the infirmity of the care recipients, explains Susan Parks, M.D., a gerontologist at Thomas Jefferson University in Philadelphia. Rather, it correlates with feeling overwhelmed. When you're overwhelmed, you develop feelings of guilt, anger, and depression. But with self-care and support, you can cope.

"Whether you call it depression or burnout, you have to deal with it," Dr. Stanford affirms. "Otherwise, you can't provide good care."

Take Action... LIFT YOUR SPIRITS

While clinical or major depression may require professional help, less severe cases often respond well to self-care. Perhaps one

---

Caregiver's Checklist

Are You at Risk for Depression?

According to the American Psychiatric Association, if you experience at least five of the following symptoms over the course of 2 weeks, you may have depression severe enough to need professional help. Consult a physician or psychiatrist as soon as possible. Treatment for depression can range from lifestyle changes to medication and counseling.

☐ Persistent feelings of sadness, hopelessness, or helplessness

☐ Severe anxiety or worry

☐ Persistent feelings of worthlessness or guilt

☐ Difficulty thinking, concentrating, remembering, or making decisions

☐ Significant weight gain or loss

☐ Headaches, abdominal distress, or other significant aches and pains

☐ Loss of interest in usual activities

☐ Loss of interest in sex

☐ Impaired sexual function

☐ Sluggishness or restlessness

☐ Insomnia or excessive sleeping

☐ Thoughts of death or suicide

FOR MORE INFORMATION

Many organizations sponsor hot lines for caregivers in crisis. Check with any of the support groups in your area—they're listed in the blue pages of your telephone directory, under "Guide to Human Services"—or call the National Institute on Aging Hot Line at **(800) 222-2225**.

of the most fundamental strategies is to build brief interludes of rest and relaxation into each day. "Our research shows that it helps," Dr. Gallagher-Thompson says. "Ten minutes here, 10 minutes there—it adds up. It's the kind of respite that just about every caregiver can work into her schedule."

Here's what else caregiving experts recommend.

- Incorporate pleasurable activities into each day, even when you don't feel like it. Rest assured, you'll appreciate it afterward. You needn't do anything elaborate, either. Listen to music, putter in the garden, engage in a hobby—whatever pastime you enjoy.

- Find ways to pamper yourself. Soak in a warm bath. Get a massage or a manicure. Hire a chef for a day. It may be an expense, but you deserve it.

- Nurture your body by eating balanced meals, exercising regularly, and sleeping at least 7 hours a night. (To learn more about each of these lifestyle factors, see chapter 29.)

- Tickle your funny bone. Buy a joke book and flip through it when you need a laugh. Rent a comedy video. Above all else, try to find the humor in everyday situations.

Caregiver's Checklist

Are You in Danger of Burnout?

The symptoms of burnout are very similar to those of depression. In fact, the two conditions often contribute to one another. You could be experiencing burnout if you notice any of the following:

- ☐ Persistent symptoms of depression
- ☐ Constant anxiety, irritability, or anger
- ☐ Persistent detachment, numbness, or exhaustion
- ☐ Continuous self-criticism

- ☐ Withdrawal from usual activities
- ☐ Negligence or hatred of caregiving responsibilities
- ☐ Trouble at work or in relationships
- ☐ Substance abuse

✗ Keep a journal. Writing down your thoughts and feelings helps provide perspective on your situation.

✗ Accept what you can't change and focus on what you can. For example, if the rest of your family declines to pitch in with your loved one's care, pressing the issue will only fuel your stress. Instead, put your energy into exploring community caregiving resources.

✗ Acknowledge your accomplishments as a caregiver, rather than dwelling on the disappointments. No one can do it all. But if you pause and reflect on your situation, you'll realize that what you have done is nothing short of amazing.

✗ Participate in a support group, either in person or online. To track down leads on groups in your area, see "For More Information" on page 350.

If you don't feel better with self-care, or if you seem to be sinking deeper into depression, see your doctor right away. Many effective treatments are available, including medications and psychotherapy.

Outlook

"Being a caregiver for a frail elder is among the greatest risk factors for developing a major depressive disorder. Recent evidence also shows a link to mortality. For some, the price is life. This is intolerable in American society. We must provide better support for families."

—LAURA CARSTENSEN, PH.D., professor of psychology and the former Barbara D. Finberg Director at the Institute for Research on Women and Gender at Stanford University

CHAPTER 27

"WHAT ABOUT ME?"

What You Need to Know

- Many caregivers feel torn between their caregiving responsibilities and their family obligations. Balancing the two takes effort, but it's important not only for preserving family relationships but also for protecting the caregiver's emotional resilience.

- As your caregiving situation evolves, your spouse and/or children may need reassurance that they, too, are priorities in your life. Perhaps the best way to demonstrate your commitment to them is to give your undivided attention to each person, even if only for a brief period every day.

- While you work to accommodate the needs of others, don't forget your own. Remember, you have only a finite amount of time and energy.

Years back, you'd see them on television variety shows—the guys who'd spin plates on poles. Remember how they'd dash from one pole to another, trying to keep each plate balanced on its tenuous perch?

Well, family life is a lot like that. Your spouse, your children, your siblings and other relatives—each person needs your full and undivided attention, and you have to deal with them all at once. Yet somehow you manage to keep all the plates spinning.

That is, until you become a caregiver. Suddenly, your carefully orchestrated balancing act seems on the verge of crashing to pieces. You're pulled in so many different directions that you're not sure you can stop it. Your family, on the other hand, expects that you will.

Some experts describe this phenomenon as the caregiver

crunch; others call it the sandwich effect. The point is, you feel caught in the middle, sandwiched between the many responsibilities of caregiving and the other legitimate demands in your life.

Still, if you want to get through your caregiving experience with the rest of your family relationships intact, you must find time to nurture those relationships. Admittedly, this can be a challenge, according to Joseph Ilardo, Ph.D., L.C.S.W., and Carole Rothman, Ph.D., coauthors of *Are Your Parents Driving You Crazy?* But while you may not be able to give everyone everything they want, you can provide them with most of the time and attention they need. It just takes a combination of forethought, planning, and ongoing communication.

Take Action... FOSTER FAMILY TIES

"Caregiving can feel overwhelming—not just for you, but for everyone in your family," says Dolores Gallagher-Thompson, Ph.D., director of the Older Adult and Family Center at the Veterans Administration Medical Center in Palo Alto, California, and associate professor of psychiatry at Stanford University. To help achieve balance in your relationships as well as in your own life, heed this advice from the experts.

X Recognize reality. You have only so much energy, and only so many hours in a day. The more of these resources you invest in your caregiving tasks, the less you can give to your non-caregiving relationships. Ideally, you and your family discussed this before you became a caregiver. If not, you should do it now. Everyone needs to understand the implications of your caregiving role. When presenting your case, temper your words with a sincere commitment to make time for your spouse, your children, and the other people in your life.

X Make caregiving part of your life, not your entire life. It has been mentioned elsewhere in this book, but it bears repeating: Caregiving is a marathon, not a sprint. If you put all your time and energy into it, to the exclusion of everything else, you're going to run out of steam fast. This is

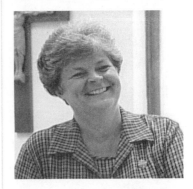

Point of View

"I think a solution to the growing need for care for the elderly is to stay networked within an intergenerational community—children with parents, grandkids with grandparents. We can't be afraid to do that; we can't put aside the elderly. Even when the elderly live together, they shouldn't interact only with each other. They need to interact with people of all ages."

—SISTER KATHERINE
of the School Sisters of Notre Dame,
Mankato, Minnesota

why you shouldn't feel guilty about taking breaks to be with your family, or just by yourself. These "pauses" keep you emotionally and physically resilient, so you can continue to provide good care.

✗ Be sensitive to the effects of a caregiving situation on other family members. In the words of Claire Berman, author of *Caring for Yourself While Caring for Your Aging Parents*, caring for a loved one triggers "a dramatic transition for the entire family." Your spouse and children have needs that won't just disappear when you become a caregiver. Even the most compassionate family members may resent losing their share of your attention. And they may feel angry or upset because of it.

Why Families Feud

When University of Nebraska researchers studied caregiving families, they found that many conflicts occur because each person has different needs. As the chart below shows, some of the variation in needs seems to be dictated by family roles. The items in each list appear in order of priority.

Caregivers Need ...	Their Spouses Need ...	Their Children Need ...
Help	Appreciation	Respect
Appreciation	Love	Love
Love	Intimacy	Age-appropriate independence
Respect	Undivided attention	Acceptance
Emotional support	Help	Money
Flexibility from other family members	Respect	Flexibility from other family members
Time with other family members	Emotional support	Emotional support
Time to be by themselves	Flexibility from other family members	Space
Control of their lives	Control of their lives	Unconditional love
Security	Patience from other family members	Age-appropriate control of their lives

✗ Set aside "quality time" for your spouse and children every day. It doesn't have to be a lot of time. You probably don't have a lot to begin with. But even little gestures can go a long way. With young children, you might read a book, play a game, or do a puzzle. With your spouse, you might take a walk, watch a favorite TV show, or just enjoy some quiet conversation after dinner.

✗ When a family conflict arises, look past the anger to the underlying cause. Research at the University of Nebraska suggests that tempers often flare simply because the parties involved have different needs. Let's suppose you and your spouse quarrel because you cancel a lunch date to accommodate your mother's rescheduled doctor appointment. Upon further reflection, you realize that you expect your spouse to be flexible, while your spouse expects you to give him your undivided attention and emotional support. Recognizing that everyone in your family has distinct needs won't necessarily prevent all conflicts, but it can help bring about swift resolutions.

✗ Seek outside assistance as necessary to preserve family time. "Initially, most families try to integrate the care recipient into their activities—another ticket to the ball game or movie, an extra bed for summer vacation," Dr. Gallagher-Thompson says. "This works up to a point. But as your loved one becomes more ill or frail, you need to get help with the caregiving tasks so you can maintain your other family relationships." You might consider placing the person in adult day care or hiring a home health aide so you can get away.

✗ Always anticipate the calm after the storm. Caregiving is a journey marked by periods of relative equilibrium and periods of crisis and transition, explains Suzanne Mintz, co-founder and president of the Kensington, Maryland–based National Family Caregivers Association. Usually, families manage all right while equilibrium prevails. But the crises command your attention, making you feel stressed and the rest of the family feel neglected. "Fortunately, the crises don't last long—a week, perhaps a month or two at most,"

FOR MORE INFORMATION

The Eldercare Locator, sponsored by the U.S. Department of Health and Human Services, offers information about federally funded eldercare resources nationwide. Call **(800) 677-1116** or visit **www.eldercare.gov**.

The National Adult Day Services Association, under the auspices of the National Council on Aging, can help locate adult day care providers in your area. Call **(800) 424-9046** or visit **www.ncoa.org/nadsa/**.

Your local office of the Visiting Nurse Associations of America can help arrange for home care services. For a referral, call the national organization at **(800) 426-2547** or visit **www.vnaa.org**.

Point of View

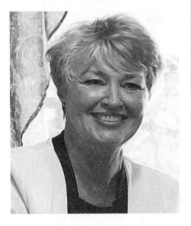

"I feel so torn. The kids have so many things going on, and I want to be there for them. But my father needs so much attention. I try to take one day at a time—no, one minute at a time. Sometimes all I can do is stop for a moment and take a deep breath."

—LORAYE BACKER,
Montevideo, Minnesota

Mintz says. "During these times, encourage your family to see the upheaval as temporary, and a return to equilibrium as not far away. It may be a different kind of equilibrium, but it will be calmer. That helps."

✗ Do your best to accommodate the needs of others without losing sight of yourself. "I wish I had words of wisdom to offer caregivers who feel caught between their caregiving responsibilities and their family commitments," says Percil Stanford, Ph.D., professor of gerontology and director of the Center on Aging at San Diego State University. "Unfortunately, I don't. Every family struggles to maintain itself in the face of caregiving's challenges. You need to find your own ways to cope."

Take Action... REINFORCE MARITAL BONDS

Of all the relationships affected by a caregiving situation, the one between caregiver and spouse may be tested the most. Often spouses become involved in the caregiving responsibilities by virtue of proximity. While some pitch in willingly, others resent having to "share" their wives and husbands with a third party— namely, the care recipient.

You can't take responsibility for your spouse's feelings. But if you do your part to nurture your marriage, perhaps your spouse will respond in kind. These tips can help.

✗ Create opportunities for the two of you to be alone together. Your spouse may be more than willing to help out with the caregiving tasks, or to take on more of the household chores so you're free to look after your loved one. In return, he or she is entitled to receive your undivided attention on a regular basis. By setting aside and safeguarding this uninterrupted "face time," you convey your commitment to your spouse and your marriage.

✗ Block out time in your calendars for one another. Spontaneity is a wonderful thing, but it seldom stands a chance in the context of caregiving. The demands of the caregiving role easily expand to take up every available minute. Scheduling dates with your spouse guarantees you private time—and as a bonus, it lets you plan ahead for respite care.

✗ Turn your "spouse time" into a special occasion. As your budget permits, you can surprise your spouse with special treats like dinner at a posh restaurant, tickets to a sporting event, or even a weekend at a bed-and-breakfast. Distancing yourselves from the caregiving situation, if only for a few hours, makes reconnecting with each other that much easier.

✗ Stay tuned in to your spouse's life. When you're caught up in your caregiving responsibilities, you can easily lose sight of everyone else's day-to-day routines. Yet your spouse is probably dealing with issues, too, especially in his or her job. By asking questions, you let the person know that you're concerned.

✗ Dig deep to understand your spouse's feelings. Certainly the person may be uncomfortable, even resentful, about com-

Caregiving around the World

England and Scotland have very different approaches to the funding of long-term care for the elderly. In Scotland, the government covers the full cost of personal and nursing care, while in England, older people must pay for most of their care themselves. Thousands have had to sell their homes to make ends meet.

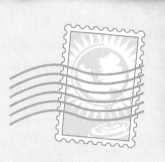

POST CARD

FROM THE
UNITED
KINGDOM

Point of View

"Shortly after Grandmother's funeral, my husband, Sang, left me. Eventually we divorced. The energy I put into caring for her was not the only reason my marriage broke up, but it was a big reason. Sang always complained, 'I'm not number one with you. Grandmother is.' It was true. I thought I had my whole life to spend with him, but little time left with Grandmother. When she was diagnosed [with Alzheimer's disease], the doctor said she had just a year, maybe two. As things turned out, I had a lot more time with Grandmother than the doctor predicted, and a lot less with Sang than I thought."

—FAITH HUNG,
Palo Alto, California

peting with the care recipient for your attention. But most marital relationships are more complicated than that, says Virginia Morris, author of *How to Care for Aging Parents*. For example, your spouse may feel guilty about not helping more with the caregiving tasks, or about not providing enough emotional support. In effect, the person is experiencing some of the same anxieties that you are. Just recognizing this can help strengthen and sustain your relationship.

✗ Keep intimacy alive. Sex can do wonders to relieve stress, and to bring couples close. But when caregiving enters the picture, libidos often suffer—for caregiver and spouse alike. Both of you must make an effort to maintain the romantic spark. Even something as simple as writing a love note or enjoying a candlelight dinner for two can fan the flames.

✗ Be open about financial matters. Caregiving is hard on the wallet, and that can add a lot of stress to a marriage, says Kay Marshall Strom, author of *A Caregiver's Survival Guide*. As the caregiver, you may need to cut back on your work hours or leave your job completely—both of which mean less income for your family. At the same time, you may be spending more to help cover caregiving expenses. Ideally, you and your spouse discussed all this before you took on the caregiving role. Either way, the two of you must work together to plan and maintain a household budget. (For advice on how to do this, see chapter 22.)

✗ Work on your marriage even when you may not feel like it. While every marital relationship has its ups and downs, they usually become more pronounced when caregiving is involved. You may get upset because your spouse isn't helping with the household chores as he said he would. Your spouse may feel slighted when you skip an important business dinner you promised you'd attend. When transgressions like these happen repeatedly, addressing them may start to seem like a waste of time and energy. It isn't. Think of it this way: Caregiving may last for weeks or even months, but marriage can endure forever.

✗ If the demands of caregiving have become more than your marriage can bear, consider seeking professional help. Perhaps a marriage counselor or someone in the clergy can help you and your spouse work through your differences.

Take Action... STAY CONNECTED WITH YOUR KIDS

If you have children living at home, their reactions to your caregiving role will depend a lot on their ages. Teenagers are old enough to realize that the care recipient's health is in decline, and they may be upset and frightened by the prospect of losing someone they love. Younger kids, on the other hand, simply may wonder why Mommy or Daddy isn't around as much.

With children, as with your spouse, your most important strategy is to just make time for them. Whether you use that time to talk with your teen about your loved one's situation or to help your 7-year-old with homework is entirely up to you. The point is, they're getting your undivided attention. In addition:

✗ See the situation from your child's point of view. Even preschoolers understand that time spent with the care recipient is time not spent with them. Under the circumstances, younger kids may become clingy and jealous, while adolescents may act aloof and sullen. Try not to take such behavior personally. Instead, let your child know in every way you can that he or she is and always will be a priority in your life.

✗ Respect your child's intelligence. Young children are more thoughtful and perceptive than they're given credit for, Morris says. Avoid shutting them out by saying, "You're too young to understand." Instead, frame the situation so they *can* understand. Every parent's instinct is to shield his or her children from life's challenges. But if you guide your children through those challenges, they can develop the necessary skills to handle similar situations in the years ahead.

✗ Let your child be a child, rather than a mini-adult. While kids may be able—and even willing—to pitch in with some caregiving tasks, they shouldn't be asked to completely forgo their friends and activities under the circumstances.

Point of View

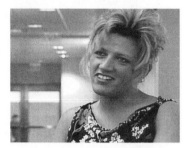

"In the summer, when the days are longer, my daughter wants to go out and play after dinner. But I'm exhausted; all I want to do is sleep. I say, 'Sorry, honey, Mama has to go to bed.' I feel bad about it, but that's the way it is."

—PAM HADDAD,
Pittsburgh

That would only breed anger and resentment. If you minimize the disruptions in your child's life, he or she may be less resistant to helping out when asked to do so.

- Keep the communication lines open. Teenagers, especially, won't open up on cue. When your child is ready to talk, you need to be ready to listen—even if it means stopping whatever else you might be doing. Encourage their questions, and be sensitive to their emotions. Your compassion and candor will help breed trust.

- Recruit other family members and family friends as stand-in parents. If you're not able to attend your child's soccer game, perhaps a favorite aunt or uncle could go in your place. It's not the same as having Mom or Dad on the sidelines, but at least your child will have a cheering section.

- Encourage interaction between your child and the care recipient. Activities like reading books, playing games, and taking walks can be stimulating for both generations. They encourage your child and the care recipient to bond with one another—which, in turn, may help your child become more accepting of your caregiving role.

FUN FOR ALL, ALL FOR FUN

Picnics, hikes, baseball games, amusement park excursions—these kinds of activities may seem dispensable in the context of a caregiving situation. In fact, they're more important than ever, because they allow you to interact with your spouse and children outside your caregiving role. Yes, they may require a bit more planning than before, and they might not happen quite as often. When they do, they can make everything else in your family life all the more manageable.

For caregivers, "manageable" is a worthy goal. As Mintz says, "Real family life isn't a TV sitcom, where crises resolve neatly in 30 or 60 minutes and everyone comes away feeling good about themselves and each other. Real family life is hard, and caregiving makes it harder. All you can do is keep plugging away, trying to make it work."

CHAPTER 28

PROTECTING YOUR PRIVATE TIME

What You Need to Know

- To thrive in your caregiving role, you need to incorporate regular breaks into your daily routine. Otherwise, you may run the risk of burning out.

- Your best bet for guaranteeing your downtime is to write it in your personal calendar. This gives it the same priority status as any other important appointment.

- You can open more "windows of opportunity" in your schedule by offloading tasks that use up time and energy without delivering any enjoyment or satisfaction in return. Those you can't delegate you can decline.

- You should never feel guilty about saying no. Taking time for yourself replenishes your mind and body. And that makes you an even better caregiver.

Many people who become caregivers accept the task philosophically: "This person sacrificed so much for me. Now I must sacrifice for her." It's a noble principle, to be sure. But it may not be a healthy one.

Caregiving does require a huge commitment in terms of time, energy, and money. It does *not* require such complete devotion that the caregiver all but forfeits her own life. Yet in all too many cases, that's exactly what happens.

"Even when they know they need it, convincing caregivers to take time for themselves is a challenge. They feel selfish and guilty," says Lois Escobar, M.S.W., a family consultant with the Family Caregiver Alliance in San Francisco. "Over and over, I find myself saying, 'If you don't take care of yourself, if you don't take time for yourself, you'll burn out physically and emotionally. And you won't be able to take care of anyone else.'"

Think 20, 30, 40 years down the road. Would you expect your children to put their lives on hold to look after you? Would you obligate them in that way? Probably not. The person you're caring for feels the same way.

"For more than 20 years, I've taken care of a husband who's disabled by multiple sclerosis," says Suzanne Mintz, cofounder

---

Caregiver's Checklist

What Is Your Caregiving Personality?

How you approach your caregiving role will determine to a large degree how it affects the rest of your life. In the list below, simply place a check mark next to the description that best fits you. The descriptions are adapted from a "continuum of caregiving" scale developed by caregiving expert Judy Bradley.

____ **1.** Supportive: You're concerned about the physical well-being of your loved one. You provide appropriate personal care freely and respectfully, but you maintain an emotional distance as a professional would.

____ **2.** Warmly supportive: You're concerned about the physical as well as the emotional well-being of your loved one. You provide appropriate personal care freely and respectfully, with compassion and love.

____ **3.** Occasionally over-involved: You are warmly supportive of your loved one, but you find yourself taking over certain aspects of the person's life while sacrificing parts of your own.

____ **4.** Often over-involved: You are warmly supportive of your loved one, but you view caregiving as a constant source of chores that you must perform at the expense of your own needs.

____ **5.** Usually/always over-involved: You are warmly supportive of your loved one, but your actions are compromised by a frantic preoccupation

with attending to the person's every conceivable need. As a result, you're devoting all your personal time to providing care—and possibly overriding your loved one's ability to do what she can for herself.

Of the five caregiving styles, #2 is considered healthiest. You're able to maintain a healthy balance between your caregiving role and the rest of your life.

If you chose #1, you're more detached from the situation than most caregivers. You may have some personal issues that are preventing you from connecting emotionally with your loved one. You may want to talk with someone about it—perhaps a counselor or a member of the clergy.

If you chose #3, #4, or #5, you're a candidate for depression, anxiety, and burnout—and the higher your number, the greater your risk. You need to make a conscious effort to set aside more time for yourself, when you can step away from your caregiving role.

and president of the Kensington, Maryland–based National Family Caregivers Association. "Take it from this longtime caregiver: You must carve out time for yourself. It's not a matter of selfishness. It's a matter of personal survival."

THE JOY OF SCHEDULING

If you allow them, your caregiving responsibilities will continue to expand until they take up virtually all your available time. And that may not amount to much to begin with, especially if other family obligations factor into the equation. Perhaps the only way to guarantee much-needed (and much-deserved) breaks in your routine is to write them into your calendar, just as you would any other important appointment.

Blocking out time for yourself might be easier if you think in terms of your loved one's schedule. Most care recipients appreciate structure—not pointless rigidity, but a reasonable flow of daily events anchored by mealtimes and enjoyable activities like a morning walk, an afternoon nap, or an evening TV show. Regular stays in adult day care, or planned visits from relatives and friends, also create a sense of stability and continuity.

Once you've identified those points in the day when you must focus all your attention on your loved one—for example, when she's bathing and dressing, or when she's eating—you can work around them to create breaks for yourself. Through this process, you also can zero in on the times that you could use extra help, and the times that your loved one might be able to manage on her own. Fostering her independence is a crucial aspect of your caregiving role.

Of course, if you're building in appointments with your spouse and children (as suggested in chapter 27), your calendar can fill up rather quickly. That's okay, as long as you honor your appointments with yourself. Explain your intentions to the care recipient, as well as to the rest of your family. Let them know that you're committed to setting aside "face time" for them—and in return, they need to allow "alone time" for you.

For a dedicated caregiver like yourself, the real challenge may lie not in convincing those around you to respect your downtime, but in convincing yourself. Perhaps formalizing your breaks by

Point of View

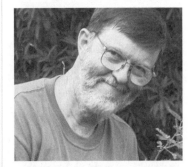

"Unlike my wife, Nancy, I'm not confined to a wheelchair. I have choices. I can get up and go out, and that takes some of the pressure off me. . . . I do need breaks. Nancy understands that, and she's good about giving that to me. And vice versa: I try to provide space for her so she can get away from me. Her physical abilities are very different from mine, but some of her feelings are very much the same."

—GEORGE MAIRS,
Tucson

Point of View

"At first, I didn't want to send Mom to adult day care. I felt guilty—like I had committed to caring for her but wasn't following through. After some adjustment, she liked it. All of us need to socialize with people our own ages, even if they're strangers. At the day care center, Mom can talk about the old days with others who lived then. We get time away from each other, which is good for both of us. And I have a chance to pay bills, go to the doctor, run errands—do all the things that I can't when I'm caring for her."

—MARY CORBETT,
Billings, Montana

writing them in your calendar will earn them the priority status they deserve.

"Scheduling is important in that it enables and encourages you to increase the number of pleasurable activities in your day," observes Dolores Gallagher-Thompson, Ph.D., director of the Older Adult and Family Center at the Veterans Administration Medical Center in Palo Alto, California, and associate professor of psychiatry at Stanford University. "That's an excellent way to prevent burnout."

Take Action... LEARN TO SAY NO

Once you establish a schedule, you must be assertive enough to stick with it. This means setting clear limits on what you're willing and able to do. You may end up having to say no more often than you'd like. This isn't easy for caregivers, who routinely put the needs of others before their own.

If you have trouble saying no, the Oregon Caregiving Resource Center—a program of the Oregon Department of Human Services—offers this advice.

✗ Determine your limits. You can do this by making three lists: one identifying the caregiving and non-caregiving tasks you enjoy; another, those tasks you feel neutral about; and the third, those tasks you complain about—the ones that make you angry, resentful, or depressed. Your goal is to decline or offload as many of the items in the third list as you can.

✗ When making your lists, be honest with yourself. Adding a task to list #1 or #2 when it really belongs in list #3 doesn't serve you or your loved one well. Caregiving can be so time-consuming that some of your day-to-day responsibilities are bound to get under your skin. Perhaps you don't like rushing home from work to pick up your mother at adult day care or to drive your daughter to her piano lessons. These are the sorts of tasks that someone else might be able to handle on your behalf, at least on occasion.

✗ If you're looking to offload certain caregiving tasks in list #3, start by exploring the support services in your community. Public agencies and private organizations offer all kinds of help, often for free or a nominal fee. Gloria Ca-vanaugh, president and chief executive officer of the San Francisco–based American Society on Aging, recommends making just one call—to your Area Agency on Aging, for example. The staff there can direct you to other resources as necessary. (If you haven't completed them already, you may want to use the Caregiver's Checklists on pages 42 and 234 to help track the information you collect.)

✗ Find out whether your church or synagogue can pitch in with the tasks in list #3. Many congregations have their own volunteer support networks. Perhaps someone could chauffeur your loved one to and from her doctor appointments, or do light housekeeping one day a week.

✗ Once you've parceled out what you can to outside resources, review the remaining tasks in list #3 and identify those that you could easily delegate. For example, since so many people drive, you may be able to recruit someone else to pick up your mother at adult day care or to drive your daughter to piano lessons. Carpooling is another option.

✗ Think about whom you want to ask for assistance. You likely will feel more comfortable approaching some people than others. Perhaps one of your friends has issued a standing invitation to call on her whenever you need to. She might be willing to sit with your loved one for a couple of hours once a week, so you can run errands, work out at the gym, window-shop at the mall—whatever you have on your agenda.

✗ When seeking help, be direct about what you need. Dancing around the issue will only add to your frustration, because in all probability, the person you're approaching won't get the message. Members of caregiving families have said that they don't pitch in because they're not asked to do so. The communication lines must be crossing somewhere.

✗ Frame your request with "I" statements. They're clear and easy to understand: "I need help taking Mom for her blood tests on Thursdays. I can manage every other week. I'd really appreciate if you could swing the off-weeks. Could you?"

FOR MORE INFORMATION

Your Area Agency on Aging can help match your caregiving needs with your community's available resources. For a telephone number, look in the blue pages of your phone directory, in the "Guide to Human Services." Or check the Eldercare Locator by calling **(800) 677-1116** or visiting **www.eldercare.gov.** Sponsored by the U.S. Department of Health and Human Services, the Eldercare Locator also provides referrals to support services nationwide.

EXPERT OPINION

"Support is so important. It makes a huge difference. I work hard to take care of myself. I haven't always succeeded, but I have gotten through. I'm okay.

"The biggest complaint among caregivers is lack of personal time. Make some. Your own good health and happiness are gifts to your loved one."

—SUZANNE MINTZ, cofounder and president of the National Family Caregivers Association, based in Kensington, Maryland

Point of View

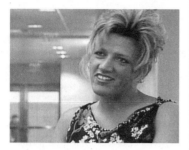

"Sunday and Monday are my days off from work. Having Mondays is wonderful. That's when I schedule doctor appointments, teacher conferences at my daughter's school, everything. The flexibility has been really important to me."

—PAM HADDAD,
Pittsburgh

✗ For the tasks in list #3 that you can't delegate, decide which you must do and which you can set aside. The fact is, some of these tasks may be unavoidable. But you might make them more tolerable by letting go of other tasks that just eat up your time and energy.

✗ When declining tasks, as when seeking help, make your case with "I" statements. Suppose your brother and his family have been coming for Sunday dinner ever since your mother moved into your home, but you just can't handle the preparations anymore. You might broach the subject this way: "I'm sorry, but I'm going to have to stop hosting the Sunday dinners. With taking care of Mom, I just don't have the time or energy to make those big meals. I'd like for you to take over. Would you?"

✗ Provide options that respect your limits. Continuing with the example, let's say your brother replies that he and his wife couldn't possibly serve dinner every Sunday. You might offer a compromise arrangement: "I understand your concerns; those dinners are a lot of work. Still, they're a wonderful family tradition. They mean so much to Mom. If I'd host the dinners two Sundays a month, could you take on the other two?"

✗ Be creative with your solutions. Perhaps neither you nor your sibling can spare several hours a week to cook a multi-course meal for the entire family. That doesn't mean your Sunday get-togethers must fall by the wayside. You might suggest switching to potluck dinners, which would divvy up the cooking among family members. Or you could turn the gatherings into dessert-only affairs.

✗ If you can't reach an agreement, acknowledge your disappointment, but stick to your guns. In the grand scheme of your caregiving situation, those Sunday dinners—which, figuratively speaking, represent any task in list #3—aren't worth sacrificing your physical and emotional health. You've done your best to offer alternatives. Now you need to just let go.

✗ If you find yourself struggling to say no, or to ask for assistance, seek the guidance of a support group. Other group members have been in situations similar to your own. They can help hone the assertiveness skills necessary to stand up for your own interests without feeling selfish or guilty about it.

RECLAIMING YOUR LIFE

By weeding out tasks that waste time and energy and focusing on those that bring joy and satisfaction, you'll shape a caregiving role that complements rather than dominates the rest of your life. You'll notice something else, too: You'll find more opportunities to break away from your daily routine and concentrate on you.

If you need a little practice in the self-indulgence department, that's perfectly understandable. After all, you probably have been concentrating on everyone *but* you. Start slowly, planning one activity at a time, suggests Escobar. If you want to see a movie, choose a showing from the theater listings in your newspaper, then write it in your calendar. If you prefer to get a massage, call to make an appointment. "Choose activities you truly look forward to," she advises. "They can help you deal with everything else."

Even if you can't get away for an hour or two, you should be able to squeeze in shorter timeouts throughout your day. "Everyone can find a half-hour to soak in a bubble bath, curl up with a novel, engage in a hobby, or call an old friend," says Mintz.

Through activities like these, you reengage with life outside your caregiving role. You see how taking time for yourself improves not only your outlook on your situation but also the quality of your care. That might be incentive to do even more just for you.

"I have a friend whose husband is a quadriplegic and needs round-the-clock care," Mintz says. "Once a year, her husband's brother comes to visit. While he's there to provide care, she goes on a long trip with a friend. Even she finds a way to take a break. In caregiving, that's your choice—either you wallow in self-pity or you become proactive about self-care."

So do what you must to protect your private time, whether that means delegating certain tasks or declining them altogether. "It's more than okay," Mintz says. "It's absolutely necessary."

FOR MORE INFORMATION

To find a support group in your area, start by looking in the blue pages of your phone directory, in the "Guide to Human Services." You might also check with the following organizations, which provide referrals to groups among other caregiving support services.

• Children of Aging Parents: **(800) 227-7294; www.caps4caregivers.org**

• Family Caregiver Alliance: **(800) 445-8106; www.caregiver.org**

• National Alliance for Caregiving: **www.caregiving.org**

• National Family Caregivers Association: **(800) 896-3650; www.nfcacares.org**

CHAPTER 29

CARING FOR YOURSELF

What You Need to Know

- Self-care might seem like a luxury to many caregivers. But once they learn to nurture themselves, they find that they're even better prepared—physically and emotionally—to nurture others.

- Managing stress, exercising regularly, eating a well-balanced diet, and getting adequate sleep are all central to a caregiver's well-being. Of these, stress management is the most important, since it has a direct impact on the others.

When people become caregivers, they expect to make compromises. Their health shouldn't be among them. If anything, it deserves even higher priority, as it must withstand the rigors of the caregiving role.

In the absence of adequate self-care, anyone's physical and emotional state can suffer. But caregivers seem especially at risk. According to statistics cited in federal hearings, some 16 percent of caregivers say their health worsened after they took on caregiving responsibilities. And compared with other people of the same age, caregivers are more likely to describe their health as "poor" and significantly less likely to perceive it as "good" or "excellent."

Research has found caregivers with full-time jobs to be especially prone to weight changes, headaches, anxiety, and depression. In fact, the use of prescription drugs for anxiety, depression, and insomnia is two to three times more common among caregivers than in the general population.

Proper self-care could help prevent many of these health problems, or at least reduce their severity. But persuading caregivers to look after their physical and emotional well-being takes work. "They don't respond well when they're told, 'Hey, you have to think about yourself,'" says Gail Hunt, executive director of the National Alliance for Caregiving, based in Bethesda, Maryland. "Typically, they'll say something to the effect of, 'This isn't about me, it's about the care recipient.' The response is natural and universal."

What caregivers must realize, Hunt says, is that if they take the time to nurture themselves, they'll have the physical and emotional stamina to provide care for their loved ones. Of course, finding that time may require some help, but caregivers shouldn't hesitate to tap into their available resources—family members, friends, and community services—for an occasional hand with day-to-day tasks. As Hunt observes, "Caregivers must be advocates not just for their loved ones' needs but also for their own."

Whether you became a caregiver by choice or by circumstance, you have stood by the care recipient out of love and respect for that person. You owe that same love and respect to yourself—and the best way to express it is to look after your own health. You can start by focusing on the four pillars of proper self-care: regular exercise, good nutrition, adequate sleep, and minimal stress. Let's explore stress management first, as it has a direct impact on the rest.

STRESS MANAGEMENT: A MATTER OF PERCEPTION

Most people think of stress as a modern phenomenon, but in fact, it has been around since prehistoric times. Back then, of course, the stressors were quite different. Instead of juggling caregiving responsibilities with family and job obligations, our ancestors were fending off wild beasts for their very survival. Their circumstances gave rise to what experts today call the fight-or-flight response.

When under stress, the human body undergoes a series of changes that prime it to either take on the threat or get out of

Point of View

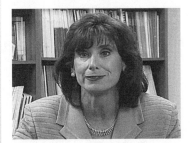

"When I look at my mother's face, I see myself in 30 years. . . . It's the first time I've faced my mortality. It's frightening not only because I'm going to lose my mother, my nurturer, the person who protected and cared for me, but also because I am at risk now. When I see my mother or my father struggling with a disability, I recognize that it could be me."

—RONA BARTLESTONE, L.C.S.W.,
Fort Lauderdale

Point of View

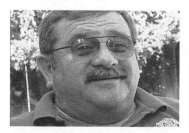

"My nickname is 911. When you become the 911 person, you're on call 24/7. It happens without your even thinking about it. Your whole life revolves around caregiving, around knowing that you have to be available. Your personal life becomes really difficult. . . . You have to find time for yourself some way, somehow."

—CHARLES FIGUEROA,
Santa Barbara, California

harm's way. The brain instructs the adrenal glands to release cortisol and adrenaline (also known as epinephrine), stimulant hormones that increase heart rate, raise blood pressure, contract muscles, and sharpen the senses. In effect, the body goes on alert, ready for whatever action a person chooses to take.

The fight-or-flight response certainly came in handy for our ancestors, who faced life-or-death situations on an almost daily basis. While we, too, must confront our share of life-altering events—divorce, a death in the family, and personal illness are the top three stressors—we're more likely to encounter routine challenges like navigating rush-hour traffic to pick up our loved ones at adult day care, or negotiating with insurance companies to pay outstanding claims. Yet regardless of the trigger, our bodies react the same.

Therein lies the problem. In occasional doses, stress can work to our advantage, helping us perform at our peak. But when it's unrelenting, as it can be for caregivers, it can seriously undermine our health. Basically, the body stays in fight-or-flight mode, with the adrenal glands churning out large amounts of cortisol and adrenaline. The more intense a situation is, the harder the adrenal glands work.

Elevated levels of the stimulant hormones not only tax the cardiovascular system, they also mobilize fat and cholesterol in the bloodstream and increase the stickiness of blood platelets—a combination that can set the stage for heart attack. Beyond the cardiovascular effects, too much cortisol and adrenaline can suppress the immune system. And cortisol, in particular, can disrupt sleep.

While stress does most of its damage at a level we can't see, over time, we feel its presence. Surveys have found that between 70 and 80 percent of doctor visits are stress-related. And doctors have observed that people under stress show measurable increases in heart rate, blood pressure, and respiratory rate—all signs of the fight-or-flight response in action.

What we need to remember about this response, and about stress in general, is that it's triggered not by a given situation but by our *perception* of a situation. Just as important, by employing proper coping skills, we can block or disrupt the biochemical chain of events that leads to physical harm.

Support Is the Best Medicine

Studies involving caregivers have established a correlation between the ability to cope and the perceived physical, emotional, and financial toll of providing care—what some experts call the caregiver burden. So which coping mechanisms are effective? One study found that "constructing a larger sense of the illness" by trying to understand it at some level, and by praying for strength to keep going, helps relieve stress. Caregivers also seem to manage better when they remind themselves that their loved ones will inevitably experience some physical decline as they age.

Not surprisingly, the perceived caregiver burden diminishes in the presence of family support—specifically, frequent visits from family members—and a strong social network. But persuading caregivers to reach out to others can be as difficult as convincing them to look after themselves. "A lot of caregivers don't acknowledge their need for assistance," says Edward M. Hallowell, M.D., instructor in psychiatry at Harvard Medical School and author of several books on the health benefits of personal relationships, including *Human Moments: How to Find Meaning and Love in Your Everyday Life.* "The term for their behavior is *counterde-*

Caregiver's
Checklist

Is Stress Getting the Best of You?

The National Alliance for Caregiving has identified the following as warning signs of stress overload. They're your cue to sharpen your coping skills—and to seek your doctor's care, if necessary.

☐ Reduced attention span and concentration

☐ Unusual or frequent memory lapses

☐ Impaired thinking and information processing

☐ Constant irritability or dulled emotions

☐ Physical aches and pains

☐ Irregular heartbeat

☐ Unusual or excessive perspiration

☐ Skin rashes

☐ Stomach problems

☐ Difficulty sleeping

☐ Withdrawal from regular activities

☐ Diminished performance or interest at work or home

For many caregivers, support groups are an invaluable source of information and comfort. But you must find one that fits your personality, lifestyle, and schedule. Many medical centers, churches, senior centers, and condition-specific organizations sponsor "live" groups. If you're not comfortable with in-person participation, or you don't have time for it, you may prefer an online group instead. Here are a few leads to start your search.

• The Family Caregiver Alliance conducts a regular online support group on its Web site, **www.caregivers.org**.

• If you're caring for an older loved one, you may want to check out the Senior Caregiver Support Group at **www.seniorcaregiversupport.com**. In addition to online support, this organization offers caregiver counseling, training, and more.

• A growing number of condition-specific organizations are reaching out to caregivers in need of support. Two that offer message boards on their Web sites are the Alzheimer's Association (**www.alz.org**) and the American Cancer Society (**www.cancer.org**).

pendent. In other words, they don't want to be taken care of, because they view it as a sign of weakness."

Unfortunately, when caregivers don't accept help, they're more likely to burn out or—even worse—to resort to unhealthy coping techniques like smoking or excessive drinking, Dr. Hallowell explains. What's more, as the perceived caregiver burden increases, so does the probability of placing a loved one in a residential care facility.

"For caregivers, the first step is to acknowledge that the need for assistance exists," Dr. Hallowell says. "From there, it's a matter of realizing that accepting help is nothing to be ashamed of. Once caregivers do that, they're ready to build their own support structures tailored to their unique situations."

In your particular case, if family members or close friends have said they're willing to pitch in with the caregiving load, take them up on their offer by identifying specific tasks they can handle. Perhaps one of them could stay with your loved one an afternoon or two every week, so you get a break. Someone else could run errands, or take on a few household chores. If a person wants to help but is too busy or too far away to provide hands-on support, maybe he'd be willing to contribute financially to your loved one's care. And don't overlook the many caregiving resources available in your community.

By reaching out to others, you are better able to deal with the demands of caregiving—and in the process, you fend off the sense of isolation that maddens and frustrates many caregivers. "They may not get any recognition for their efforts, but that's only part of the problem," Hunt says. "Often they just feel alone, not knowing where to turn for information and advice."

But if caregivers play their cards right, their circumstances actually might bring them closer to the people around them. The caveat is, they must be willing to make the first move. "Especially if you're feeling angry or upset with other family members, now is the time to do something about it," Dr. Hallowell says. "You can use humor or adopt a low-key approach—whatever suits the situation. The key is to connect openly and honestly with the other person. You owe it to yourself as a caregiver and to the loved one in your care. You will feel better and stronger for it."

Take Action... HONE YOUR COPING SKILLS

Of course, for those caregivers accustomed to doing everything on their own, the very act of opening up to others and requesting assistance from them can be stressful in itself. The following strategies—developed with input from physicians, scientists, and the National Family Caregivers Association—can defuse stress and thwart the fight-or-flight response, regardless of the trigger.

✗ Engage in any activity that enables you to escape the stressful situation by shifting your focus inward. "Your goal is to achieve deep relaxation," explains Karen Koffler, M.D., director of integrative medicine at Evanston Northwestern Health Care in suburban Chicago. "I compare it to the feeling you have when you're just coming out of a sleep state but you're not completely awake. Once you experience deep relaxation, you'll know which activities can get you there and which cannot." Experiment by taking a walk, soaking in a comfortably warm bath, or getting a massage— all of which can bring about the desired effect.

✗ Practice deep breathing for on-the-spot stress relief. Dr. Koffler recommends a simple technique she learned from Andrew Weil, M.D., director of the program in integrative medicine and clinical professor of medicine at the University of Arizona College of Medicine in Tucson. Called four-square, it involves inhaling for a count of four, holding for a count of four, exhaling for a count of four, then holding again for a count of four. Repeat three times, and you should notice a difference in your stress level. As Dr. Koffler explains, "This breathing technique creates space for a brief respite, which can alter your perception of a situation." Remember, it's your perception of a situation, not the situation itself, that leads to stress and the fight-or-flight response.

✗ Schedule "worry time." William T. Riley, Ph.D., senior researcher for Personal Improvement Computer Systems, a Reston, Virginia–based company that specializes in self-improvement programs, recommends setting aside a half-hour each day just for worrying. Then as issues arise, you can mentally defer them, knowing that you can dwell on

---

FOR MORE INFORMATION

Left unchecked, chronic stress can contribute to depression, a common condition among caregivers. In fact, it affects some 46 percent of those who seek professional help for caregiving-related problems. To learn more about symptoms and treatment, contact one of the following organizations.

• National Foundation for Depressive Illness: **(800) 239-1265**

• National Mental Health Association: **(800) 969-6642**

• National Institute of Mental Health: **(301) 443-4513**

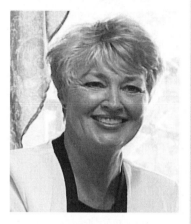

Point of View

"You have to take one day at a time—sometimes not even a day but a minute at a time. Stop and take a deep breath; try to put yourself in the care recipient's place. After all, one day all of us will be in that same place."

—LORAYE BACKER,
Montevideo, Minnesota

them later on. Dr. Riley theorizes that by concentrating your concerns in this way, you simply exhaust yourself thinking about them. Mentally, you're ready to move on.

✗ Put your thoughts into words. Some researchers and psychotherapists suggest that talking with a family member or close friend about a stressful situation can help alleviate any tension and anxiety you're experiencing. If you're not comfortable opening up to someone else, try writing in a journal instead.

✗ If your loved one requires care because of a specific health problem, educate yourself about it. Knowledge is empowering; when you're informed, you discover options and opportunities for dealing with a situation that otherwise might seem beyond your control.

✗ Organize the rest of your life as much as you can. This helps minimize the sort of everyday chaos that keeps the fight-or-flight response simmering below the surface. Just try not to be too rigid with your routine. It only adds to your stress, especially when something unexpected happens. In caregiving, "unexpected" is the norm.

✗ Know your limits. As a caregiver, you're more than willing to lend a hand when someone else needs it. But you have only so much time and energy to go around. You can conserve these resources by offloading some tasks and saying no to others. (For guidance on which tasks to keep and which to let go, see chapter 28.)

EXERCISE: BENEFITS FOR MIND AND BODY

In the midst of a stressful situation—at any point in a caregiving relationship, for that matter—working out can quickly sink to the bottom of your to-do list, if it's there at all. Yet physical activity is more important now than ever. It not only offsets the effects of the fight-or-flight response, it also appears to minimize symptoms of depression, which occurs in greater proportion among caregivers than in the general population. In short, exercise is just as good for your mind as for your body.

The scientific evidence linking regular physical activity with better health and longer life continues to grow. For example, the landmark Framingham Heart Study found that walking for an hour every day, or engaging in other forms of exercise to burn an extra 2,000 calories a week, can extend life span by 2 years. And the 1996 Surgeon General's Report on Physical Activity and Health made a case for the positive effects of exercise on practically every organ and system in the body.

Most people think of physical activity in connection with weight loss. But it does so much more. Besides trimming body fat, it reduces the risk of certain cancers, protects against type 2 (adult-onset) diabetes, lowers blood pressure and cholesterol, slows bone loss, sharpens memory, and enhances sleep, digestion, and sexual function. With benefits like these, exercise is almost too good for anyone to pass up.

Yet a lot of people do. Government statistics indicate that one-quarter of the American population, and one-third of those age 50 and older, are completely sedentary. What's more, 60 percent of our nation's adults don't get even the minimum recommended amount of exercise—30 minutes of moderate physical activity most days, and ideally every day, of the week.

Heart and Sole

Scientists once believed that people had to exercise at 70 to 80 percent of their maximum heart rate to experience health benefits like weight loss and heart disease prevention. But the latest research suggests that staying between 50 to 60 percent is just as effective.

To calculate your maximum heart rate, subtract your age from 220. Then multiply that figure by 0.5 and 0.6 to determine your workout range. As an example, a 45-year-old woman has a maximum heart rate of 175 beats per minute (220 − 45 = 175), with a workout range of 87 to 105 beats per minute (175 x 0.5 = 87.5; 175 x 0.6 = 105).

To monitor your heart rate while you're exercising, periodically take your pulse (with your index and middle finger on your wrist) for 10 seconds. Then multiply the count by 6.

You can also keep tabs on your intensity level through what's known as rate of perceived exertion. In fact, many exercise scientists favor this measure over heart rate. To check your rate of perceived exertion, all you need to do is rank the intensity of your workout on a scale of 1 (easy) to 10 (difficult). If you're just starting an exercise program, you should aim for an intensity of 5. At this level, you should be able to carry on a conversation while you're working out without getting winded.

Caregivers should meet this standard, too. "But we know they aren't exercising enough," Hunt says.

In today's world, carving 30 minutes out of a day's schedule for exercise can be a tall order for anyone, especially for caregivers. The good news is, you may not need to do all 30 minutes at once. A growing number of scientists believe that engaging in physical activity in small increments throughout the day can produce big changes in body composition (more muscle, less fat) and chemistry (less cholesterol, more mood-enhancing brain chemicals).

The evidence has proven so pervasive that in 1998, the American College of Sports Medicine modified its recommendation for 30 minutes of exercise a day to include three 10-minute sessions. More recent research indicates that even six 5-minute sessions can change a person's health for the better.

If these short bouts of physical activity still seem like more than you can manage, perhaps you should take a closer look at your daily routine. That's standard procedure for clients of Andrea Dunn and her colleagues at the Cooper Institute in Dallas. "We get people thinking about how they spend their days by asking them to complete a personal time study for 2 weekdays and 1 weekend," explains Dunn, a senior exercise researcher. "Usually, people are shocked at how much they sit—up to 14 hours a day. Everyone can find ways to sit less."

Take Action... MAKE MOVEMENT PART OF YOUR DAY

Remember that "exercise" doesn't necessarily mean a formal fitness program. Anything that involves moving your body counts toward your 30 minutes a day. You could try conventional activities like walking, running, cycling, or swimming. Or you could look for opportunities to add movement to your daily routine. For example, researchers have found that climbing stairs for 15 minutes a day (in 2½-minute sessions) can significantly improve health. So if you have a choice between riding an elevator and taking the stairs, opt for the latter.

By finding ways to be active in everyday life, you'll easily accumulate your 30 minutes of exercise—and then some. Be creative, and have fun! These ideas can get you moving.

✗ Take your dog for a walk. After all, he needs exercise, too—and he's likely to keep you moving at a brisk pace. If you don't have a canine companion of your own, perhaps you could borrow a neighbor's for a quick trip around the block. You might also consider volunteering as a dog-walker at your local animal shelter.

✗ When you drive somewhere, park as far as you can from your destination. The extra steps add up over time.

✗ On trips to the mall or the supermarket, take a nonstop lap around the inside before you start shopping. You can use the time to collect your thoughts and scan your choices.

✗ Every week, identify one errand that you can do on foot or by bicycle rather than by car. You cross an item off your to-do list and squeeze in a short bout of exercise to boot.

✗ Divvy up household chores so that you're doing one or two each day. You might find them more bearable if you think of them as workouts rather than as just plain work.

✗ Putter in your garden whenever you get a chance. Studies have found gardening to be therapeutic for mind and body.

✗ When taking a break from your caregiving role to be with family or friends, suggest active alternatives to dining out and other sedentary pastimes. For example, you could go to a community dance, or tour a museum, or stroll through a local park.

✗ If you have young children, make play dates with them. A rousing game of tag, hide-and-seek, or Frisbee gets you moving and lets you spend quality time with your kids.

✗ On your next visit to the video store, check out the offerings in the fitness section. Videos allow you to work out in the privacy of your own home, and they just might tempt you to try a new activity like yoga or tai chi. When you find a tape that piques your interest, commit to working out to it before the return date.

Point of View

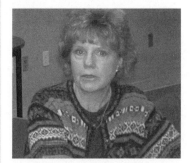

"If you can take a 10-minute walk—just a timeout—it makes a world of difference. The day care my husband is going to literally saved my life. That may sound overly dramatic, but it's true. Just getting away from caregiving for a few hours a day saved my life."

—MARY ANN NATION,
Franklin, Ohio

Don't Forget to S-t-r-e-t-c-h

As you increase your activity level throughout the day, you might want to make a point of incorporating some stretching into your routine. It not only relaxes your mind and body but also primes your muscles for the physical demands of providing care.

For example, stretching can help minimize the risk of lower back pain, a common complaint among caregivers. According to David Upton, spokesperson for the American Council on Exercise, some 80 percent of all American adults experience lower back pain sometime in their lives. Often it results not from a structural problem, such as a slipped disk, but from a combination of tight hamstrings (located at the backs of the thighs), tight hip flexors, and weak abdominals. Stretching these muscles regularly can help preserve their flexibility and protect against injury.

If you want to learn proper stretching technique, your best bet is to schedule at least one session with a personal trainer or a physical therapist. Either professional can identify areas of tension or weakness and recommend exercises that target the affected muscles.

For now, you can get a taste of stretching's benefits by trying this modified yoga pose, which you can perform on the floor or on a firm mattress. You should feel a good stretch in your neck, lower back, and hips.

1. Lie on your back with your knees bent and your feet flat on the ground. Move your arms into a T position, with your palms facing up.

2. Let your hips and knees gently fall to one side. Turn your head so that it's facing the opposite side. If your knees don't touch the floor at first, don't worry; that may take time. You may notice a mild pulling sensation in your lower back, which is normal. But if you feel pain, stop.

3. Hold for 15 seconds to start, then return to the starting position. You can work toward 20 to 30 seconds over time.

4. Repeat steps 2 and 3, this time changing the direction of your hips, knees, and head.

You also can take quick stretch breaks throughout the day, whenever you need to relax and recharge your batteries. The following

---

FOR MORE INFORMATION

If you need help finding a qualified personal trainer or physical therapist in your area, try contacting either of the following organizations.

• American Council on Exercise, 4851 Paramount Drive, San Diego, CA 92123. Phone: **(800) 825-3636**; Internet address: **www.acefitness.org**.

• American Physical Therapy Association, 111 North Fairfax Street, Alexandria, VA 22314. Phone: **(800) 999-2782**; Internet address: **www.apta.org**.

exercise is especially good for relieving tension in your shoulders, chest, and abdominal muscles.

1. Stand in a doorway. Place your hands on either side of the door at about shoulder height, with your palms facing forward.

2. Slowly lean your upper body forward until you feel a comfortable stretch in your arms and chest. Keep your head and chest up, and your knees slightly bent.

3. Hold for 15 to 20 seconds before returning to the starting position.

At least one study suggests that the longer you're able to hold a stretch, the more it will improve flexibility and range of motion—important for preventing injury. Still, you need to be careful not to overdo, especially if you're new to stretching. If you feel any pain, stop right away.

The Benefits of Strength Training

If fitness experts had to name one activity that provides the greatest return on investment, chances are good that a majority would choose strength training. It may demand a bigger time commitment than other forms of exercise, and it usually involves some out-of-pocket expenses for equipment and/or training. But the payoff is better health, physically and emotionally.

Various studies have shown strength training to be helpful for lowering blood pressure, controlling blood sugar (a risk factor for diabetes), and easing depression. Of course, it's considered an important component of any weight-loss plan. Researchers at Tufts University found that women who engaged in strength training shed 44 percent more body fat than women who didn't, even though all of them were following the same diet. This is partly because muscle burns more calories than fat, even at rest.

For caregivers, in particular, strength training can build the necessary muscle to perform physically challenging tasks like helping a loved one out of a chair. If you're thinking, "I don't have the time or money to go to a gym!" you may not need to anyway. Many personal trainers say you can get a good workout at home, using dumbbells and resistance bands.

Ideally, you should receive instruction from a certified personal trainer when you're just starting out, so you learn proper lifting technique and avoid injury. A good trainer can customize a workout to your needs and lifestyle. And it may not take as much time as you think: Some experts say lifting for just 20 minutes two or three times a week produces good results.

NUTRITION: YOU ARE WHAT YOU EAT

Like exercising regularly, eating healthfully is beneficial for both mind and body. The right foods in the right amounts deliver a wealth of key nutrients that help protect against potentially debilitating conditions like heart disease, cancer, diabetes, and osteoporosis. Equally important for caregivers, some of these nutrients are converted to fuel that replenishes the body's energy supply, while others are used in the manufacture of brain chemicals that enhance mood and mental performance.

But maintaining sound dietary habits often is a struggle for caregivers, who may make unhealthy food choices or skip meals altogether because they're so pressed for time. Unfortunately, good nutrition falls by the wayside precisely when it's needed most. Research has shown that chronic stress can deplete the body's supply of essential vitamins and minerals. On the other hand, certain nutrients—like beta-carotene and vitamins C and E—help repair the physical damage caused by the fight-or-flight response.

Take Action... STICK WITH THE FUNDAMENTALS

For a basic primer on eating nutritiously, you can look to the USDA's Food Guide Pyramid, which appears on the labels of many packaged foods. Following the pyramid's recommendations helps control calorie and fat intake—important for maintaining proper weight—while delivering the mix of nutrients necessary for good health.

Because the Food Guide Pyramid applies to the population as a whole, it usually needs some tweaking to match the nutrition needs of specific demographic groups. For caregivers, experts advise paying special attention to the following:

X Aim for at least five servings of fruits and vegetables every day. This is consistent with the pyramid's recommendations, but it's worth emphasizing because most of us come up short in the produce department. And that's not good, considering that fruits and veggies contain an abundance of antioxidants, nutrients that offset the physical effects of stress. To get more servings, buy precut produce at the supermarket and store it in resealable plastic bags for on-the-go snacks.

✗ Increase your fiber intake to between 25 and 35 grams per day. Fiber supports healthy function of the digestive system, which can suffer under stress. As a bonus, it may bind with cholesterol and help escort it out of the body. Fruits and vegetables contain some fiber, but the best sources are whole grains and beans. Just read labels carefully: A bread that's described as "wheat," for example, may not be whole grain.

✗ Eat two servings of fish per week—not just any fish, but a species rich in omega-3 fatty acids, such as salmon, mackerel, or sardines. Omega-3's are good fats that appear to not only boost levels of HDL cholesterol (the heart-healthy kind) but also combat emotional distress.

✗ As much as possible, steer clear of foods made with white flour and/or white sugar. Both are common ingredients in cookies, crackers, and other processed foods. Occasional munching on these manufactured snacks won't do any harm. But when they become a steady diet, they can widen your waistline and sap your energy reserves.

✗ Make time for breakfast. The brain and body need food first thing in the morning to replenish blood sugar levels depleted during the night. What's more, the right combination of foods can deliver an energy boost that just might last for hours. That means eating a mix of complex carbohydrates and protein, with just a bit of fat. A high-fiber, low-sugar cereal with nonfat milk would do, as would a whole-grain bagel topped with peanut butter.

✗ Enjoy nutritious snacks at regular intervals. Snacking prevents the dips in blood sugar that can bring on feelings of fatigue—and in the process, it discourages the overeating that's common during periods of stress. Stock your kitchen with containers of yogurt, mini-boxes of raisins, microwave popcorn, and sliced cheese and crackers so you can reach for something healthful when you're ready to nibble.

✗ Drink at least eight 8-ounce glasses of water a day. It may seem like a lot, but your body needs every last drop to stay properly hydrated. Without enough fluids, you might notice your energy level beginning to flag. Your ability to think and concentrate could be affected as well.

Take Action... SIMPLIFY MEALTIMES

For nutrition-conscious caregivers, perhaps the real concern is not what to eat but how to squeeze meal preparation into an already hectic schedule. After a day of juggling caregiving responsibilities, family obligations, and job demands, anyone would be tempted to head for the nearest fast-food drive-thru or call for Chinese takeout.

But making healthful meals needn't be complicated or time-consuming. It just requires a bit of creativity and advance planning on your part. These tips can help.

X Set aside a few hours each weekend to cook for the week ahead. That might seem like a significant commitment up-front, but it can save time and hassle in the long run. Entrées and soups can be stored in the freezer, then defrosted and reheated in the microwave. Pair each entrée with a side dish or two, each soup with a salad or sandwich, and you have a week's worth of complete meals.

X For those occasions when you can't cook ahead, fill your freezer with frozen vegetables. Dietitians say that in most cases, frozen veggies are nutritionally comparable to fresh. They thaw quickly and can be added directly to boiling pasta or stir-fries.

X Be inventive with leftovers. For example, rather than just reheating last night's ham or chicken, you can use it as an ingredient in a salad or as filling for a pita or wrap. Baked potatoes can be mashed; mashed potatoes can become potato pancakes.

X Once in a while, let the oven and microwave rest. Some people get very attached to the idea that a meal isn't a meal unless it's hot. But a sandwich-and-salad combination, or a fresh fruit plate, is perfectly healthful and satisfying. And nothing could be simpler to prepare—especially if you buy precut salad greens or fruit at the supermarket, or you cut your own ahead of time.

✗ Get a jump start on breakfast by doing the prep work the night before. Pour your cereal into a bowl and clean the berries to top it. If you're having oatmeal, cook it and store it in the refrigerator for a quick reheating in the morning. And put your toast, English muffin, or bagel in the toaster, so all you need to do is push the button.

SLEEP: REST FOR THE WEARY

While good nutrition can be a potent energizer, it can't possibly take the place of deep, restful slumber. These days, though, few people get as much shut-eye as they should. Caregivers, in particular, tend to shortchange themselves. The more they have on their plates, the more they stretch their days to accommodate the extra work. Sometimes they just can't sleep—a byproduct of the stress they're experiencing.

Perhaps you're willing to tolerate a little daytime fatigue. But the effects of inadequate rest extend far beyond that. In one revealing study, University of Chicago researchers were able to link chronic sleep deprivation—averaging less than 7 hours per night—with increases in the stress hormone cortisol and decreases in human growth hormone, which is vital to tissue growth and repair. After just 2 weeks, the study participants—all men in their twenties—had levels of the two hormones that matched those of men who are decades older.

Another study focusing specifically on people caring for cancer patients found lost sleep to be a factor in raising the caregivers' risk of depression. It also impairs memory and motor skills, which can affect a caregiver's ability to perform certain tasks.

Take Action... TAKE A NAP

As a general rule, sleep experts recommend aiming for 8 hours of shut-eye a night. Some people might do fine with a little less; others may need more. Your body will tell you how much is enough.

FOR MORE INFORMATION

The National Sleep Foundation has a number of publications with information and advice on getting a good night's sleep. To find out what's available, call **(202) 347-3471** or visit **www.sleepfoundation.org**.

Keep in mind, too, that a nap can help satisfy your body's sleep requirement. But it must be done right. Some guidelines:

✗ Limit your nap time. Ten to 20 minutes is considered sufficient to reduce physical and mental fatigue. Snoozing longer than that during the day could disrupt your body's sleep/wake cycle, setting the stage for a sleepless night.

✗ Avoid napping too close to bedtime. Dozing off in the early evening—say, right after dinner—could keep you awake at night. Plan your nap for the afternoon instead. In fact, research has pinpointed 3:00 P.M. as our sleepiest daytime hour.

✗ Use trial and error to determine when and how long you should sleep. You want to wake up from your nap feeling refreshed, not groggy. If even 20 minutes of shut-eye isn't enough, your nighttime sleep habits may need some tweaking. (For tips on getting a good night's sleep, see chapter 13.)

✗ If napping doesn't come naturally, skip it. Trying to force yourself to sleep only adds to your stress. Let your body be your guide.

CHAPTER 30

WORKING 9 TO 5, CARING 'ROUND THE CLOCK

What You Need to Know

- **The Family and Medical Leave Act of 1993 allows employees to take up to 12 weeks of unpaid leave a year to care for a sick family member, including a spouse or an elderly parent.**

- **Many companies offer other caregiving benefits that employees may not be aware of, including referral services, flextime policies, and on-site support groups.**

- **The number of companies offering caregiving benefits grew rapidly in the 1990s and is expected to increase even more dramatically through the first decade of the 21st century.**

- **Supervisors may be willing to bend to accommodate working caregivers. But informing your boss of your circumstances is absolutely essential.**

Balancing personal obligations with professional responsibilities is among the most challenging tasks that working caregivers face. At times, it may feel like an impossible one, as those who have felt forced to choose between family and career will attest.

Companies vary widely in their caregiving policies and practices. Some allow up to a year of unpaid leave to care for aging or ill loved ones; others implicitly discourage even a few hours off to handle unforeseen caregiving crises. Many fall somewhere in between: They're supportive of the caregivers on their payrolls, but they don't offer many benefits or resources to ease the workers' load.

Incidentally, a company's size has little bearing on its caregiving philosophy. Large firms can be extremely flexible and progressive, or rigid and bureaucratic. Small businesses may take pride in their ability to accommodate unexpected changes in caregivers' work schedules, or they may balk at the need to find someone who can take over key functions in a caregiver's absence.

Of course, regardless of your employer's official stance, your relationship with your supervisor may have an even greater impact on your approach to handling caregiving tasks while on the job. Some bosses are naturally empathic; they understand that when an employee is overwhelmed with responsibilities but has little leeway to deal with them, her productivity declines—sometimes significantly so. What's more, some bosses are caregivers themselves. They know all too well that situations arise over which an employee has no control. Perhaps their own supervisors treated them kindly—or harshly, as the case may be—and they've learned from their experiences.

Even in the most trying workplace environment, you can take steps to improve your circumstances. Most important is adapting coping mechanisms to maintain your equilibrium. Otherwise, stress could get the best of you—and both your caregiving role and your job performance will suffer.

Another essential step is to read your employment manual, paying special attention to the sections on personal and vacation days, family leave, and anything else that may be relevant to your caregiving situation. Get to know your legal rights, too: Though limited, existing federal law requires employers to make certain accommodations for caregivers. (We'll explore this government mandate a bit later in the chapter.)

CAREGIVING'S IMPACT ON THE WORKPLACE

When you think about it, employees who care for aging or ill loved ones face many of the same issues as their colleagues who have young children. Yet for the most part, employers have been much more aggressive about instituting child care benefits, ranging from pretax day care spending accounts to on-site day care facilities. These companies recognize the financial and logistical advantages of supporting employees who must juggle parental and professional claims on their time and energy.

But according to a study published in the *Academy of Man-*

FOR MORE INFORMATION

The Family Caregiver Alliance provides support for people coping with the dual demands of work and caregiving. You can contact the organization at **(800) 445-8106** or visit the Web site at **www.caregiver.org**.

agement Journal, eldercare demands may undermine workplace performance even more so than child care responsibilities. Employees who care for aging or ill loved ones are at greater risk for anxiety, depression, and physical illness, especially if they feel unable to discuss their situations with their colleagues.

In light of such findings, you might imagine that employers would be as forward-thinking about eldercare as they have been about child care. Unfortunately, that hasn't been the case. In a survey conducted by the consulting firm Hewitt Associates, 47 percent of big employers offered some form of eldercare benefits in 1999. While that's an improvement over the 20 percent tallied 6 years earlier, it lags far behind the 90 percent providing child care benefits in 1999.

While companies have been slow to recognize and address the eldercare issue, experts predict a sea change similar to the one that precipitated the child care "movement" of the 1980s and 1990s. As the U.S. population ages, more and more workers will be taking on caregiving roles. For their employers, the financial impact could be tremendous.

In fact, a 1997 study cosponsored by the Metropolitan Life Insurance Company—widely acknowledged as one of the most comprehensive studies on eldercare costs to businesses—came up with an estimated price tag for caregiving of $29 billion a year. When researchers recalculated their numbers using only data from employees who provide extensive care—defined as helping with at least two activities of daily living (such as bathing and feeding) and at least four instrumental activities of daily living (such as shopping, finances, preparing meals, and transportation)—the costs remained at $11.5 billion a year.

Interestingly, almost $5 billion of this amount went toward replacing employees who left their jobs because of their caregiving responsibilities. The $5 billion reflects the costs of recruiting and training workers, as well as the losses associated with the learning curve of the new hires.

Among the study's other findings was that 10.5 percent of working caregivers missed at least 3 days of work in the prior 6 months for reasons tied to their caregiving situations. The total cost to their employers: $398 million. Businesses suffered even more when employees came in late, dashed out for an hour, or

EXPERT OPINION

"In today's world, employers are competing to identify, recruit, hire, and retain qualified talent. And the talent pool is shrinking more and more. The smart company is going to look at the individual as a whole person and address all of that person's needs, whether they're professional or personal. . . . The end result is that the company will have happy, productive, long-term employees."

—**BRIAN CLOYD,** director of North American human resources at Steelcase, Inc., in Grand Rapids, Michigan

EXPERT OPINION

"The employer's attitude makes a huge difference in how well people juggle work and caregiving. If employees feel understood and cared for, they're very appreciative and very committed to maintaining their productivity. But many people are afraid to bring up [caregiving] issues. They're afraid their employers will get mad at them for receiving too many phone calls or taking too much work time to coordinate services. And while employers can be very sympathetic in times of acute illness, they may not be so understanding about Alzheimer's or Parkinson's or another illness that can last for years and years.

"You have to help your employer understand that some aspects of your situation are within your control, and some are not. Those things beyond your control don't make you a bad employee."

—DONNA SCHEMPP, L.C.S.W., clinical supervisor at Family Caregiver Alliance in San Francisco

left early. About one-fifth of these people couldn't make up the time, costing their employers another $488 million.

Even the occasional phone call and similar workday interruptions to handle caregiving tasks add up to about an hour a week for each working caregiver, which translates to about $3.8 billion a year for businesses. And $805 million a year is the price tag for the number of hours supervisors spend dealing with the fallout of their employees' caregiving crises.

Subsequent research appears to confirm the Metropolitan Life study's bottom line: Caregiving costs employers, and the national economy, dearly. And the financial burden will continue to grow as more people need care and more working caregivers provide it.

WHAT EMPLOYERS CAN DO

Even when companies understand caregiving's financial implications, often they feel stymied in their search for an appropriate response. They have plenty of options. Consider the kinds of benefits already offered by some employers, either on their own or as members of a consortium or industry group.

- Resources and referrals for employees who need medical or legal advice, or other caregiving information—by far the most common caregiving benefit

- On-site support groups, seminars, and caregiver fairs

- An in-house social service professional who can assess a caregiving situation and provide case management if necessary

- Flexible spending accounts, which allow employees to set aside pre-tax income for dependent care

- Long-term care insurance for employees and their immediate family members, including parents

- Reimbursement or subsidies for skilled nursing care and other home care services

- Leaves of absence and flexible work schedules

- Transportation services for care recipients

- On-site adult day care—probably the least common caregiving benefit

At the very least, many—though not all—employers must comply with the provisions of the Family and Medical Leave Act of 1993, signed into law during the Clinton Administration. Also known as FMLA, it allows employees to take 12 weeks of unpaid leave per year if they themselves are sick or if they need to care for an infant, a newly adopted child, or an immediate family member—including a parent—who is seriously ill. Companies must continue to provide health insurance while employees are on leave; when they return to work, they're guaranteed either the same job or another position with equal status, salary, and benefits.

The provisions of the FMLA are not without conditions. For example, while the law applies to all public agencies, private businesses with fewer than 50 employees are exempt. In addition, employees must have worked for a company for at least a year, putting in at least 1,250 hours in the previous 12 months, to qualify for leave. Those employees who are caring for sick rela-

Businesses That Care about Caregivers

In recent years, some employers have made real strides in providing innovative caregiving benefits for their employees. A few current examples:

• Fannie Mae, which has a long-standing reputation for being sensitive to family matters, contracted with a local social service agency to provide a full-time in-house eldercare case manager. Employees can ask the case manager to assess an elderly loved one's physical and mental health. Based on her evaluation, the case manager recommends a plan for the person's care and identifies public and private resources to help carry out the plan. The case manager also offers advice on common caregiving issues like evaluating adult day care centers, finding quality in-home care, and holding family meetings.

• AT&T introduced a liberal policy on unpaid leave to accommodate working caregivers. The program allows employees to take off a full year during any 2-year period to care for elderly or ill loved ones. Employees continue to receive complete medical benefits for the first 6 months of their leave. The company also offers access to a referral service that helps locate caregiving resources and information.

• In 1995, several businesses in the San Francisco Bay Area launched a program that provides emergency in-home care for both children and the elderly. An agency contracted by the consortium of companies is on call around-the-clock to provide care on short notice, should employees experience an unexpected schedule change or a conflict between personal obligations and professional responsibilities. In many cases, the companies cover part or all of the fees for this service.

FOR MORE INFORMATION

If you have questions about the provisions of the Family and Medical Leave Act, or if you wish to file a complaint against an employer that isn't complying with the law, you can contact the U.S. Department of Labor. The local offices are listed in the blue pages of the telephone directory, under "United States Government."

FOR MORE INFORMATION

If you have Internet access, you can print the text of the Family and Medical Leave Act of 1999 directly from the Web site for the U.S. Department of Labor. Go to **www.dol.gov/dol/ esa/fmla.htm** and click on "The Family and Medical Leave Act." You also can request a copy of the law by calling **(866) 4-USA-DOL.**

tives may opt to schedule their leave in chunks, or to work fewer hours each week, instead of taking their 12 weeks all at once.

Companies that fail to conform to the FMLA guidelines can face legal action. The U.S. Department of Labor is responsible for investigating complaints about violations; if necessary, it can file papers in court to force a company into compliance. Similarly, a private citizen could seek damages against a recalcitrant employer through a civil suit.

Take Action... DISCUSS YOUR NEEDS WITH YOUR SUPERVISOR

If your employer falls under FMLA jurisdiction, just knowing that you have the law behind you might make your caregiving situation a little bit easier. Still, many people feel uncomfortable even mentioning their caregiving responsibilities at work—not just because the issue is so personal, but also because it could draw mixed reactions from supervisors and colleagues alike.

While some coworkers may resent what they perceive as "special" treatment, many others will sympathize with your situation—and may even offer their assistance. Your supervisor, in particular, can help navigate occupational red tape to secure the necessary time and resources on your behalf. But he needs to know what's going on, especially if your caregiving role begins to affect your job performance.

When you're ready to approach your boss, use these tips to help make the conversation go smoothly.

✗ First, learn your rights as an employee. This was mentioned before, but it bears repeating. The fact is, many people have never read their companies' employment manuals and are not familiar with their entitlements and obligations. If your company has a human resources department, someone there should be able to provide the information you need and answer any questions you have. Remember, too, that if your company employs at least 50 people, it must comply with the FMLA. Get a copy of the law and read through it as well.

✗ If you belong to a union, find out if your contract makes any provisions for caregiving benefits. In addition, ask your union representative whether other employees of the same company have been in situations similar to yours, so you can refer to those cases as precedents. If you don't belong to a union, you might want to research the caregiving policies and practices of other employers. Then when you talk with your supervisor, you'll be in a position to make positive suggestions.

✗ Respect your company's concerns. Even a sympathetic boss is likely to worry about the impact of your caregiving role on your job performance. Approach your conversation with him not as a time to make demands but as an opportunity to work together toward a solution that accommodates your caregiving responsibilities while minimizing workplace disruptions.

✗ Make a list of the issues that you need to cover with your supervisor, including any points and questions that you plan to raise. If you feel comfortable doing so, you can review your list with a coworker whom you trust and solicit input from that person on the best way to approach your supervisor. You might even recruit a colleague as a stand-in for your boss to run through your conversation.

✗ Find the right moment to initiate a discussion. You probably don't want to approach your supervisor when he's putting together the departmental budget for next year or he's trying to finish an important report by 5 o'clock. You're better off waiting until both of you are in a calm and open frame of mind. Often caregivers don't mention anything about their situations until they're dealing with a crisis on the home front. Being in an emotional state only complicates efforts to hold a productive conversation.

✗ When you finally sit down to talk, be as direct as possible. The more information your supervisor has, the more likely your request will be met with understanding. Explain your current circumstances and the general course of your loved

Outlook

"We've studied the costs associated with the disruption in work that caregivers often face—that is, whether they leave their jobs entirely or cut back on their hours, or fail to take promotions and miss extra training. We found that when people leave the workforce to provide care, especially when they are fairly advanced in their careers, there is a substantial increase in the opportunity costs. We hope that in the future, employers can increase work schedule flexibility, and technological advances might allow employee caregivers to monitor the person for whom they're caring while they're on the job, so there is less need to disrupt work."

—PHYLLIS MUTSCHLER, PH.D., executive director of the National Center on Women and Aging, Heller School of Social Policy and Management, at Brandeis University in Waltham, Massachusetts

one's condition. But make clear that you cannot fully predict how the situation will unfold or what the demands on your time will be.

✗ Whether during your first or subsequent conversations, work with your supervisor to develop a course of action. Be proactive in making suggestions. Offer to switch to another shift, or to cover days others don't want, such as weekends and holidays. If your company has a flextime policy, discuss that as an option. If not, perhaps you could go in early some days and work late other days to make up for lost time. Or you could shorten your lunch break, do some work at home, or—if necessary—reduce your hours.

✗ Once you and your supervisor agree on a course of action, suggest implementing it for a trial period of several weeks or months. This might help your boss feel more comfort-

---

Caregiver's Checklist

Are You Ready to Talk with the Boss?

Make a copy of this checklist and take it to work with you. It can help you prepare to discuss your caregiving responsibilities with your supervisor.

☐ Find out what caregiving benefits are available at your company and how management has previously handled situations similar to your own.

☐ Familiarize yourself with the Family and Medical Leave Act.

☐ If you belong to a union, check whether your contract contains any provisions for caregiving benefits.

☐ Make a list of the issues you need to discuss with your supervisor.

☐ If appropriate, seek the advice of coworkers on the best way to approach your supervisor.

☐ Wait for the right time to initiate the conversation, when both you and your supervisor are calm and rational.

☐ Be direct and honest, and provide as much information about your situation as is comfortable or possible.

☐ Be proactive; suggest ways to make up lost time or complete unfinished work.

☐ Agree on a course of action, even if it takes more than one conversation.

☐ Send your supervisor a memo outlining the key points the two of you have agreed to.

able with your plan. Then do your best to hold up your end of the bargain. If you're successful, persuading your supervisor to continue the arrangement for as long as necessary will be that much easier.

✗ After your conversation, draft a memo to your supervisor outlining what the two of you have agreed to, how you will make up any time you miss, which corporate benefits you intend to take advantage of, and so on. Then both of you have a written record of your plan, in case you need to revisit any points down the road.

✗ If your supervisor seems unsympathetic to your situation or resists any changes in your job functions or schedule, consider your options for transferring to another department or division within your company. This must be handled tactfully, of course, and it might be too stressful on top of your caregiving responsibilities. But a little investigation could lead to another, less demanding position or to a supervisor known for dealing fairly with employees in caregiving roles.

Take Action... SHARPEN YOUR WORKPLACE SURVIVAL SKILLS

Even if you're able to modify your job functions and schedule to accommodate your caregiving responsibilities, you'll need to do some juggling to manage your workload and avoid overextending yourself. The following strategies can help maintain your equilibrium without sacrificing your job performance.

✗ Do as much advance planning as you can. Suppose your loved one has a doctor appointment one morning next week. You know you'll be in late that day, so make arrangements to work through lunch or to stay an extra hour or two to make up the time.

✗ Recruit family members, friends, and neighbors to help out when you can't get away from your job. Often parents establish networks of people to look after their children on

Outlook

"If I had to choose just one thing to focus on, it would be the enactment of paid family leave. The federal Family and Medical Leave Act protects workers' jobs but does not provide for their compensation. Many employees cannot afford to take unpaid leave to care for their loved ones.

Many states across the country have been expanding and enhancing the provisions of the federal Family and Medical Leave Act. But so far, none requires employers to offer paid leave. Eight weeks of paid leave, with the continuation of health benefits, would allow people to care for those they care about without jeopardizing their health status at the same time."

—**DONNA WAGNER, PH.D.**, director of gerontology at Towson University in Maryland

EXPERT OPINION

"The caregiver has always been a part of Hopi culture. . . . We have our elders, and we have a sense of responsibility that we should take care of them. We want to take care of them. But times are changing; now we have men and women who are working. Sometimes providing care isn't possible."

—AURELIA NEHOITEWA,
ombudsman for the Office of Hopi
Elderly Services, Kykotsmovi, Arizona

short notice. You could make similar arrangements for your loved one. Just be sure she feels safe and comfortable with the people you choose.

✕ If you're comfortable doing so, ask colleagues who are or have been in caregiving situations how they cope. Based on their experiences, they may be able to offer practical suggestions that you hadn't thought of before. Perhaps they'd be willing to trade off caregiving responsibilities on occasion.

✕ If a colleague pitches in for you when you're called away, let the person know that you're grateful for his support and assistance. You might want to treat him to lunch or buy him a small gift as a token of your appreciation. The point is, don't take his kindness for granted.

✕ Offer to pitch in yourself when you're able. Caregiving responsibilities tend to come in waves, leaving some periods not quite as hectic as others. During the "lulls," you might be able to take on an extra project or otherwise assist your supervisor or colleagues.

✕ When you're on the job, try to find moments to relax. Close your eyes for a few minutes or take a walk on your break, particularly if you feel stressed. If you work yourself to exhaustion, neither you nor your employer will benefit.

✕ When you need to make personal calls or attend to other caregiving responsibilities while at work, try to wait until lunchtime or another break. If you can't, explain the situation to your supervisor and outline your plan for making up the time. Offer to reimburse the company for long-distance calls or other expenses.

✕ If your caregiving situation changes to such an extent that you no longer can meet your job's demands, talk with your supervisor as soon as possible. Depending on the circumstances, you might be able to manage with additional modifications in your job functions or schedule. Or you may need to explore other employment opportunities within your company or elsewhere.

CHAPTER 31

PREPARING FOR YOUR FUTURE

What You Need to Know

- Most Americans—including caregivers who understand the challenges of obtaining quality long-term care—are unprepared for the possibility that they may become care recipients themselves.

- It is never too early to begin planning for the future. Adults of all ages should organize their legal and financial affairs, evaluate their long-term care options, and discuss their decisions with everyone likely to be involved in their care.

- Planning ahead is not an act of selfishness. Rather, it's a gift to the people you love, who one day may be in the position of making decisions about your care. Letting them know your wishes now can shield them from anguish and heartbreak down the road.

Sometime during your tenure as a caregiver, you likely will start contemplating your own future as a potential care recipient. Where will you live? How will you pay for your care? What must you do to ensure that your wishes are carried out?

They're difficult questions, to be sure. And they're so easy to put off, especially when we're young and healthy—seemingly years away from needing care. Yet this is precisely when we should be making plans. After all, illness and disability don't follow a set schedule. Aging is a bit more predictable, but until science can say with certainty who will get cancer, or suffer a stroke, or develop Alzheimer's, we have no idea what our elder years will hold.

What we do know from our collective caregiving experience is that while we can't predict the future, we can prepare for it.

We've seen firsthand how meticulously detailed plans spare family members from making painful decisions about a loved one's care—and how lack of planning tears families apart. As a caregiver, how many times have you said to yourself, "If only we had discussed this sooner . . ."?

Remember, if you suddenly become incapacitated, your immediate family will need to make decisions about your care, whether or not they're ready to do it. That's why discussing your wishes now, while you're healthy and independent, is so important. In fact, it's one of the greatest gifts you can give to the people you love the most.

A sudden illness or injury would affect not just you as the patient but everyone around you. Your immediate family may be so distressed by your situation that they're unable to make tough medical and financial decisions with a clear head. Having to choose without knowing your wishes can be all the more devastating.

For your family's sake as well as your own, start making plans for your care now, while it's on your mind. Think of it this way: You've been given an opportunity to shape your destiny, at least to some degree. Take advantage of it!

Take Action... ANSWER KEY QUESTIONS ABOUT YOUR CARE

Like most caregivers, you probably are programmed to pay more attention to other people's needs than to your own. So you may have a hard time focusing on yourself and thinking about your wishes for your future care. If so, remind yourself that planning ahead is not an act of selfishness or egotism. On the contrary, it's an act of caring and compassion, carried out on behalf of those you love.

Of course, even if you're mentally ready to contemplate your future, you may be wondering: "When will I find the time?" If you can scrounge up a spare hour or two, you may prefer to spend it reading a book, or taking a bike ride, or going out with friends. Pleasurable activities like these are important; they make the rest of your day-to-day routine all the more bearable.

But contemplating your future needn't be as unpleasant, or as time-consuming, as it might seem. Yes, it may require some hard thinking, a bit of research, and a few potentially uncomfortable discussions with your family. But people who've been through the process find that they're not nearly as overwhelmed by it as they expected. In fact, they're relieved by it, because they finally have their personal affairs in order.

So where do you begin? The following strategies are a good jumping-off point.

✗ Organize and review key personal documents. If you wish, you can use the Caregiver's Checklist on page 107 to track what you have and what you need. And make sure what you have is up-to-date—particularly wills, insurance policies, and other documents that name their beneficiaries. Do they still reflect your wishes? If not, they'll need to be changed.

✗ Consider who should make financial decisions on your behalf in the event you become incapacitated. Many people choose a relative, such as a grown child. But you might prefer your attorney or financial planner. Once you appoint someone—talk with the person first, to make sure he's willing—you must make it official with a document known as a durable power of attorney for finances. It authorizes the person to pay bills, submit insurance claims, file taxes, and handle other financial transactions in your name. (To learn more about durable powers of attorney, see chapter 25.)

✗ Also pick someone to make medical decisions on your behalf, in case you can't do it yourself. You could go with the same person who'll be managing your finances, but you don't have to. You want someone who has earned your complete trust and who will act in your best interests, because he understands your preferences in particular medical situations. You need to officially appoint this person through a durable power of attorney for health care.

✗ Think carefully about whether you would want medical personnel to use aggressive measures to sustain your life—and if so, to what extent. For example, do you want to be fed intravenously? Or hooked up to a respirator? The more explicit you make your instructions, the more easily your

FOR MORE INFORMATION

AARP sponsors a legal program that offers advice on planning for long-term care, including tips on preparing wills, powers of attorney, advance directives, and other documents. To learn more, you can contact the legal program at **(202) 234-0970** or visit the AARP Web site at **www.aarp.org**. In addition, be aware that some states' AARP affiliates run their own legal hot lines.

EXPERT OPINION

"All of us may be care recipients one day, so we really should take an active role in planning for our care. This includes filling out powers of attorney, buying long-term care insurance, making sure we have burial [insurance] so our kids don't have to worry about it, and other measures. We really have to think about all these things. If we do, I believe we'll treat our elders with more respect and dignity. And hopefully, we'll support them through the rest of their years."

—JANET MORRIS,
elder law attorney for Bet Tzedek
Legal Services in Los Angeles

family and health care providers can determine the right course of treatment. All of the particulars should be spelled out in a living will. (For more information on living wills, refer to chapter 25.)

✗ To make your living will as specific and complete as possible, discuss available treatments with your physician and other health care providers. Ask questions about the various approaches to pain relief, about the procedure for resuscitating a patient who's in cardiac arrest, about the process of evaluating a person's chances for full or partial recovery—whatever piques your interest. This information can be helpful in deciding which measures you'd want used should certain medical situations arise.

✗ Determine your preferences for funeral and burial arrangements. Some people want to go in style, so to speak; others have little desire for a grand memorial. Making arrangements in advance—and paying for them, if possible—can ease the burden on your family. They won't need to think about coffins and headstones at a time when they're grappling with grief.

Take Action... ASSESS YOUR FINANCES

Perhaps the most important aspect of preparing for your future care is making sure you have adequate financial resources to pay for it. With some exceptions, most kinds of residential and in-home care are not covered by Medicare or by standard health insurance policies. You'll be footing most of the caregiving bill, which could amount to tens of thousands of dollars a year, depending on where you live and which services you require.

Through extremely diligent planning, you can muster the wherewithal to pay for quality care without jeopardizing your future financial security. In general, the simplest and wisest approach involves comparing potential sources of income—Social Security, bank accounts, investments, real estate holdings, and so on—against the potential costs of long-term care. Having more than one source of income helps offset the impact of almost certain economic fluctuations, as well as unanticipated caregiving expenses.

While you can do your own financial planning (and you'll get some basic how-to advice below), you might want to consider consulting a professional, such as an elder law attorney or a certified financial planner. Many social service agencies offer financial counseling for a nominal fee or free to those with limited resources.

Sizing Up Your Income

Most people think of income as a weekly paycheck. Actually, it's much broader than that. For your purposes here, think of it as any resource that can be converted to cash to cover caregiving expenses. For a list of resources that might fall into this category, see the Caregiver's Checklist on page 298. Then use the following strategies to get as clear a picture of your income as possible.

✗ Tally all your anticipated retirement and pension benefits, including Social Security, employer-based pension plans, IRAs, and 401(k)s. Since the size of your benefits payments can vary according to the age at which you begin collecting them, among other factors, you might want to calculate payment amounts for a variety of scenarios. If you're named as a beneficiary for any of your spouse's retirement or pension benefits, calculate those payments as well.

✗ Make sure you have up-to-date information on your income sources. To estimate your Social Security payments, for example, you can obtain worksheets from the Social Security Administration. Your employer's human resources department should be able to explain your pension payments. And a financial planner or tax advisor can help navigate the eligibility requirements and payment options for IRAs and other retirement accounts.

✗ Round up other assets—bank accounts, certificates of deposit, investments, real estate holdings—and figure out their contributions to your bottom line. Their value can be more unpredictable than retirement and pension benefits, so when doing your calculations, err on the conservative side.

FOR MORE INFORMATION

The National Academy of Elder Law Attorneys, a professional association, can provide a wealth of information on the legal questions related to long-term care. The organization can also help locate a qualified lawyer in your area, should you need one. On their Web site, **www.naela.org**, you can find an extensive list of links to a wide variety of associations, agencies, and other resources.

You can also contact the organization by calling **(520) 881-4005**, or writing to 1604 North Country Club Road, Tucson, AZ 85716.

FOR MORE INFORMATION

The Social Security Administration's Web site features a benefits calculator that allows you to estimate your benefits based on certain variables, such as how much you expect to earn when you plan to retire. To check it out, go to **www.ssa.gov/planners** and click on "Calculators."

You can also request benefits worksheets from your local Social Security office. It should be listed in the blue pages of your telephone directory, under "United States Government."

Aligning Your Insurance Benefits

You can stretch your anticipated income by making the most of public and private insurance coverage. While no single policy covers every caregiving expense, a combination of policies could make a substantial dent in your caregiving bills. Now is the time to size up your coverage, to make sure you're not over- or under-insured. These tips can help.

✗ Remember that Medicare kicks in only when you turn 65. Even then, it likely won't cover all of your medical expenses, let alone caregiving costs. Many people purchase what are known as Medigap policies, which—as their name suggests—often pick up the tab when Medicare won't. But they tend to be limited in their caregiving coverage, too. (To learn more about Medicare and Medigap, see chapter 24.)

✗ Check whether you'll be eligible for any post-retirement health insurance coverage provided by your employer, including benefits offered under the federal Comprehensive Omnibus Budget Reconciliation Act (COBRA). Then find out how you go about signing up for it, when the time comes. Explore other health insurance options as well, such as group plans offered through fraternal organizations, church associations, and professional societies. Compare benefits, costs, and cancellation requirements before settling on a specific policy.

✗ Determine whether you have disability coverage through an employer and, if so, under what circumstances you become eligible for benefits. If you aren't already covered, you might want to consider enrolling in a private plan that would pay benefits in the event you become incapacitated.

✗ Research the various kinds of life insurance policies, such as term life and whole life, to identify the one that best suits your needs. If you have coverage through an employer, be sure to read up on the benefits. You may decide that you want to invest in an individual policy, too.

✗ Consider whether you're a candidate for long-term care insurance. As explained in chapter 24, this type of coverage isn't for everyone. But it can be a sound investment if you're in reasonably good health and you have financial assets you want to protect. Keep in mind that the younger you are when you purchase a long-term care policy, the lower your premiums may be. Still, policies can vary widely in price as well as benefits, so take the time to shop and compare. A good insurance broker should be able to recommend coverage that matches not only your long-term care plans but also your budget.

Estimating Long-Term Care Costs

When looking into long-term care insurance—when doing any sort of long-range financial planning, for that matter—you should have a reasonably good sense of what you expect to be paying by the time you're ready for care. Expenses tend to rise every year, with the cost of living; they'll also vary according to the type and duration of services you require. Since all of these factors are beyond your control, your best bet may be to consider your options and preferences for several possible scenarios. Use the following strategies as your guide.

✗ Contemplate your future living arrangements. If you're like most people, you envision yourself staying at home for as long as you're able. That's more possible today than ever, given all the in-home support services you can take advantage of. But suppose your health declined to the point that you couldn't live by yourself. Would you want to move in with another family member? Or would you feel more comfortable in a residential care facility? In general, home care is less expensive than residential care. But cost isn't the only issue. You also need to think about things like whether you want to stay in the same geographic area, and how you get along with your relatives.

✗ Familiarize yourself with the kinds of residential care available. Even if you no longer can manage on your own, you may not need the round-the-clock care that's typical of nursing homes. Why pay for services that you aren't using? You may be better off with the on-call support of an assisted living facility, which tends to be less expensive. Another option is continuing care, in which one residential

EXPERT OPINION

"[In a survey of caregivers,] the high incidence of insufficient financial planning held true regardless of age, income, or the level of caregiving burden. It is well-known that Americans in general have not done much long-term care planning and that boomers in particular have been criticized for not saving or investing for their retirement. But since the women in our survey have been caring for an older person, we expected that they would have begun to plan for their own futures. This does not appear to be true.

"What's more, very few of these caregivers feel they are 'well' prepared. Over half report feeling 'a little or not at all' prepared. Nearly all believe that their own long-term care will be paid for by either their own savings and investments or government insurance. The notion that Medicare and Medicaid will pay for long-term care probably reflects the common lack of knowledge about the financial and medical conditions required to qualify for government coverage."

—**GAIL HUNT,** executive director of the National Alliance for Caregiving, based in Bethesda, Maryland

EXPERT OPINION

"What people need to do is plan early for long-term care and have the wherewithal to pay privately. That way, they're ready. They can go into a nursing home or assisted living facility, get respite care, get services in the community for which there's a fee. They're financially prepared and financially responsible for a crisis when it occurs.

"The difficulty with long-term care is that planning for it takes a long time. You can't buy fire insurance when your house is in flames. Likewise, you can't buy long-term care insurance when you have Alzheimer's disease. You need to think about that 10, 15, 20 years—preferably 25 or 30 years—ahead, before care becomes necessary."

—**STEPHEN MOSES**, president of the Center for Long-Term Care Financing in Seattle

community offers several living arrangements, including independent housing, an assisted living facility, and a nursing home. Continuing care can be very costly, but its flexibility may be worth the price. (To learn more about your options in residential care, see chapter 21.)

X When making decisions about your future housing, take into account your personal habits and lifestyle. For example, you may prefer having private accommodations rather than sharing your living space with someone else. Or you might want a place that accepts pets. Make a list of your preferences, then prioritize them. This might help narrow your choices, especially when considered in context with your financial circumstances.

X Keep in mind that no single insurance policy or benefits plan covers all the costs of long-term care. To limit out-of-pocket expenses, you likely will need to utilize a combination of resources. Find out now what benefits you'll be entitled to, whether through Medicare, an employer-sponsored retirement package, or private insurance. Then you can use that information, along with your projected long-term care costs, to develop a spending and saving plan that will support your future care and safeguard your financial interests. (For advice on creating a personal budget, see chapter 23.)

Take Action... TALK WITH YOUR FAMILY

You needn't have made all your long-term care decisions before you call a family meeting to discuss them. But doing as much advance preparation as possible helps set your agenda and ease what can be a stressful situation. Of course, some issues will be resolved only after your family offers its input; others will need to wait until care becomes necessary.

What's important now is that you at least initiate the conversation. You want to make your wishes known while you're healthy rather than after you become sick, when a sense of urgency can cloud the decision-making process. Consider, too, that the longer you wait, the less preparation time you have; the less time you have, the more limited your options will be.

While you might see the wisdom in talking about your long-term care sooner rather than later, your family could require some convincing. The following tips can help facilitate the conversation.

✗ Call everyone together at a time when you expect them to be relatively calm and open-minded. If you try to hold a meeting while the participants are preoccupied with other matters, you may not get the attention and cooperation you need to thoughtfully discuss your long-term care. For the same reason, avoid extending a meeting about a loved one's care to address your own. It might seem like a good idea, since the same people are involved. But you're better off scheduling separate meetings, so your situation—and your loved one's—gets the consideration it deserves.

✗ If anyone in your family balks at your invitation to discuss your long-term care, be respectful of their reluctance. After all, this may be the first time they've faced the possibility of your becoming a care recipient one day, and they may not be comfortable with it. What's more, if you're in good health, they may view your preparations as premature. Let them know you understand how they feel, but be firm about moving forward. Explain that you want to protect them from the emotional turmoil of making decisions about your care without knowing your wishes.

✗ Approach the meeting as an opportunity to explore how your family might handle various situations in the event you required care. All of you may need time to contemplate your options or do more research before making any commitments. If you must reconvene at a later date, that's okay. At least everyone will be thinking about the issues you raise.

✗ Before your meeting, carefully consider family relationships and try to anticipate any potential emotional minefields, such as sibling rivalries. As you might imagine, family dynamics will play a critical role in determining how any discussion of your long-term care progresses. Given the seriousness of the matter, longstanding or unspoken conflicts easily could emerge. Consider how to frame your comments in a way that minimizes the potential of inflaming these conflicts.

✗ Depending on your family situation, consider inviting a non-family member to attend your meeting. An objective but sympathetic "outsider" can help navigate sensitive issues and resolve disagreements. This person could be a trusted family friend, a member of the clergy, or even a professional mediator. Just be sure it's someone whom all the meeting participants feel comfortable with.

✗ During the meeting, encourage family members to express their opinions, even if theirs differ from your own. Disagreement can cultivate insightful, productive discussion; it shouldn't be construed as a lack of love or respect on your family's part. They may have knowledge or experience that gives them a unique perspective on a certain issue or situation. Hear them out, and let them know that what they say matters.

✗ While your family is together, take the opportunity to explain the legal and financial documents you already have in place and those you plan to prepare, like durable powers of attorney and a living will. If you've completed the Caregiver's Checklist on page 107, as recommended earlier, you may want to make a copy for each family member. Note where you've filed the documents, in case someone needs to find them in an emergency.

✗ Also consider reviewing the provisions of your will. This can be an especially delicate matter, so be sure to weigh your family situation before you proceed. But disclosing your plans for the distribution of your assets may help prevent the sorts of surprises that could cause conflicts among your survivors after your death. What's more, it gives everyone a chance to indicate which mementos or keepsakes they'd like for themselves.

✗ If you've appointed someone as executor of your will, or as your representative through a durable power of attorney, be prepared to explain why that person is appropriate for the role. Otherwise, family members who are overlooked may feel slighted by your decision, which could worsen any underlying rivalries. When you discuss your rationale, focus

FOR MORE INFORMATION

Nolo Press publishes a wide range of do-it-yourself books that include sample forms for wills, powers of attorney, and other documents. You can visit the company's Web site at **www.nolo.com**, call **(800) 728-3555**, or write to 950 Parker Street, Berkeley, CA 94710-2524.

your comments on the person's qualifications, rather than pointing out everyone else's shortcomings.

✗ If tensions arise—and they likely will, at some point—confront them directly. Rather than blaming those involved, try to understand what they're angry or upset about. Then work with them to come up with a solution that everyone feels comfortable with. Addressing troublesome issues now is much better than letting them fester until they begin to erode family relationships, especially if you're counting on your family to oversee your long-term care.

✗ Before you adjourn your meeting, make plans for a follow-up to discuss any unresolved issues. If a particular issue requires further research, come to an agreement on who should do what before you get together again. The assignments should be as clear and specific as possible. That way, you collect the information you need—and everyone feels they've contributed to the decision-making process.

✗ If possible, follow the meeting with an activity that creates an atmosphere of connectedness and solidarity. It could be a family potluck dinner, a volleyball game, or a night out at the movies. Choose something that helps alleviate any remaining tensions and reinforces familial bonds.

A TIME TO GRIEVE

For caregivers, the idealism of planning for their own long-term care often is juxtaposed against the reality of being responsible for someone else's. They're keenly aware of the complex and challenging issues that have defined their caregiving situations. By looking to the future, they're able to make peace with the present.

That's especially true when eventually, inevitably, they must grieve the loss of their loved ones. Grief is a chaotic and confusing emotion—or more precisely, a complex of emotions, since someone who's in mourning can swerve from despair to rage to relief with unexpected swiftness. Often the trigger is something as simple as a sound or smell that evokes sharp memories of the person who has passed on.

While grieving is a universal experience, it takes everyone

Outlook

"The oldest baby boomers are seeing parents caught off-guard by the lack of public coverage for necessary services, and they're taking more personal responsibility and putting together private funding plans. As a result, the baby boomers will catapult highly personalized long-term care services into existence. We'll see assisted living residences adapting to changing tastes. Maybe on-site ice cream parlors will be replaced by gourmet coffee shops, and physical therapy will be expanded to include spa- and salon-type treatments. The baby boom generation will drive the demand for things they value during their active years, like more intellectual stimulation, not just arts and crafts."

—**NANCY P. MORITH, CLU,** president of N P Morith, Inc., in Princeton, New Jersey

down a unique path. So any emotions that bubble to the surface should be viewed as perfectly normal and appropriate. Grieving doesn't come with an instruction book; it has no rules, no "right" or "wrong."

That said, some responses to grief do seem to occur rather routinely—though the order in which they occur can vary widely. Initially, shock and numbness certainly are common. So are acute and debilitating pain, extreme exhaustion, disorientation, and an inability to concentrate. Many people lose their appetites or have trouble sleeping. Some report flashbacks to prior losses in their lives.

Grief can affect personal relationships, too. Some people may feel alienated from family members and friends, and so try to isolate themselves by engaging in solitary pursuits. Others may reach out for comfort—surrounding themselves with loved ones, renewing old acquaintances, even getting involved in a whirlwind of activities.

No matter how grief manifests itself, those who endure it can take comfort in knowing that the emotional roller-coaster ride does come to an end. As they adjust to and accept their losses, they gradually ease out of mourning and back into their "normal" lives, though often with a profoundly different perspective of themselves and the world around them. Grief has changed them.

Interestingly, many people who've gone through the grieving process have found that the very act of contemplating their own long-term care helps them cope with the pain of loss and begin to move beyond it. For one thing, looking ahead distracts them from focusing exclusively on the past. For another, it allows them to take the lessons of their caregiving situations and apply them to their own lives. Through this process, people feel their departed loved ones are still guiding and advising them. It can be quite comforting.

Of course, not everyone feels at ease thinking about the future in the wake of a loved one's death. You must decide if and when you want to take that step. Remember, though, that just as planning ahead is a gift to those who one day may be responsible for your care, it can be a private and loving tribute to the person who is gone.

PART EIGHT

Resources

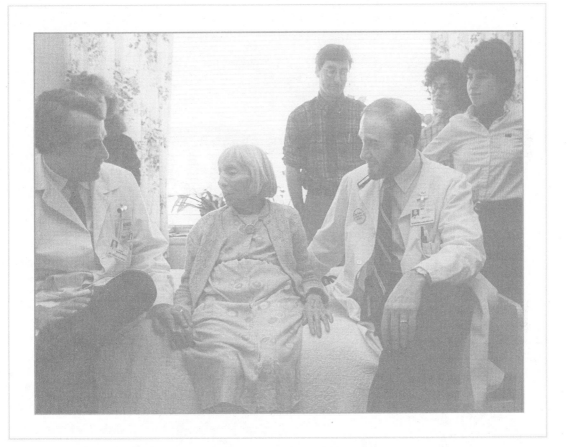

AND THOU SHALT HONOR

COMPANION WEB SITE

Throughout this book, we've made every effort to provide comprehensive, up-to-date information on the key issues that matter most to caregivers. If you'd like to learn more about anything presented in these pages, or in the PBS special *And Thou Shalt Honor*, you're invited to visit our companion Web site, **www.thoushalthonor.org**.

In addition to profiles of the caregivers, care recipients, and caregiving professionals from the PBS broadcast, thoushalthonor.org lists almost 100,000 community resources that may be helpful to caregivers. The site also features links to additional research, training, and support materials, as well as online forums for laypeople and professionals alike. You'll have the opportunity to share experiences and exchange insights and inspiration with others in situations similar to your own.

If you're looking for additional references, thoushalthonor.org has an extensive e-commerce section. You'll find books, audiotapes, and DVDs of interest to anyone involved in caregiving.

OTHER WEB SITES

The following independent Web sites offer all kinds of information relevant to caregivers, including questionnaires and assessment tools, expert advice, directories of local resources, and links to public health organizations and services. Many of these sites also feature online support groups and chat rooms, where visitors can take part in ongoing discussions of caregiving issues.

www.access-able.com

Access-Able Travel Source offers helpful advice for elderly and disabled travelers.

www.acsu.buffalo.edu/~drstall/

At this site, Robert S. Stall, M.D., an internist and geriatrician, provides numerous resources for caregivers, including assessment tools, information on working with the elderly and terminally ill, and contacts for online discussion groups of caregiver-related topics.

www.agelessdesign.com

Ageless Design provides information and advice on home modifications and resources, especially for people with Alzheimer's disease.

www.asktransitions.com

This Minneapolis firm's site offers a glossary of the official terms used in caregiving, a sample form for evaluating residential care facilities, and a section of tips and tools for the caregiver.

www.benefitscheckup.org

The National Council on Aging sponsors this free online service, which allows you to quickly assess your loved one's eligibility for benefits. You'll be asked for some basic information, like the person's age and ZIP code (but not name or Social Security number, as the service is anonymous). Based on this personal profile, the site produces a list of programs that match your loved one's needs, interests, and location.

www.bestcaregiverinfo.com

This site includes only those resources that adhere to its own standards of care. Its purpose is to provide visitors with access to the businesses, government agencies, and not-for-profit organizations responsible for providing caregiving services and information in their local communities.

www.care-givers.com

Founded by Gail Mitchell following her own caregiving experience, this site offers articles and interactive opportunities for caregivers, with a focus on supporting spiritual growth and coping with end-of-life issues.

www.caregivers.com

Part of the AgeNet Eldercare Network, this resource offers information on medical, legal, financial, and other caregiving-related issues, along with a members-only chat room and a toll-free number for a phone consultation with an eldercare specialist.

www.caregiversmarketplace.com

This is the Internet home of the Caregivers Marketplace, which offers an array of resources—including product rebates and discounts—specifically for family caregivers.

www.caregiving.com

Caregiving Online is the electronic version of a newsletter for people who provide care for aging loved ones. It's the Internet home for *Today's Caregiver* magazine and offers online support groups.

www.carescout.com

This Miami-based Web site offers state-by-state information on nursing homes, assisted living facilities, home health care providers, and hospice facilities.

www.cms.hhs.gov

This Web site offers information about Medicaid, including benefits and eligibility requirements.

www.ec-online.net

ElderCare Online is an Internet community that allows caregivers to chat with each other and with caregiving professionals. The site also posts a bimonthly newsletter.

www.eldercare.gov

This Web site, sponsored by the U.S. Administration on Aging, can direct you to a variety of community services to support your older loved one.

www.eldercorner.com

This site functions primarily as an online marketplace for specialty products designed to help seniors live more active lives. Visitors can check out the site's Health Message Board to exchange information with others.

www.eldernet.com

This site serves as a seniors' guide to the World Wide Web, directing visitors to information on health, housing, legal and financial issues, retirement, lifestyles, news, and entertainment.

www.elderweb.com

This site is a valuable resource for information on eldercare as well as legal, financial, and public policies concerning the elderly. You'll find state-by-state links to support services, plus more than 6,000 reviewed links to long-term care information. The site also features an expanding library of articles and reports, news, and events.

www.familycareamerica.com

Visitors can use this site to find caregiving resources in their area, including residential care facilities, adult day care services, and hospice care. The site also offers solution sharing and discussion forums.

www.healthfinder.gov

Supported by the U.S. Department of Health and Human Services, this site provides a search engine to locate information on various health issues. It also offers a directory of health-related Web sites from government agencies, clearinghouses, nonprofit organizations, and universities.

www.hiicap.state.ny.us/home/hiassist.htm

Run by the state of New York, this Web site features contact information for health insurance counseling programs in many other states.

www.mayoclinic.com

The Mayo Clinic maintains an impressive online library of health information, including profiles of prescription and over-the-counter drugs, herbal remedies, and nutritional supplements.

www.mentalhelp.net/selfhelp

The American Self-Help Clearinghouse Self-Help Sourcebook is designed to be a starting point for exploring support groups and networks in your community and around the world. The site also offers advice on starting your own self-help group.

www.nationalsharedhousing.org

The National Shared Housing Resource Center publishes a directory of programs that help older people establish shared housing arrangements.

www.pueblo.gsa.gov

This is the official Web site for the Federal Consumer Information Center (FCIC). Here you can read or print out the current *Consumer Information Catalog* and the full text of all the publications listed in it. You can also search for specific subjects.

www.seniorlaw.com/hotlines.htm

This site contains a listing of telephone hot lines that will answer legal questions for people over age 60. Though some charge a fee, most are free.

www.thirdage.com

This free membership site caters to the interests and needs of first-wave baby boomers, adults in their mid-forties through fifties. In addition to a section on caregiving, it offers information on a broad range of topics, including family, health and fitness, money and work, news, technology, and travel.

www.travelsource.com

The information on this site is useful for caregivers who are planning vacations with their loved ones.

www.usc.edu/dept/gero/hmap/library/drhome

This Web site provides instructions for making home modifications, such as installing handrails, to create safe living environments for care recipients.

BOOKS

For additional information and perspectives on all aspects of caregiving, including financial, legal, and medical advice, consult one or more of the following books.

Abrams, William. *Merck Manual of Geriatrics.* Merck and Company, 2000.

Berg, Adriane G. *Warning: Dying May Be Hazardous to Your Wealth.* Career Press, 1995.

Berman, Claire. *Caring for Yourself While Caring for Your Aging Parents: How to Help, How to Survive.* Owl Books, 2001.

Bornstein, Robert, and Mary A. Languirand. *When Someone You Love Needs Nursing Home Care: The Complete Guide.* Newmarket, 2001.

Bove, Alexander A., Jr. *The Medicaid Planning Handbook.* Little, Brown, and Company, 1996.

Burger, Sarah. *Nursing Homes: Getting Good Care There.* Impact Publishers, 2001.

Cason, Ann. *Circles of Care: How to Set Up Quality Home Care for Our Elders.* Shambhala, 2001.

Esperti, Robert A., et al. *The Living Trust Workbook.* Penguin USA, 2001.

Irving, Shae. *The Financial Power of Attorney Workbook.* Nolo Press, 1997.

Karpinski, Marion. *Quick Tips for Caregivers.* Healing Arts Communications, 2000.

Lebow, Grace, et al. *Coping with Your Difficult Older Parent.* Avon Books, 1999.

Lieberman, Trudi, and Consumer Reports Editors. *Consumer Reports Guide to Health Services for Seniors.* Three Rivers (Crown), 2000.

Mace, Nancy, and Peter V. Rabins. *The 36-Hour Day: The Family Guide to Caring for Persons with Alzheimer Disease, Related Dementing Illnesses, and Memory Loss in Later Life.* Warner Books, 2001.

Matthews, Joseph L. *Beat the Nursing Home Trap: A Consumer's Guide to Choosing and Financing Long-Term Care.* Nolo Press, 2001.

McLeod, Beth Witrogen. *Caregiving: The Spiritual Journey of Love, Loss, and Renewal.* John Wiley and Sons, 2000.

Meyer, Maria M., et al. *The Comfort of Home: An Illustrated Step-by-Step Guide for Caregivers.* CareTrust Publications LLC., 1998.

Morris, Virginia. *How to Care for Aging Parents.* Workman, 1996.

Morse, Sarah, and Donna Quinn Robbins. *Moving Mom and Dad.* Lanier Publishing, 1998.

Perry, Angela (ed.). *American Medical Association Guide to Home Caregiving.* Wiley, 2001.

Rhodes, Linda Colvin. *The Complete Idiot's Guide to Caring for Aging Parents.* Alpha (Macmillan), 2000.

Schumacher, Vickie, and Jim Shumacher. *Understanding Living Trusts: How You Can Avoid Probate, Save Taxes, and Enjoy Peace of Mind.* Schumacher and Company, 1999.

Shannon, Joyce Brennfleck (ed.). *Caregiving Sourcebook.* Omnigraphics, 2001.

Shenkman, Martin M. *The Complete Book of Trusts.* John Wiley and Sons, 1997.

Strong, Maggie. *Mainstay: For the Well Spouse of the Chronically Ill.* Bradford Books, 1997.

Susik, D. Helen. *Hiring Home Caregivers: The Family Guide to In-Home Eldercare.* Impact Publishers, 1995.

Warner, Mark L. *The Complete Guide to Alzheimer's Proofing Your Home.* Purdue University Press, 2000.

Williams, Mark E. *The American Geriatrics Society's Complete Guide to Aging and Health.* Harmony Books, 1995.

ORGANIZATIONS

A number of national organizations provide helpful services for caregivers and their loved ones, including education, advocacy, referrals, and support. We offer a selection here (in alphabetical order), based on the topics covered in this book. Many of these groups have established Web sites; if you have Internet access, the sites are a good place to start gathering information.

AAA Foundation for Traffic Safety

Web site: www.seniordrivers.org
1440 New York Avenue NW, Suite 201
Washington, DC 20005
(202) 638-5944

The Web site for this organization offers senior driving self-assessments, safe driving tips, emergency information, and more.

AARP

Web site: www.aarp.org
601 E Street NW
Washington, DC 20049
(800) 424-3410

AARP provides information and advice on every aspect of caregiving, ranging from home modifications to legal and financial issues.

Abledata

Web site: www.abledata.com
8630 Fenton Street, Suite 930
Silver Spring, MD 20910
(800) 227-0216

ABLEDATA is a federally funded project that provides information on assistive technology and rehabilitation equipment to consumers, professionals, and organizations.

Accreditation Commission for Health Care

Web site: www.achc.org
Grove Towers
1110 Navaho Drive, Suite 500
Raleigh, NC 27609
(919) 785-1214

This agency provides accreditation for home health agencies, home care aide programs, home medical equipment suppliers, specialty pharmacies, and hospices.

Administration on Aging

Web site: www.aoa.gov
330 Independence Avenue SW
Washington, DC 20201
(202) 619-7501

This federal agency sponsors the Eldercare Locator, which identifies Area Agencies on Aging by geographic location. You can access the Eldercare Locator through the agency's Web site or directly at www.eldercare.gov or (800) 677-1116 (Monday through Friday from 9:00 A.M. to 8:00 P.M. EST). The agency's Web site also features a helpful guide to caregiving called *Because We Care*.

Alliance for Retired Americans

Web site: www.retiredamericans.org
888 16th Street NW
Washington, DC 20006
(888) 373-6497

This advocacy organization, launched by a national coalition of AFL-CIO affiliated unions and community organizations, participates in government policymaking on aging issues. Anyone who isn't a retired member of an affiliated union can join the organization for an annual fee.

Alzheimer's Association

Web site: www.alz.org
919 North Michigan Avenue, Suite 1100
Chicago, IL 60611-1676
(800) 272-3900 or (312) 335-8700

The association's Web site includes a listing of local chapters, online versions of the association's brochures, and links to other Alzheimer's Web sites.

Alzheimer's Disease Education and Referral Center

Web site: www.alzheimers.org
PO Box 8250
Silver Spring, MD 20907-8250
(800) 438-4380

A service of the National Institute on Aging, this center provides information about Alzheimer's disease and related disorders, its impact on families, and research into possible causes and cures.

American Association of Daily Money Managers (AADMM)

Web site: www.aadmm.com
PO Box 8857
Gaithersburg, MD 20898-8857
(301) 593-5462

The AADMM can explain the services provided by daily money managers and provide referrals to money managers in your area.

American Association of Homes and Services for the Aging

Web site: www.aahsa.org
2519 Connecticut Avenue NW
Washington, DC 20008-1520
(202) 783-2242

This organization's mission is to promote high-quality, affordable, and ethical long-term care for older Americans. Its Web site includes tips on choosing facilities and services, information on types of care, and other resources.

American Bar Association (ABA)

Web site: www.abanet.org
750 North Lake Shore Drive
Chicago, IL 60611
(312) 988-5522

The ABA's Lawyer Referral and Information Service can help you find a lawyer in your area who's knowledgeable in eldercare issues.

American Cancer Society

Web site: www.cancer.org
National Office
1599 Clifton Road Northeast
Atlanta, GA 30329-4251
(800) 227-2345

The American Cancer Society offers information on cancer and sponsors support groups for cancer patients and their families.

American College of Gastroenterology

Web site: www.acg.gi.org
4900 B South 31st Street
Arlington, VA 22206
(703) 820-7400

This organization provides information on digestive diseases and offers referrals to physicians who specialize in this field of medicine.

American Council on Life Insurance

Web site: www.acli.com
1001 Pennsylvania Avenue NW
Washington, DC 20004-2599
(800) 589-2254 or (202) 624-2000

On this organization's Web site, you can find information on financial and retirement security products as well as a state insurance department directory.

The American Foundation for AIDS Research

Web site: www.amfar.org
120 Wall Street, 13th Floor
New York, NY 10005-3902
(212) 806-1600

This nonprofit organization provides support for AIDS research, prevention, treatment, education, and advocacy. By visiting the group's Web site and adding your name to the mailing list, you can receive regular e-mail updates on all aspects of the disease.

American Foundation for the Blind

Web site: www.afb.org
11 Penn Plaza, Suite 300
New York, NY 10001
(212) 502-7600

This organization's Web site provides information on blindness and low vision, a directory of organizations that help the blind and visually impaired in the United States and Canada, and online message boards.

American Gastroenterological Association

Web site: www.gastro.org
7910 Woodmont Avenue, 7th Floor
Bethesda, MD 20814
(301) 654-2055

This organization advocates for biomedical research and scientific training in gastroenterology. Its Web site offers a wealth of information on a variety of digestive diseases and message boards for discussions of digestive health.

American Heart Association

Web site: www.americanheart.org
National Center
7272 Greenville Avenue
Dallas, TX 75231
(800) 242-8721

This organization's Web site features information on the warning signs of heart attack, facts on heart-related diseases and conditions, and updates on the latest research in the field. The site also provides access to local chapters.

American Institute of Certified Public Accountants
Personal Financial Planning Division
Web site: www.cpapfs.org
1211 Avenue of the Americas
New York, NY 10036
(888) 777-7077

This organization offers information on financial planning and referrals to accountants.

American Medical Association (AMA)
Web site: www.ama-assn.org
515 North State Street
Chicago, IL 60610
(312) 464-5000

The AMA maintains a database of almost every M.D. and D.O. in the country. Check the organization's Web site for a list of board-certified primary care physicians in your area.

American Pharmaceutical Association
Web site: www.pharmacyandyou.org
2215 Constitution Avenue NW
Washington, DC 20037-2985
(202) 628-4410

This organization provides all kinds of information on the field of pharmacy. Its Web site features helpful advice on medication use, including adverse reactions.

American Red Cross
Web site: www.redcross.org
In addition to providing disaster relief, the American Red Cross sponsors a variety of health and safety education programs. You can find your local chapter in the blue pages of your telephone directory, in the "Guide to Human Services."

American Stroke Association
Web site: www.strokeassociation.org
National Center
7272 Greenville Avenue
Dallas, TX 75231
(888) 478-7653

A division of the American Heart Association, this organization specializes in stroke research, education, fundraising, and advocacy. Its Web site provides information on caring for someone who has suffered a stroke.

Amyotrophic Lateral Sclerosis Association
Web site: www.alsa.org
27001 Agoura Road, Suite 150
Calabasas Hills, CA 91301-5104
(800) 782-4747

The Web site for this organization offers news, research updates, and consumer support for people with ALS (Lou Gehrig's disease) and their families.

ARCH National Respite Network and Resource Center
Web site: www.chtop.com
Chapel Hill Training-Outreach Project
800 Eastowne Drive, Suite 105
Chapel Hill, NC 27514
(888) 671-2594 or (919) 490-5577

Through this organization's Web site, you can find respite care providers in your state or local area.

Arthritis Foundation
Web site: www.arthritis.org
PO Box 7669
Atlanta, GA 30357-0669
(800) 283-7800

This organization is devoted to raising public awareness of arthritis and other joint diseases through education, research, advocacy, and support. It publishes a bimonthly magazine, *Arthritis Today*, that's available by subscription or online.

Assisted Living Federation of America
Web site: www.alfa.org
11200 Waples Mill Road, Suite 150
Fairfax, VA 22030
(703) 691-8100

This organization represents more than 7,000 for-profit and not-for-profit providers of senior housing. Its Web site features a list of assisted living facilities that can be searched by state, county, or city.

Association of Jewish Family and Children's Agencies

Web site: www.ajfca.org

557 Cranbury Road, Suite 2

East Brunswick, NJ 08816-5419

(800) 634-7346

This national organization offers faith-based services for older adults and their families. Its online Elder Support Service Directory lists service providers and contact information by state.

Canadian Association for the Fifty-Plus

Web site: www.50plus.com

27 Queen Street East, Suite 1304

Toronto, ON Canada

M5C 2M6

(416) 363-8748

Also known as CARP, this nonprofit organization works to promote the rights of older Canadians. Member benefits include a free newsletter and discounts on health insurance and financial services.

CareGuide, Inc.

Web site: www.careguide.com

12301 NW 39th Street

Coral Springs, FL 33056

(888) 389-8839

CareGuide is a care management company with a national network of care managers and a toll-free caregiver support center.

Carescout/National Eldercare Referral Systems

Web site: www.NursingHomeReports.com

36 Washington Street, Suite 250

Wellesley Hills, MA 02481

(800) 571-1918 or (781) 431-7033

These sister organizations offer a wealth of information about assisted living facilities. They also conduct nursing home inspections.

Catholic Charities USA

Web site: www.catholiccharitiesusa.org

1731 King Street, Suite 200

Alexandria, VA 22314

(703) 549-1390

This faith-based organization sponsors a variety of caregiving services, including adult day care and support groups. It also offers referrals to local chapters.

Centers for Medicare and Medicaid Services (CMS)

Web site: www.cms.hhs.gov

7500 Security Boulevard

Baltimore, MD 21244-1850

(410) 786-3000

Previously known as the Health Care Financing Administration, this government agency administers Medicare and Medicaid. You can find information about these programs on the CMS Web site.

Certified Financial Planner Board of Standards

Web site: www.cfp-board.org

1700 Broadway, Suite 2100

Denver, CO 80290-2101

(888) CFP-MARK

Through this organization's Web site, you can locate a certified financial planner in your area. You'll also find a list of questions to ask during your initial interview.

Children of Aging Parents

Web site: www.caps4caregivers.org

1609 Woodburne Road, Suite 302A

Levittown, PA 19057

(800) 227-7294 or (215) 945-6900

This organization's mission is to assist people who care for elderly loved ones by giving them reliable information, referrals, and support.

Community Health Accreditation Program

Web site: www.chapinc.org

61 Broadway

New York, NY 10006

(800) 656-9656 or (212) 480-8828

This organization provides accreditation for home care agencies.

Consumer Consortium on Assisted Living

Web site: www.ccal.org

2342 Oak Street

Falls Church, VA 22046

(703) 533-8121

This organization offers resources to prospective residents of assisted living facilities, including a checklist for evaluating facilities.

Continuing Care Accreditation Commission

Web site: www.ccaconline.org
2519 Connecticut Avenue NW
Washington, DC 20008-1520
(202) 783-7286

This agency provides accreditation for continuing care facilities.

Deaf and Disabled Telecommunications Program

Web site: www.ddtp.org
1939 Harrison Street, Suite 520
Oakland, CA 94612
(800) 867-4323

This organization can help caregivers obtain special telephone equipment for loved ones who are hearing impaired.

Department of Veterans Affairs

Web site: www.va.gov
Department of Veterans Affairs
Washington, DC 20011
(800) 827-1000

This government agency offers a variety of benefits and services for veterans and their beneficiaries. Its Web site features a facilities locator that can help you find the nearest VA offices, medical centers, and clinics.

Division of Aging and Seniors

Web site: http://www.hc-sc.gc.ca/seniors-aines/seniors/english/division.htm
Population Health Directorate
Health Canada
Address Locator 1908A1
Ottawa, ON Canada
KIA 1B4
(613) 952-7606

This agency serves in an advisory capacity to the Canadian government, offering education and research on issues affecting the country's senior population. It also provides operational support for the National Advisory Council on Aging.

Division of HIV/AIDS Prevention

Web site: http://www.cdc.gov/hiv/dhap.htm
Part of the Centers for Disease Control and Prevention, this division's Web site includes fact sheets on transmission, testing, treatment, and prevention of HIV/AIDS.

Family Caregiver Alliance

Web site: www.caregiver.org
690 Market Street
Suite 600
San Francisco, CA 94104
(800) 445-8106

This organization's Web site includes an information clearinghouse, archives of the group's newsletter, online conferences, and an online support group.

Financial Planning Association

Web site: www.fpanet.org
1615 L Street NW
Suite 650
Washington, DC 20036
(800) 282-7526

This organization can provide names of qualified financial planners in your area.

Friends' Health Connection

Web site: www.48friend.org
PO Box 114
New Brunswick, NJ 08903
(800) 483-7436 or (732) 418-1811

This nonprofit organization administers support networks for people with similar health problems and their caregivers.

Home Care Companions

Web site: www.homecarecompanions.org
1320 Divisadero Street
San Francisco, CA 94115
(415) 824-3269

This organization offers training to those who provide home care for people with cancer, AIDS, and brain tumors.

Homecare University

Web site: www.homecareuniversity.org
228 Seventh Street SE
Washington, DC 20003
(202) 547-3576

This organization provides accreditation for home care agencies.

Hospice Education Institute

Web site: www.hospiceworld.org

3 Unity Square

PO Box 98

Machiasport, ME 04655-0098

(800) 331-1620

Contact this organization for information on hospice care and referrals to hospice programs in your area.

Hospice Foundation of America

Web site: www.hospicefoundation.org

2001 S Street NW #300

Washington, DC 20009

(800) 854-3402 or (202) 638-5419

This organization provides information on hospice and end-of-life care. Through its Web site, you can find a hospice program in your area.

Internal Revenue Service (IRS)

Web site: www.irs.gov

(800) 829-1040

The IRS has several programs for seniors, including Tax Counseling for the Elderly and the Volunteer Income Tax Assistance Program.

International Hearing Society

Web site: http://www.pitt.edu/~uclid/ihs.htm

20361 Middlebelt

Livonia, MI 48152

(800) 521-5247

Contact this organization to learn more about treatments and support services for people with hearing loss.

Joint Commission on Accreditation of Healthcare Organizations

Web site: www.jcaho.org

One Renaissance Boulevard

Oakbrook Terrace, IL 60181

(630) 792-5000

This agency provides accreditation for home health care agencies.

Lutheran Services in America

Web site: www.lutheranservices.org

700 Light Street

Baltimore, MD 21230

(800) 664-3848

This faith-based organization sponsors a variety of caregiving services, including senior centers, adult day care, telephone reassurance, and transportation. It also operates nursing homes.

Meals on Wheels Association of America

Web site: www.mowaa.org

1414 Prince Street, Suite 302

Alexandria, VA 22314

(703) 548-5558

This organization can refer you to meal delivery programs in your loved one's community.

Medicare

Web site: www.medicare.gov

(800) 633-4227

Visit the Medicare Web site for information on Medicare eligibility requirements and benefits. The site also features a list of participating physicians and information on dialysis facilities, nursing homes, and prescription assistance programs.

National Academy of Elder Law Attorneys, Inc.

Web site: www.naela.com

1604 North Country Club Road

Tucson, AZ 85716

(520) 881-4005

This nonprofit organization assists lawyers and others in the legal profession who work with elderly clients and their families. Through its Web site, you can find an elder law attorney in your area.

National Adult Day Services Association

Web site: www.ncoa.org/nadsa

409 Third Street SW

Washington, DC 20024

(866) 890-7357

This organization maintains information on adult day care facilities nationwide and offers a checklist for evaluating them.

National Alliance for Caregiving

Web site: www.caregiving.org

4720 Montgomery Lane, Suite 642

Bethesda, MD 20814

This organization provides information and support for caregivers and their families. The Web site features links to many helpful organizations.

National Association for Continence

Web site: www.nafc.org
PO Box 8310
Spartanburg, SC 29305-8310
(800) 252-3337

Formerly known as Help for Incontinent People (HIP), this nonprofit organization is dedicated to improving the quality of life of people with incontinence.

National Association for Home Care

Web site: www.nahc.org
228 Seventh Street SE
Washington, DC 20003
(202) 547-7424

This is the nation's largest trade association, representing the interests and concerns of home care agencies, home care aide organizations, medical equipment suppliers, and hospice programs. On the Web site, you'll find information on choosing a home care provider, as well as a home care/hospice locator.

National Association of Area Agencies on Aging (N4A)

Web site: www.n4a.org
927 15th Street NW, 6th Floor
Washington, DC 20005
(202) 296-8130

N4A is the umbrella organization for the nation's 655 Area Agencies on Aging and more than 230 Title VI Native American aging programs. It advocates on behalf of these government entities to ensure that services are available to older Americans.

National Association of Insurance Commissioners

Web site: www.naic.org
2301 McGee, Suite 800
Kansas City, MO 64108-2604
(816) 842-3600

This organization offers a selection of consumer publications, which can be ordered for a nominal fee.

National Association of Personal Financial Advisors

Web site: www.napfa.org
355 West Dundee Road, Suite 200
Buffalo Grove, IL 60089
(888) 333-6659

This organization has more than 750 members and affiliates who provide financial advice on a "fee-only" basis, meaning that their compensation is not based on the sale of financial products. The Web site features a listing of fee-only advisors nationwide.

National Association of Professional Geriatric Care Managers

Web site: www.caremanager.org
1604 North Country Club Road
Tucson, AZ 85716
(520) 881-8008

Through this organization's Web site, you can find a geriatric care manager in your area.

National Association of Social Workers

Web site: www.socialworkers.org
750 First Street NE, Suite 700
Washington, DC 20002
(800) 638-8799

This organization offers referrals to qualified social workers nationwide.

National Association of State Units on Aging

Web site: www.nasua.org
1201 15th Street NW, Suite 350
Washington, DC 20005
(202) 898-2578

The membership of this nonprofit organization consists of the 57 state and territorial government agencies on aging. Together, they work to promote public policy on behalf of the nation's diverse aging population.

National Association of the Deaf

Web site: www.nad.org
814 Thayer Avenue
Silver Spring, MD 20910-4500
(301) 587-1788
TTY: (301) 587-1789

This organization's programs include grassroots advocacy for the hearing impaired, captioned media, and certification of American Sign Language professionals. Check the Web site for information on the legal rights of the hearing impaired.

National Cancer Institute

Web site: www.cancer.gov
NCI Public Inquiries Office
Building 31, Room 10A31
31 Center Drive, MSC 2580
Bethesda, MD 20892-2580
(800) 4-CANCER (Cancer Information Service)
(301) 435-3848

The Web site for this government agency—a branch of the National Institutes of Health—offers information on cancer risk factors, screening and testing, treatments, and clinical trials. Consumers with specific questions should call the toll-free number listed above.

National Center for Vision and Aging

Web site: www.lighthouse.org
111 East 59th Street
New York, NY 10022-1202
(800) 334-5497

Operated by The Lighthouse International, this organization provides information and support for people with vision loss.

National Center on Elder Abuse

Web site: www.elderabusecenter.org
1225 I Street NW, Suite 725
Washington, DC 20005
(202) 898-2586

Visit the center's Web site to learn what constitutes elder abuse, how to prevent it, and how to report it.

National Citizens' Coalition for Nursing Home Reform

Web site: www.nccnhr.org
1424 16th Street NW, Suite 202
Washington, DC 20036
(202) 332-2275

This consumer organization advocates the development of public policy that will improve life and care for residents of nursing homes.

National Consumers League

Web site: www.fraud.org
PO Box 65868
Washington, DC 20035
(800) 876-7060

This organization runs the National Fraud Information Center, which seeks to help consumers recognize and report various types of fraud. A complaint form is available online.

National Council on the Aging

Web site: www.ncoa.org
409 Third Street SW, Suite 200
Washington, DC 20024
(202) 479-1200

This organization works with professionals and community organizations to improve the lives of the elderly. Visit its Web site to learn about its wide-ranging advocacy role and to access its journal, *Innovations*.

National Family Caregivers Association

Web site: www.nfcacares.org
10400 Connecticut Avenue, Suite 500
Kensington, MD 20895-3944
(800) 896-3650 or (301) 942-6430

This nonprofit membership organization provides information and support for caregivers with aging parents, ill spouses, or disabled children.

National Foundation for Depressive Illness

Web site: www.depression.org
PO Box 2257
New York, NY 10116
(800) 239-1265

Contact this organization for information on depression's symptoms and available treatments.

National Hospice and Palliative Care Organization

Web site: www.nhpco.org

1700 Diagonal Road

Arlington, VA 22314

(703) 837-1500 or (800) 658-8898

This is the nation's largest membership organization representing hospice and palliative care programs and professionals. Its Web site can direct you to programs in your area.

National Institute of Mental Health

Web site: www.nimh.nih.gov

NIMH Public Inquiries

6001 Executive Boulevard, Room 8184, MSC 9663

Bethesda, MD 20892-9663

(301) 443-4513

Contact this government organization to learn about the various types of depression, as well as their diagnosis and treatment.

National Institute on Aging

Web site: www.nia.nih.gov

Building 31, Room 5C27

31 Center Drive, MSC 2292

Bethesda, MD 20892

(800) 222-2225 or (301) 496-1752

This agency, a branch of the National Institutes of Health, conducts research on age-related diseases and issues. Check out the Web site for updates on the latest findings.

National Kidney and Urologic Diseases Information Clearinghouse

Web site: www.niddk.nih.gov/health/kidney/nkudic.htm

3 Information Way

Bethesda, MD 20892-3580

(800) 891-5390 or (301) 654-4415

This government agency produces a number of publications on diseases of the kidneys and urologic system. Its toll-free consumer hot line is available Monday through Friday, 8:30 A.M. to 5:00 P.M. EST.

National Mental Health Association

Web site: www.nmha.org

1021 Prince Street

Alexandria, VA 22314-2971

(800) 969-6642

Contact this organization for information on the diagnosis and treatment of mental illness, as well as referrals to local treatment services.

National Osteoporosis Foundation

Web site: www.nof.org

1232 22nd Street NW

Washington, DC 20037-1292

(202) 223-2226

This nonprofit organization is dedicated to promoting life-long bone health. Its Web site features a directory of member physicians as well as information on the prevention, diagnosis, and treatment of osteoporosis.

National Pressure Ulcer Advisory Panel (NPUAP)

Web site: www.npuap.org

SUNY at Buffalo, Beck Hall

3435 Main Street

Buffalo, NY 14214

(703) 464-4849

This organization provides booklets and other resources for the prevention and treatment of bedsores.

National Reverse Mortgage Lenders Association

Web site: www.reversemortgage.org

1625 Massachusetts Avenue NW

Washington, DC 20036

(202) 939-1760

Contact this organization to learn more about reverse mortgages and to locate lenders in your area.

National Self-Help Clearinghouse

Web site: www.selfhelpweb.org

365 5th Avenue, Suite 3300

New York, NY 10016

(212) 817-1822

This organization offers helpful resources for people who want to launch their own support groups.

National Sleep Foundation

Web site: www.sleepfoundation.org

1522 K Street NW, Suite 500

Washington, DC 20005

(202) 347-3471

This organization offers information on diagnosing and treating sleep disorders, as well as advice on getting a good night's sleep.

Parkinson's Disease Foundation

Web site: www.pdf.org
William Black Medical Building
Columbia-Presbyterian Medical Center
710 West 168th Street
New York, NY 10032-9982
(800) 457-6676 or (212) 973-4700

This nonprofit organization supports and promotes Parkinson's research worldwide. On its Web site, experts answer questions about the disease.

Partnership for Caring

Web site: www.partnershipforcaring.org
1620 Eye Street NW, Suite 202
Washington, DC 20006
(800) 989-9455

This nonprofit organization offers free state-specific sample forms for durable powers of attorney and living wills.

Pioneer Network

Web site: www.pioneernetwork.net
PO Box 18648
Rochester, NY 14618-0648
(585) 271-7570

This nonprofit organization is spearheading a grassroots movement to transform eldercare and build elder-focused communities.

Rosalynn Carter Institute for Human Development

Web site: www.rosalynncarter.org
Georgia Southwestern State University
800 Wheatley Street
Americus, GA 31709
(229) 928-1234

The institute promotes the health and well-being of family and professional caregivers through research, education, and training.

Shepherd's Centers of America

Web site: www.shepherdcenters.org
One West Armour Boulevard, Suite 201
Kansas City, MO 64111
(800) 547-7073 or (816) 960-2022

These centers train senior citizen volunteers to provide part-time respite care. Currently, more than 100 centers operate in communities throughout the United States.

Simon Foundation for Continence

Web site: www.simonfoundation.org
Box 835-F
Wilmette, IL 60091
(800) 237-4666

This organization provides assistance to people with incontinence and their families. It also reviews relevant legislation and encourages medical professionals to learn about the condition.

Social Security Administration

Web site: www.ssa.gov
Office of Public Inquiries
6401 Security Boulevard
Room 4-C-5 Annex
Baltimore, MD 21235-6401
(800) 772-1213

On this government agency's Web site, you can find benefits information, obtain claims forms, and view publications. Call the national toll-free number or your local Social Security office with any questions.

Society of Financial Service Professionals

Web site: www.financialpro.org
270 South Bryn Mawr Avenue
Bryn Mawr, PA 19010-2195
(800) 392-6900 or (610) 526-2500

This organization can help you find a financial professional in your area.

Visiting Nurse Associations of America

Web site: www.vnaa.org
11 Beacon Street, Suite 910
Boston, MA 02108
(800) 426-2547 or (888) 866-8773 or (617) 523-4042

This organization provides information and referrals for home health care and hospice programs.

Well Spouse Foundation

Web site: www.wellspouse.org
PO Box 30093
Elkins Park, PA 19027
(800) 838-0879

This organization offers information and support to people who are providing care for their spouses.

INDEX

Underscored page references indicate boxed text and tables.

A

Underscored page references indicate boxed text and tables.

Underscored page references indicate boxed text and tables.

L

M

Underscored page references indicate boxed text and tables.

R

S

Underscored page references indicate boxed text and tables.